HEMATOPATHOLOGY IN ONCOLOGY

Cancer Treatment and Research

Steven T. Rosen, M.D., *Series Editor*

Muggia, F.M. (ed): *Concepts, Mechanisms, and New Targets for Chemotherapy.* 1995.
ISBN 0-7923-3525-2.
Klastersky, J. (ed): *Infectious Complications of Cancer.* 1995. ISBN 0-7923-3598-8.
Kurzrock, R., Talpaz, M. (eds): *Cytokines: Interleukins and Their Receptors.* 1995. ISBN 0-7923-3636-4.
Sugarbaker, P. (ed): *Peritoneal Carcinomatosis: Drugs and Diseases.* 1995. ISBN 0-7923-3726-3.
Sugarbaker, P. (ed): *Peritoneal Carcinomatosis: Principles of Management.* 1995.
ISBN 0-7923-3727-1.
Dickson, R.B., Lippman, M.E. (eds.): *Mammary Tumor Cell Cycle, Differentiation and Metastasis.*
1995. ISBN 0-7923-3905-3.
Freireich, E.J, Kantarjian, H. (eds): *Molecular Genetics and Therapy of Leukemia.* 1995.
ISBN 0-7923-3912-6.
Cabanillas, F., Rodriguez, M.A. (eds): *Advances in Lymphoma Research.* 1996. ISBN 0-7923-3929-0.
Miller, A.B. (ed.): *Advances in Cancer Screening.* 1996. ISBN 0-7923-4019-1.
Hait , W.N. (ed.): *Drug Resistance.* 1996. ISBN 0-7923-4022-1.
Pienta, K.J. (ed.): *Diagnosis and Treatment of Genitourinary Malignancies.* 1996. ISBN 0-7923-4164-3.
Arnold, A.J. (ed.): *Endocrine Neoplasms.* 1997. ISBN 0-7923-4354-9.
Pollock, R.E. (ed.): *Surgical Oncology.* 1997. ISBN 0-7923-9900-5.
Verweij, J., Pinedo, H.M., Suit, H.D. (eds): *Soft Tissue Sarcomas: Present Achievements and Future
Prospects.* 1997. ISBN 0-7923-9913-7.
Walterhouse, D.O., Cohn, S. L. (eds.): *Diagnostic and Therapeutic Advances in Pediatric Oncology.*
1997. ISBN 0-7923-9978-1.
Mittal, B.B., Purdy, J.A., Ang, K.K. (eds): *Radiation Therapy.* 1998. ISBN 0-7923-9981-1.
Foon, K.A., Muss, H.B. (eds): *Biological and Hormonal Therapies of Cancer.* 1998. ISBN 0-7923-9997-8.
Ozols, R.F. (ed.): *Gynecologic Oncology.* 1998. ISBN 0-7923-8070-3.
Noskin, G. A. (ed.): *Management of Infectious Complications in Cancer Patients.* 1998.
ISBN 0-7923-8150-5.
Bennett, C. L. (ed.): *Cancer Policy.* 1998. ISBN 0-7923-8203-X.
Benson, A. B. (ed.): *Gastrointestinal Oncology.* 1998. ISBN 0-7923-8205-6.
Tallman, M.S., Gordon, L.I. (eds): *Diagnostic and Therapeutic Advances in Hematologic Malignancies.*
1998. ISBN 0-7923-8206-4.
von Gunten, C.F. (ed): *Palliative Care and Rehabilitation of Cancer Patients.* 1999. ISBN 0-7923-8525-X
Burt, R.K., Brush, M.M. (eds): *Advances in Allogeneic Hematopoietic Stem Cell Transplantation.* 1999.
ISBN 0-7923-7714-1.
Angelos, P. (ed.): *Ethical Issues in Cancer Patient Care* 2000. ISBN 0-7923-7726-5.
Gradishar, W.J., Wood, W.C. (eds): *Advances in Breast Cancer Management.* 2000. ISBN 0-7923-7890-3.
Sparano, Joseph A. (ed.): *HIV & HTLV-I Associated Malignancies.* 2001. ISBN 0-7923-7220-4.
Ettinger, David S. (ed.): *Thoracic Oncology.* 2001. ISBN 0-7923-7248-4.
Bergan, Raymond C. (ed.): *Cancer Chemoprevention.* 2001. ISBN 0-7923-7259-X.
Raza, A., Mundle, S.D. (eds): *Myelodysplastic Syndromes & Secondary Acute Myelogenous Leukemia* 2001.
ISBN: 0-7923-7396.
Talamonti, Mark S. (ed.): *Liver Directed Therapy for Primary and Metastatic Liver Tumors.* 2001.
ISBN 0-7923-7523-8.
Stack, M.S., Fishman, D.A. (eds): *Ovarian Cancer.* 2001. ISBN 0-7923-7530-0.
Bashey, A., Ball, E.D. (eds): *Non-Myeloablative Allogeneic Transplantation.* 2002. ISBN 0-7923-7646-3.
Leong, Stanley P.L. (ed.): *Atlas of Selective Sentinel Lymphadenectomy for Melanoma, Breast Cancer and
Colon Cancer.* 2002. ISBN 1-4020-7013-6.
Andersson , B., Murray D. (eds): *Clinically Relevant Resistance in Cancer Chemotherapy.* 2002.
ISBN 1-4020-7200-7.
Beam, C. (ed.): *Biostatistical Applications in Cancer Research.* 2002. ISBN 1-4020-7226-0.
Brockstein, B., Masters, G. (eds): *Head and Neck Cancer.* 2003. ISBN 1-4020-7336-4.
Frank, D.A. (ed.): *Signal Transduction in Cancer.* 2003. ISBN 1-4020-7340-2.
Figlin, Robert A. (ed.): *Kidney Cancer.* 2003. ISBN 1-4020-7457-3.
Kirsch, Matthias; Black, Peter McL. (ed.): *Angiogenesis in Brain Tumors.* 2003. ISBN 1-4020-7704-1.
Keller, E.T., Chung, L.W.K. (eds): *The Biology of Skeletal Metastases.* 2004. ISBN 1-4020-7749-1.
Kumar, Rakesh (ed.): *Molecular Targeting and Signal Transduction.* 2004. ISBN 1-4020-7822-6.
Verweij, J., Pinedo, H.M. (eds): *Targeting Treatment of Soft Tissue Sarcomas.* 2004. ISBN 1-4020-7808-0.
Finn, W.G., Peterson, L.C. (eds.): *Hematopathology in Oncology.* 2004. ISBN 1-4020-7919-2.

HEMATOPATHOLOGY IN ONCOLOGY

Edited by

William G. Finn
University of Michigan Medical School, Ann Arbor, Michigan

LoAnn C. Peterson
Northwestern University Feinberg School of Medicine, Chicago, Illinois

Kluwer Academic Publishers
Boston/Dordrecht/London

Distributors for North, Central and South America:
Kluwer Academic Publishers
101 Philip Drive
Assinippi Park
Norwell, Massachusetts 02061 USA
Telephone (781) 871-6600
Fax (781) 681-9045
E-Mail: kluwer@wkap.com

Distributors for all other countries:
Kluwer Academic Publishers Group
Post Office Box 322
3300 AH Dordrecht, THE NETHERLANDS
Telephone 31 786 576 000
Fax 31 786 576 254
E-Mail: services@wkap.nl

 Electronic Services <http://www.wkap.nl>

Library of Congress Cataloging-in-Publication Data

A C.I.P. Catalogue record for this book is available
from the Library of Congress.

Hematopathology in Oncology
William Finn and LoAnn Peterson
ISBN 1-4020-7919-2
e-Book ISBN: 1-4020-7920-6

The Publisher offers discounts on this book for course use and bulk purchases.
For further information, send email to <Laura.Walsh@wkap.com>.

Dedication

This book is dedicated

to Cindy and Ellen, who give
my life meaning

-WGF

to Lance, Kari, Anja, and Kyle,
who give me inspiration and
support

-LCP

Contents

Contributing Authors

Stephanie R. Brockman, B.A., C.L.Sp.(C.G.), Cytogenetics Laboratory, Mayo Clinic, Rochester Minnesota

Gerald M. Davis, M.P.H., M.T.(A.S.C.P.), Department of Pathology, University of Michigan Medical School, Ann Arbor, Michigan

Gordon W. Dewald, Ph.D., Cytogenetics Laboratory, Mayo Clinic, Rochester, Minnesota

William G. Finn, M.D., Department of Pathology, University of Michigan Medical School, Ann Arbor, Michigan

John L. Frater, M.D., Department of Clinical Pathology, Division of Pathology, Cleveland Clinic Foundation, Cleveland, Ohio

Charles L. Goolsby, Ph.D., Department of Pathology, Northwestern University Feinberg School of Medicine, and Robert H. Lurie Comprehensive Cancer Center, Chicago, Illinois

Timothy C. Greiner, M.D., Department of Pathology and Microbiology, University of Nebraska Medical Center, Omaha, Nebraska

Eric D. Hsi, M.D., Department of Clinical Pathology, Division of Pathology, Cleveland Clinic Foundation, Cleveland, Ohio

Ameet R. Kini, M.D., Ph.D., Cardinal Bernardin Cancer Center & Stritch School of Medicine, Loyola University Chicago, Maywood, Illinois

Aseem Lal, M.D., Department of Pathology, Northwestern University Feinberg School of Medicine, Chicago, Illinois

Kay Lynne Lantis, M.T.(A.S.C.P.), SH, Department of Pathology, University of Michigan Medical School, Ann Arbor, Michigan

Laura Marszalek, M.T.(A.S.C.P.), Northwestern Memorial Hospital, Chicago, Illinois

Ritu Nayar, M.D., Department of Pathology, Northwestern University Feinberg School of Medicine, Chicago, Illinois

Sarah F. Paternaster, B.S., C.L.Sp.(C.G.), Cytogenetics Laboratory, Mayo Clinic, Rochester, Minnesota

Mary Paniagua, M.T.(A.S.C.P.)S.I., Robert H. Lurie Comprehensive Cancer Center, Northwestern University Feinberg School of Medicine, Chicago, Illinois

Martin S. Tallman, M.D., Northwestern University Feinberg School of Medicine, and Robert H. Lurie Comprehensive Cancer Center, Chicago, Illinois

James W. Vardiman, M.D., Department of Pathology, University of Chicago, Chicago, Illinois

Carla S. Wilson, M.D., Ph.D., Department of Pathology, University of New Mexico Health Sciences Center, Albuquerque, New Mexico

Preface

Hematologist/oncologists rely heavily upon the discipline of hematopathology for the care and management of their patients. Whether interpreting a lymph node or bone marrow biopsy, directing a high throughput automated hematology laboratory, or translating testing modalities from the research bench to the clinical laboratory, hematopathologists and other laboratory medicine specialists provide a steady stream of critical data for the clinical practitioner. Recently the rapid advances in diagnosis and treatment of hematologic disorders including the need to evaluate patient eligibility for, and monitor responses to, rapidly evolving targeted therapies have made the close collaboration between pathologists and clinician practitioners even more essential. We hope that this book will enable the reader to learn about the emerging role of the pathologist and clinical laboratory in the dynamic and rapidly evolving field of clinical hematology and oncology.

The topics covered in this book are not comprehensive, but were selected to give the reader a glimpse into the ongoing interplay in day to day practice between tried and tested histopathologic principles and rapidly changing concepts in translational hematopathology. Several chapters provide overviews of established and emerging disease entities, with an eye toward the future of diagnostic laboratory medicine. The chapter by Schnitzer and Valdez covers the history and basic histologic principles of Hodgkin lymphoma, with a state-of-the art update on the application of new classifications and technologies that are useful not only in enriching our understanding of this complex disease, but also in its application to diagnosis and management. Vardiman reviews the myeloproliferative/myelodysplastic overlap syndromes, a recently defined category of diseases that was first formally published with the new World Health Organization classification of hematopoietic neoplasms. Likewise, Wilson updates us on important advances in the classification and management of plasma cell dyscrasias, and Hsi and Frater discusses current approaches to the diagnosis and classification of chronic lymphoproliferative disorders. Lal and Nayar tackle the timely and perhaps controversial topic of the role of fine needle aspiration cytology in the diagnosis of lymphoma, and Tallman provides a "clinician's-eye view" on the role that pathologic classifications of acute leukemia play in the design of clinical trials for acute leukemia, and in the day-to-day management of these patients.

Established topics are covered with a new twist. Goolsby, Paniagua and Marszalek take a technology familiar to practicing hematologists, flow cytometry, and update us on exciting new applications to clinical diagnosis and monitoring of patients treated with emerging therapeutic modalities. Davis, Lantis, and Finn open up the world of automated laboratory hematology to introduce us to the expanding potential of automated methods for hematologic diagnosis. Kini addresses historical and emerging concepts of the importance of angiogenesis in the pathophysiology and management of leukemia and lymphoma.

Molecular hematopathology has exploded in recent years with the rapid development of DNA based methods in both research and clinical practice. Dewald, Brockman, and Paternaster provide an outstanding primer on the use of fluorescence in situ hybridization (FISH) in the diagnostic laboratory, while Greiner informs us of the exciting emergence of functional genomics and cDNA microarray technology as pathways to expand our understanding of leukemia and lymphoma.

Our goal in putting together this volume was to provide outstanding reviews of selected topics in hematopathology in a format that would provide both general and historical background, but that would also provide an overview of the state-of-the-art in diagnostic hematopathology, with an eye on future potential and future developments. You will be the final judge as to our success or failure in this endeavor.

William G. Finn, M.D.
LoAnn C. Peterson, M.D.

Chapter 1

mRNA MICROARRAY ANALYSIS IN LYMPHOMA AND LEUKEMIA

Timothy C. Greiner
University of Nebraska Medical Center, Omaha, Nebraska

1. INTRODUCTION

The analysis of gene expression in lymphoma and leukemia has been previously characterized by the analysis of single genes or proteins, whether by Western or Northern blots, reverse transcriptase-polymerase chain reaction (RT-PCR), or *in situ* hybridization. Advances in the last decade have led to the ability to analyze the expression of thousands of known and unknown genes by the use of microarrays on filters, glass slides, or other substrate devices. These analyses have been pursued to aid in the identification of unique expression profiles of the tumors, the molecular subclassification of hematologic cancers, the discovery of new proteins to diagnose lymphoma and predict prognosis, and the cloning of new genes involved in the pathogenesis of lymphoma/leukemia.

2. CLUSTERIN: A DIAGNOSTIC PROTEIN DISCOVERED BY MICROARRAY

After using a small filter based microarray with 588 probes, Wellman demonstrated the first novel protein finding that now assists in the diagnosis of a subtype of lymphoma.[1] Clusterin was found to be solely expressed in anaplastic large cell lymphoma cell lines, and secondly was shown by immunohistochemistry to be expressed almost exclusively in clinical cases of anaplastic large cell lymphoma.[1] This observation has been confirmed in two immunohistology studies on paraffin embedded tissue where the highest frequency of clusterin expression was seen in anaplastic large cell lymphoma.[2, 3]

3.   LANDMARK STUDIES IN LEUKEMIA AND LYMPHOMA

The reports by Golub on leukemia and Alizadeh on lymphoma illustrated the potential for high density gene expression arrays to contribute to the understanding of hematologic malignancies.[4, 5] While two different microarray platforms were chosen in the two studies, powerful results were obtained by both methods. Golub et al demonstrated that the major subtype of acute myeloid leukemia (AML) could be distinguished from acute lymphoid leukemia (ALL) while using an oligoprobe microarray designed by Affymetrix (Figure 1-1).[4] In Alizadeh's study, a spotted cDNA microarray Lymphochip slide was utilized to separate diffuse large cell lymphoma into two subgroups, germinal center B-cell and activated B-cell (Figure 1-2).[5, 6] Since 1999, there have been a number of microarray studies analyzing subtypes of leukemias and lymphomas.

4.   VARIABLES IN MIRCOARRAY STUDIES IN LYMPHOMA

A comparison of the different studies of microarray analysis in lymphoma will demonstrate that there are variables in the type of platform used, the number of probe targets present, the control (if any) RNA source utilized, the number of cases studied, and the type of software used to analyze the data (Table 1-1). Variables in tissue preservation, percent of tumor cells, and normalization of the data also likely exist, but will not be further detailed here as these data were variably reported. The two major platforms are cDNA microarrays, popularized by Pat Brown, and the oligoprobe microarray developed by Affymetrix. The number of targets in the published studies in lymphoma have ranged from 588 to approximately 18,000. The source of control RNA included cell lines, reactive lymph nodes, isolated germinal centers, sorted cells from tonsils, or another subtype of lymphoma. Software analysis methods are characterized into two broad categories of unsupervised and supervised clustering, including ratio ranking, hierarchal clustering, self-organized mapping and others. The number of cases studied per subtype of lymphoma has ranged from 5 to 240.[1, 5, 7-13]

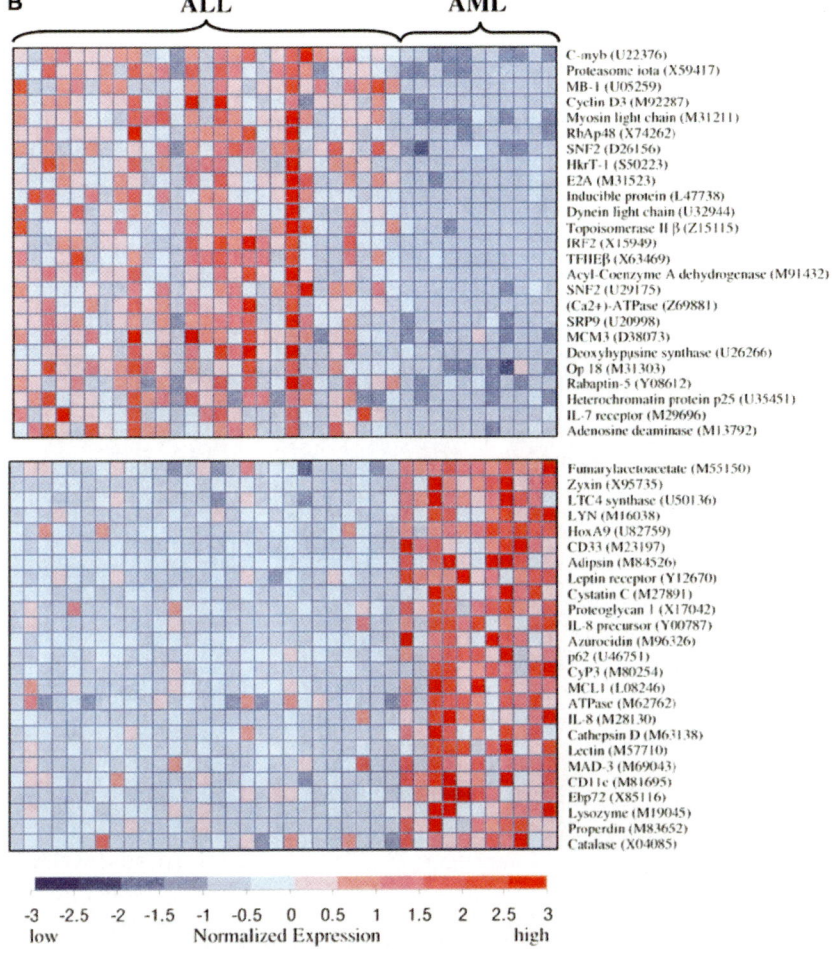

Figure 1-1. Identification of leukemia subtypes by oligonucleotide array (from Golub[4])

5.   ADVANCES IN LYMPHOMA

What are some of the conclusions that can be derived from microarray analysis in lymphoma? First, morphologic subtypes of lymphoma do cluster together in microarray analysis. Second, large numbers of tumor cases are needed for proper analysis and subsequent validation of the data. Third, cell lineage subgroups have been biologically validated by other assays, (e.g., identification of t(14;18) translocations in only the germinal center B-cell subgroup of diffuse large cell lymphoma).[9, 14] Fourth, prognostic models for survival can be generated by gene expression analyses; resulting in the construction of a predictor model on a subset of genes.[5, 9, 12, 13] Fifth, the gene components in predictor models vary between studies of diffuse large B-cell lymphoma.

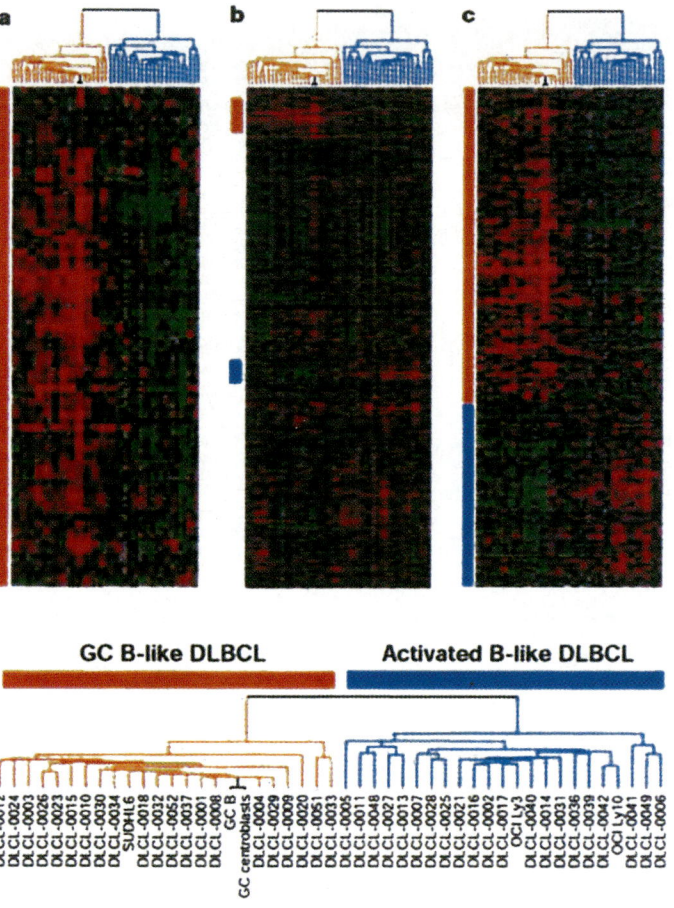

Figure 1- 2. Identification of diffuse large B-cell lymphoma subtypes by cDNA array (from Alizadeh et al[5])

Table 1-1. Microarray Analysis of mRNA Gene Expression in Lymphoma

Author	Year	Method	Genes	Control	Cases	Subtype	Ref.
Wellman	2000	cDNA[c]	588	Cell lines	31	Anaplastic	1
Alizadeh	2000	CDNA	17,800	9 cell lines	42	Large B cell	5
Hofmann	2001	Oligo[a]	5,600	Reactive LN	5	Mantle cell	17
Husson	2002	cDNA[c]	588	Tonsil GC	6	Follicular	8
Shipp	2002	Oligo[a]	6,800	Follicular	58	Large B cell	12
Rosenwald	2002	CDNA	17,800	9 cell lines	240	Large B cell	9
Ek	2002	Oligo	12,700	Tonsil sorted	7	Mantle cell	11
Zhu	2002	cDNA[c]	406	Tonsil	18	Mantle cell	19
Nishiu	2002	CDNA	18,432	Reactive LN	15	Large B cell	10
de Vos	2003	Oligo[a]	5,600	NA	5	Follicular/ Large B cell	20
Rosenwald	2003	CDNA	17,800	9 cell lines	92	Mantle cell	13

a-Affymetrix, c-Clontech membrane array, GC-germinal centers, LN-lymph node, NA-not available

5.1 Diffuse Large B-cell Lymphoma

Using the Lymphochip with 17,800 spotted probes, diffuse large cell lymphoma was easily separated from cases of chronic lymphocytic leukemia and follicular lymphoma.[5] In that study approximately 100 genes could be used to separate the germinal center B-cell group from the activated B-cell group. The germinal center B-cell subgroup of diffuse large B-cell lymphoma was characterized by overexpression of genes, such as CD10, CD38, A-myb, and OGGI, found predominantly in germinal derived B-cells.[5] The germinal center B-cell group had a much better survival than the activated B-cell subgroup identified with the Lymphochip.[5] Later, Huang et al showed in a subset of large cell lymphoma cases that the t(14;18) was only identified in the germinal center B-cell group.[14] This restriction of the t(14;18) to the germinal center B-cell group and the better survival in this subgroup was later confirmed in the much larger study of 240 cases of diffuse large B-cell lymphoma.[9] Rosenwald went on to show that c-rel amplification was also restricted to the germinal center B-cell group.[9] In addition, Lossos et al showed hypermutation of the immunoglobulin heavy chain gene, a feature of B-cells in germinal centers, is largely restricted to the germinal center B-cell group of large cell lymphoma.[15] This finding, along with the localization of the two oncogenic events (bcl-2, c-rel) in the germinal center B-cell subgroup, serve to provide biological validity to the subclassification generated by the cDNA microarray analysis in diffuse large B-cell lymphoma.

In a comparative analysis of high stage versus low stage disease, Nishui et al found that genes promoting cell proliferation (MPHOSPH1, RUVBL1, CHN2, PSA, AND CD10) were overexpressed in high stage lymphoma.[10] Confirmatory studies by RT-PCR correlated with overexpression of RUVBL1 and PSA.[10]

5.2   Predictor Models in Diffuse Large Cell Lymphoma

The genes identified in predictor models for prognosis in diffuse large cell lymphoma are significantly different in the two major studies published to date (Table 1-2).   One of the major reasons the lists of genes in the predictor models do not overlap is because the probe sets of gene targets and the two platforms were not the same.   Future studies with common probe sets will help clarify the predictive role of the significant genes from the two studies.   Bcl-6, centerin and M17 appear to be highly predictive of good prognosis in the germinal center B-cell subgroup, while BMP-6 is the most predictive of poor outcome.[9]   In Shipp's study, protein kinase C-β (PKC-β) expression was identified as one of the most predictive genes for poor survival.   The   expression   of   PKC-β   was   confirmed   by immunohistochemistry in refractory cases of large cell lymphoma.[12]   The identification of PKC-β-1 has led to the development of a chemotherapeutic protocol to target this gene in large cell lymphomas.   Similarly, the National Cancer Institute has begun a protocol which targets the overexpression of NFκB, a finding in the activated B-cell group via the Lymphochip.[16]

Table 1-2. Comparison of Genes in Predictor Models for Survival in Diffuse Large B-Cell Lymphoma

Rosenwald[9]	Shipp[12]
Bcl-6	Dystrophin rel prot 2
Centerin	3UTR of unk prot
M17	Uncharacterized
DP alpha	Prot kinase C gamma
DQ alpha	5-Hydroxytrypta 2B Rec
DR alpha	H731
DR beta	Transducin-line enhancement
Alpha actin	Uncharacterized
Collagen type IIIa	Prot kinace C beta 1
Connec tissue gr factor	Oviductal glycoprot
Fibronectin	Zinc fing prot C2H2-150
KAA0233	
Plasminogen activ	
c-myc	
E21G3	
Nucleophosmin	
BMP6	

The identification of the predictor genes was based on the analysis of lymphoma cases treated during the past decade, largely prior to the advent of Rituximab chemotherapy. It is unknown whether the same gene subsets will be predictive of response to chemotherapy and survival in patients treated with Rituximab.

5.3   Mantle Cell Lymphoma

Hoffmann's study in five cases of mantle cell lymphoma suggested that altered apoptotic pathways occurred in mantle cell lymphoma.[17] The authors demonstrated preliminary correlation by RT-PCR with the overexpression of 10 selected genes in the validation set of other cases of mantle cell lymphoma. In another study, Ek et al, in an analysis of seven cases of mantle cell lymphoma, demonstrated lymphoproliferative signal pathways were highly active, including genes such as IL10Rα, IL8 and oncogenes Bcl-2, and MERTK.[11] Cyclin D1 was uniformly expressed in all cases.[11] In an alternative approach using RT-PCR, work by Korz et al supported the findings of enhancement of proliferation genes in mantle cell lymphoma.[18] In a comparison of the blastoid variant, Zhu et al found that oncogenes CMYC, BCL2, and PIM1 were upregulated more frequently than in typical mantle cell lymphoma.[19] Along with these three genes, TOP1, CD23, CD45, CD70, and NFATC were used to create a classifier to separate blastoid from typical mantle cell cases.[19] In a definitive study, Rosenwald et al have shown in 92 cases that a signature of overexpressed proliferation genes characterizes mantle cell lymphoma.[13] The degree of expression of the proliferation signature appears to correlate with deletion of the cell cycle control gene p16, but not with ATM or p53 deletions.[13]

5.4   Follicular Lymphoma

One preliminary study showed the ability to separate the follicular lymphomas from diffuse large cell lymphoma and chronic lymphocytic leukemia.[5] Husson et al examined the gene expression profile in follicular lymphoma compared to normal germinal center B-cells.[8] Confirmation of overexpressed genes was performed by RT-PCR, however, with only six cases analyzed, the data are preliminary. De Vos suggested that novel genes (ABC2, NEK2) were increased and PDCD1 and VOUP1 were decreased in follicular lymphoma which had transformed to diffuse large cell lymphoma.[20]

6.   ADVANCES IN ACUTE AND CHRONIC LEUKEMIA (TABLE 1-3)

Golub et al were the first to show that the two major subgroups of acute leukemia, lymphoid and myeloid, could be separated by expression profiles of an oligoprobe array study of 38 cases.[4] Using a 50 gene set as a predictor of classification into AML and ALL, a high accuracy was observed in an independent set of 34 other cases of acute leukemia. Important genes in this predictor set included S-phase cell cycle genes (cyclin D3, Op18, MCM3) chromatin remodeling (RbAp48 and SNF2) transcription (TF11EB) cell adhesion (ZYXIN, CD11c) and oncogene (c-MYB, E2A and HOXA9).[4] HOXA9 overexpression was the most predictive for treatment failure in AML.[4]

Table 1-3. Microarray Analysis of Gene Expression in Leukemia

Author	Year	Method	Genes	Type	Cases	Ref
Golub	1999	Oligo[a]	6,817	ALL/AML	72	4
Chen	2001	cDNA[b]	4,132	ALL	4	25
Virtaneva	2001	Oligo[a]	6,606	AML	20	21
Armstrong	2002	Oligo[a]	12,600	ALL	37	28
Yeoh	2002	Oligo[a]	12,600	ALL	360	27
Schoch	2002	Oligo[a]	12,600	AML	37	22
Moos	2002	CDNA	4,608	ALL/AML	51	23
Rosenwald	2001	CDNA	17,856	CLL	33	30
Stratowa	2001	CDNA	1,024	CLL	54	36
Klein	2001	Oligo[a]	12,600	CLL	34	29
Wiestner	2003	CDNA	13,868	CLL	107	31

a-Affymetrix, b-radiolabelled, ALL-acute lymphoblastic leukemia, AML-acute myelogenous leukemia, CLL-chronic lymphocytic leukemia.

6.1   Acute Myeloid Leukemia

Virtaneva, et al showed that AML with normal cytogenetics and AML with trisomy 8 could be separated from normal CD34 positive cells.[21] Schoch et al showed specific gene expression profiles existed with the three major subgroups of acute myelogenous leukemia: AML-M2 t(8;21); AML-M3 t(15;17); and AML M4EO inv (16).[22] Thirty six genes were identified which performed accurate class prediction of the three cytogenetic subtypes of AML[22] Moos demonstrated that as few as 20 genes could be used to discriminate leukemia subsets.[23]

Other studies have compared myelodysplastic syndrome with AML,[7, 24] and showed a selective overexpression of Delta-like (DLK) protein in myelodysplastic syndrome.[24]

6.2   Acute Lymphoblastic Leukemia

What discoveries have been made in acute lymphoid leukemia (ALL) since Golub's study? While few cases of B-ALL were studied, Chen identified seven proteins (CD58, creatine kinase B, ninjurin, Ref-1, calpastatin, HDJ-2 and annexin VI), that were overexpressed in B-lineage ALL, compared to normal CD19 and CD10 positive B-cell progenitors.[25] They went on to show that CD58 coexpression by flow cytometry could be used to demonstrate residual ALL disease in 9 of 104 bone marrow samples.[25] CD58 overexpression has been previously described in leukemic cells.[26] Confirmatory correlation of residual disease detected by CD58 expression with positive PCR results of immunoglobulin heavy chain rearrangements was seen.[25] This is the first example of a microarray discovery leading to a discovery of protein expression useful in the follow-up of residual disease.

Yeoh et al, in a study of 360 cases of acute lymphoblastic leukemia (ALL), showed that specific subgroups localize with specific gene translocations including T-ALL, E2A-PBXI, BCR-ABL, TEL-AML1, MLL, and hyperdiploid (>50 chromosomes).[27] The gene expression profile correlated more with the primary genetic abnormality present than the immunophenotypic subclassification (e.g., pre-B, etc.).[27] HOXA9 was exclusively seen in the MLL cases. A novel new subgroup with overexpression of PTP-RM and LHF-PL2 was identified,[27] although no specific genetic lesion is known. No single expression profile could predict relapse across all six subtypes of ALL, but a predictive profile could be delineated within each subgroup.[27] Similar to Golub, a validation set of cases was used to show a high accuracy in predicting the subgroup of ALL.[4, 27]

Armstrong et al showed specific gene expression profiles can be seen with a subgroup of acute leukemia harboring translocations with the mixed lineage leukemia (MLL/HRX/ALL1) gene on chromosome 11q23.[28] Underexpression of genes seen in early B-cells (MME, CD-79B, CD24, CD22, and DNTT) and overexpression of adhesion molecules (LGALSI, ANXAI, ANXA2, CD44 and SPN) were seen in ALL with MLL translocations. Compared to ALL or AML, MLL cases expressed high levels of hematopoietic progenitors (PROMLI, LM02, FLT3). They suggest that MLL cases, since they have high expression of SPN and CD44, and low

CD24 and CD79B expression, are arrested at an earlier stage of development compared to regular B-ALL.[28]

6.3 Chronic Lymphocytic Leukemia

Klein suggested that the profile in CLL is related to that seen in memory B-cells more than to other B-cell populations. They also showed that expression profiles in 23 genes could be used to distinguish immunoglobulin mutated versus unmutated cases of CLL.[29]

Rosenwald et al also showed a correlation of expression profile with the mutation status of CLL and constructed a 50 gene predictor model useful for identifying the subgroups.[30]

Zap-70 was found to be expressed most differentially in the IgH unmutated cases.[30] This utility of ZAP-70 in predicting mutated cases of CLL was recently confirmed.[31] ZAP-70 was expressed 5-fold higher in IgH mutated cases than in unmutated cases and predicted mutated status in 93% of CLL patients.[31]

7. SUMMARY

We have reviewed the ability of gene expression microarrays to characterize subgroups of lymphoma and leukemia, identify expression profiles that correlate with known cytogenetic abnormalities, demonstrate that expression profiles can predict prognosis, new proteins identified for diagnosis and followup, and provided new therapeutic targets for chemotherapy. We can expect that new prognostic models will be designed and tested, incorporating the pathologic diagnosis based on morphology, the molecular gene expression profile, and the clinical assessment (e.g. International prognostic index). In addition, the gene expression profiles will be used to generate correlative and ultimately predictive data for response to particular chemotherapeutic regimens. Translation for clinical usage is likely in a diagnostic fashion in both lymphoma and leukemia.[32-35]

REFERENCES

1. Wellmann A et al. Detection of differentially expressed genes in lymphomas using cDNA arrays: identification of clusterin as a new diagnostic marker for anaplastic large-cell lymphomas. Blood 2000; 96(2): 398-404.

2. Lae ME, Ahmed I, Macon WR. Clusterin is widely expressed in systemic anaplastic large cell lymphoma but fails to differentiate primary from secondary cutaneous anaplastic large cell lymphoma. Am J Clin Pathol 2002; 118(5): 773-779.
3. Saffer H et al., Clusterin expression in malignant lymphomas: a survey of 266 cases. Mod Pathol 2002; 15(11): 1221-1226.
4. Golub TR et al. Molecular classification of cancer: class discovery and class prediction by gene expression monitoring. Science 1999; 286(5439): 531-537.
5. Alizadeh AA et al. Distinct types of diffuse large B-cell lymphoma identified by gene expression profiling. Nature 2000; 403(6769): 503-511.
6. Alizadeh, A et al. The lymphochip: a specialized cDNA microarray for the genomic-scale analysis of gene expression in normal and malignant lymphocytes. Cold Spring Harb Symp Quant Biol 1999; 64: 71-78.
7. Hofmann, WK et al. Characterization of gene expression of CD34+ cells from normal and myelodysplastic bone marrow. Blood 2002; 100(10): 3553-3560.
8. Husson H et al., Gene expression profiling of follicular lymphoma and normal germinal center B cells using cDNA arrays. Blood 2002; 99(1): 282-289.
9. Rosenwald A et al. The use of molecular profiling to predict survival after chemotherapy for diffuse large-B-cell lymphoma. N Engl J Med 2002; 346(25): 1937-1947.
10. Nishiu M et al. Microarray analysis of gene-expression profiles in diffuse large B-cell lymphoma: Identification of genes related to disease progression. Jpn J Cancer Res 2002; 93: 894-901.
11. Ek S et al. Mantle cell lymphomas express a distinct genetic signature affecting lymphocyte trafficking and growth regulation as compared with subpopulations of normal human B cells. Cancer Res 2002; 62(15): 4398-4405.
12. Shipp MA et al. Diffuse large B-cell lymphoma outcome prediction by gene-expression profiling and supervised machine learning. Nat Med 2002; 8(1): 68-74.
13. Rosenwald A et al. The Proliferation Gene Expression Signature is a Quantitative Integrator of Oncogenic Events That Predicts Survival in Mantle Cell Lymphoma. Cancer Cell 2003; in press.
14. Huang JZ et al. The t(14;18) defines a unique subset of diffuse large B-cell lymphoma with a germinal center B-cell gene expression profile. Blood 2002; 99(7): 2285-2290.
15. Lossos IS et al., Ongoing immunoglobulin somatic mutation in germinal center B cell-like but not in activated B cell-like diffuse large cell lymphomas. Proc Natl Acad Sci USA 2000; 97(18): 10209-10213.
16. Davis RE et al. Constitutive nuclear factor kappaB activity is required for survival of activated B cell-like diffuse large B cell lymphoma cells. J Exp Med 2001; 194(12): 1861-1874.
17. Hofmann WK et al. Altered apoptosis pathways in mantle cell lymphoma detected by oligonucleotide microarray. Blood 2001; 98(3): 787-794.
18. Korz C et al. Evidence for distinct pathomechanisms in B-cell chronic lymphocytic leukemia and mantle cell lymphoma by quantitative expression analysis of cell cycle and apoptosis-associated genes. Blood 2002; 99(12): 4554-4561.
19. Zhu Y et al. Investigatory and analytical approaches to differential gene expression profiling in mantle cell lymphoma. Br J Haematol 2002; 119(4): 905-915.
20. de Vos S et al. Gene expression profile of serial samples of transformed B-cell lymphomas. Lab Invest 2003; 83(2): 271-285.
21. Virtaneva K et al. Expression profiling reveals fundamental biological differences in acute myeloid leukemia with isolated trisomy 8 and normal cytogenetics. Proc Natl Acad Sci USA 2001; 98(3): 1124-1129.

22. Schoch, C., et al., Acute myeloid leukemias with reciprocal rearrangements can be distinguished by specific gene expression profiles. Proc Natl Acad Sci USA 2002; 99(15): 10008-10013.

23. Moos PJ et al. Identification of gene expression profiles that segregate patients with childhood leukemia. Clin Cancer Res 2002; 8(10): 3118-3130.

24. Miyazato A et al. Identification of myelodysplastic syndrome-specific genes by DNA microarray analysis with purified hematopoietic stem cell fraction. Blood 2001; 98(2): 422-427.

25. Chen JS et al. Identification of novel markers for monitoring minimal residual disease in acute lymphoblastic leukemia. Blood 2001; 97(7): 2115-2120.

26. De Waele M et al. Different expression of adhesion molecules on CD34+ cells in AML and B-lineage ALL and their normal bone marrow counterparts. Eur J Haematol 1999; 63(3): 192-201.

27. Yeoh EJ et al. Classification, subtype discovery, and prediction of outcome in pediatric acute lymphoblastic leukemia by gene expression profiling. Cancer Cell 2002; 1(2): 133-143.

28. Armstrong SA et al. MLL translocations specify a distinct gene expression profile that distinguishes a unique leukemia. Nat Genet 2002; 30(1): 41-47.

29. Klein U et al. Gene expression profiling of B cell chronic lymphocytic leukemia reveals a homogeneous phenotype related to memory B cells. J Exp Med 2001; 194(11): 1625-1638.

30. Rosenwald A et al. Relation of gene expression phenotype to immunoglobulin mutation genotype in B cell chronic lymphocytic leukemia. J Exp Med 2001; 194(11): 1639-1647.

31. Wiestner A et al. ZAP-70 expression identifies a chronic lymphocytic leukemia subtype with unmutated immunoglobulin genes, inferior clinical outcome, and distinct gene expression profile. Blood 2003; 101(12): 4944-4951.

32. Mohr S et al. Microarrays as cancer keys: an array of possibilities. J Clin Oncol 2002; 20(14): 3165-3175.

33. Ramaswamy S, Golub TR. DNA microarrays in clinical oncology. J Clin Oncol 2002; 20(7): 1932-1941.

34. Staudt LM. Gene expression profiling of lymphoid malignancies. Annu Rev Med 2002; 53: 303-318.

35. Chan WC, Huang JZ. Gene expression analysis in aggressive NHL. Ann Hematol 2001; 80(Suppl 3): B38-41.

36. Stratowa C et al. cDNA microarray gene expression analysis of B-cell chronic lymphocytic leukemia proposes potential new prognostic markers involved in lymphocyte trafficking. Int J Caner 2001; 91(4): 474-480.

Chapter 2

MYELODYSPLASTIC/MYELOPROLIFERATIVE DISEASES

James W. Vardiman
University of Chicago Department of Pathology, Chicago, Illinois

1.   INTRODUCTION

The chronic myeloproliferative diseases (CMPDs) are generally regarded as clonal hematologic disorders that arise in a pluripotent or multipotent bone marrow stem cell. There is proliferation of cells of one or more of the bone marrow lineages, and the marrow becomes hypercellular as the neoplastic clone expands to replace normal bone marrow cells. The neoplastic hematopoiesis shows maturation and is often "effective", so that there is a corresponding increase in the number of one or more of the cell lines in the peripheral blood. Hepatosplenomegaly, marrow fibrosis, and genetic evolution associated with progressive disease are common.

Myelodysplastic syndromes (MDSs) also originate in a pluripotent or multipotent stem cell, and there is also maturation of the neoplastic cells. Expansion of the abnormal clone usually results in marrow hypercellularity, but, in contrast to the CMPDs, in MDSs the maturing cells exhibit dysplastic morphology and undergo premature apoptosis, resulting in ineffective hematopoiesis and cytopenia(s) in the blood. Organomegaly, at least to the degree observed in CMPD, is uncommon in MDSs. However, genetic evolution is often associated with disease progression, and 25-30% of patients develop overt acute leukemia. Thus, although there are biological, clinical, and laboratory differences between CMPD and MDS, they share a number of features. It is therefore not surprising that some patients initially present with hematologic diseases that seem to be a "hybrid" of MDS and CMPD. This poses a dilemma as to how they should be categorized. Perhaps chronic myelomonocytic leukemia (CMML) is the best example of such an entity. The finding of morphologic dysplasia similar to that observed in MDS and the tendency for patients to evolve to AML were considered by the French-American-British (FAB) investigators as reasons to include CMML in the FAB classification of MDS.[1] However, some patients have marked leukocytosis and hepatosplenomegaly, and therefore other authors have questioned whether CMML is a CMPD rather than MDS.[2, 3]

In the World Health Organization (WHO) classification of myeloid neoplasms, a separate category, Myelodysplastic/ Myeloproliferative Diseases (MDS/MPD), has been introduced to accommodate disorders that appear to "bridge" MDS and CMPD.[4] The concept of "MDS/MPD" is not unique to the WHO classification. Hematologists and hematopathologists have recognized for some time that juvenile myelomonocytic leukemia (JMML) and BCR/ABL-negative atypical chronic myeloid leukemia (aCML) have many similarities to CMML.[5-7] The WHO category, MDS/MPD, includes each of these three diseases.

The "MDS/MPD" category may be viewed as one which encompasses diseases that truly "bridge" MDS and CMPD. On the other hand, it might also be considered as a collection of diseases for which current knowledge is not sufficient for distinguishing patients with a mainly myeloproliferative disease from those whose disease will behave more as a myelodysplastic process. At the least, the creation of this category should remind physicians that patients with one of the MDS/MPD disorders may not always be best served by therapy designed for other subtypes of MDS or CMPD.

2.   PATHOGENESIS OF MDS/MPD

A single pathogenetic abnormality common to all of the disease entities in this category has not been discovered. Even within the same diagnostic category, the symptoms and the clinical and laboratory findings are heterogeneous; therefore, it is likely that a number of diverse molecular defects underlie the MDS/MPD diseases. There are no cytogenetic or molecular genetic abnormalities that are currently known to be specific for any of the MDS/MPD diseases. However, as detailed in the paragraphs that follow, two broad categories of genetic lesions have been described that probably play an important role in their pathogenesis. The first category includes mutations of genes encoding proteins that are important in the regulation of the RAS/MAPK pathway of signal transduction. These abnormalities often render the leukemic cell "hypersensitive" to specific growth factors. The second category includes chromosomal translocations involving genes that encode specific growth factor receptors. These abnormalities lead to abnormal receptors that are constitutively activated with subsequent, constant downstream activation of a number of different signaling pathways.[4, 6, 8-15]

2.1 Juvenile Myelomonocytic Leukemia (JMML)

Although JMML is less common than CMML, the molecular defects that contribute to its pathogenesis are better understood. This understanding comes in part from the association of some cases of JMML with two inherited diseases for which the underlying genetic defects are known, namely, neurofibromatosis type 1 (NF1) and Noonan syndrome.[6, 10, 11, 16] In addition, a hallmark of JMML is the marked hypersensitivity of progenitor cells to granulocyte-macrophage colony-stimulating factor (GM-CSF), which accounts for their ability to form spontaneous colonies in vitro in the absence of exogenous growth factors. This consistent hypersensitivity of JMML progenitor cells to GM-CSF, but not to other growth factors, provided an important clue that pathways of signal transduction from the GM-CSF receptor to the nucleus were likely to be deregulated.[16-18] There is no evidence that the GM-CSF receptor is abnormal. Therefore, downstream pathways that are activated by the binding of GM-CSF with the receptor, such as the Ras-mediated signaling pathway, seem more likely to be the points of deregulation.[19, 20]

The Ras family of proteins is involved in relaying signals from surface receptors to the nucleus. Ras activation is essential for the proliferative response by myeloid cells to a number of hematopoietic growth factors, particularly GM-CSF.[6, 16] The function of the Ras proteins is regulated by their ability to cycle between an activated, GTP-bound state, Ras-GTP, that activates mitogen-activated kinase (MAPK), and an inactive, GDP-bound state, Ras-GDP (Figure 2-1). Somatic RAS mutations are common in myeloid malignancies. Activating point mutations of N-RAS or K-RAS increase intracellular levels of Ras-GTP, and they keep the Ras pathway of signal transduction "switched on." Such activating mutations have been reported in up to 25% of patients with JMML.[21, 22]

The Ras pathway is down-regulated by GTPase-activating proteins that hydrolyze active Ras-GTP to inactive Ras-GDP. One of the GTPase-activating proteins is neurofibromin, a tumor-suppressor protein encoded by the gene NF1. Approximately 15% of patients with JMML have clinical findings of neurofibromatosis type 1, a disease characterized by mutations of NF1.[6, 16] In JMML, the mutations of NF1 are loss-of-function mutations, which are usually accompanied by loss of heterozygosity at the NF1 allele as well. In such cases, the negative regulatory effect of neurofibromin on the Ras pathway is lost, and increased levels of Ras-GTP can be detected in the bone marrow cells of affected children.[23] Furthermore, up to 15% of patients with JMML but no clinical evidence of neurofibromatosis, have been reported to harbor loss-of-function mutations of NF1.[10] Therefore, mutations of NF1 may contribute to leukemogenesis in up to 30% of patients with JMML.

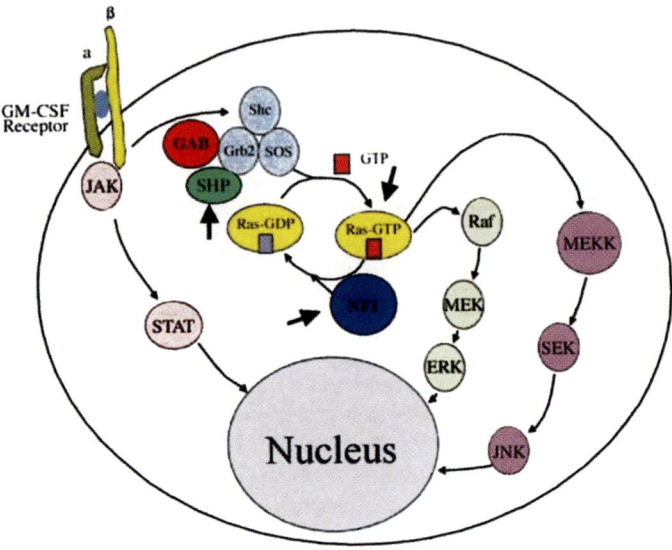

Figure 2-1. Diagram of abnormalities in RAS pathway of signal transduction known to occur in JMML. The arrows indicate points of deregulation of the Ras pathway due to mutations in K-Ras or N-Ras genes, the Nf1 gene that encodes neurofibromin, and the PTPN11 gene that encodes SHP2. These abnormalities are detailed in the text.

Recently, the rare association of JMML with another inherited developmental disorder, Noonan syndrome, has led to the discovery of abnormalities in another protein important in the regulation of the RAS pathway, SHP-2. Germline mutations of the gene PTPN11, which encodes the tyrosine phosphatase SHP-2, have recently been reported in patients with Noonan syndrome. In patients with JMML and Noonan syndrome, the germline mutations of PTPN11 lead to activation of the Ras pathway.[11] Additionally, in a study of 62 patients with JMML who had no clinical evidence of Noonan syndrome, more than one-third also showed de novo somatic mutations of PTPN11.[11] Thus, abnormalities in genes affecting the

RAS signaling pathway, i.e, N-RAS, K-RAS, NF1, and PTPN11, are found in the great majority of children with JMML (Figure 2-1). To date, these mutations seem to be mutually exclusive, which supports the interpretation that they play some role in the pathogenesis of the disease. Whether additional cooperating lesions are necessary for establishing the disease is not yet known.

In JMML, the abnormalities in regulation of the RAS/MAPK pathway account for the marked hypersensitivity of the myeloid progenitor cells to GM-CSF, and for the proliferation in the leukemic clone. There is maturation of the leukemic cells, particularly in the monocytic lineage. However, the mature cells are abnormal, and they may produce cytokines such as interleukin 1 (IL-1) and GM-CSF, which potentiate the proliferation of the neoplastic cells, as well as the production of other cytokines, such as tumor necrosis factor alpha (TNF-alpha, which inhibits normal hematopoiesis. The abundance of mature neutrophils and monocytes results in infiltration of a variety of tissues that contributes to the morbidity associated with JMML.[6, 16]

2.2   Chronic Myelomonocytic Leukemia (CMML)

There are many similarities between CMML and JMML, the most obvious being the effective proliferation of the monocytic lineage and the frequent finding of hepatosplenomegaly. CMML, however, is clinically more heterogeneous than JMML. For example, although all patients with CMML have absolute monocytosis, some have high WBC counts with neutrophilia, whereas others have lower WBC counts, sometimes associated with neutropenia.[24] Such diversity suggests that all patients with CMML are unlikely to have identical underlying molecular and genetic defects, although they may share events that deregulate some key pathways. Unfortunately, many of the studies investigating the pathogenesis of CMML have provided scant details of the laboratory and clinical features of the patients studied. Thus, it is difficult to know whether the defects described pertain to those with mainly myeloproliferative or those with mainly dysplastic disease, or to both groups.

In contrast to JMML, in CMML the ability of progenitor cells to form spontaneous colonies *in vitro*, and their responsiveness to GM-CSF, is reported to be variable.[25-27] The variability may be related to whether the defect is in the regulation of a pathway that requires GM-CSF activation, or whether a leukemia-associated chromosomal translocation produces a tyrosine kinase fusion gene (see below) that leads to constitutive activation of alternate pathways.

The most common genetic defects in CMML are activating mutations of N-RAS or K-RAS, reported in 20-40% of patients.[9, 28] In these cases, hypersensitivity to GM-CSF would be expected, based on a model similar to that for JMML. Other abnormalities that might lead to deregulation of Ras have not yet been delineated. In contrast to the finding in JMML, adults with the NF1 phenotype are not predisposed to CMML.[10]

Cytogenetic abnormalities occur in 20-40% of cases of CMML, although none are entirely specific.[28-30] Chromosomal translocations involving PDGFRbeta, on chromosome band 5q33, are reported to be most commonly associated with CMML with eosinophilia[12-15] Although they are found in fewer than 1-2% of patients with CMML, these translocations serve as an important model of leukemogenesis. Several different partner genes have been reported for PDGFRbeta. The most common translocation is t(5;12)(q33;p13), which results in the fusion of the PDGFRbeta with ETV6 on chromosome 12.[12,15] Other partner genes reported in CMML include HIP1, at 7q11, and RAB5, at 17p13.[31,32] These translocations result in fusion genes that lead to the constitutive activation of the platelet-derived growth factor (PDGF) receptor, and that render the cell growth-factor-independent. The mechanism of activation is most likely through STATs 1 and 5, members of the STAT family of cytoplasmic transcription regulators[14, 33] Therefore, in the case of tyrosine kinase fusion oncogenes, such as the t(5;12), hypersensitivity to growth factors may not be present or necessary for expansion of the neoplastic clone[14]

2.3   Atypical Chronic Myeloid Leukemia (aCML)

The mechanisms of pathogenesis of aCML are probably very similar to those described for CMML, but only a few patients have been studied to date. As is the case for CMML and JMML, there are no specific cytogenetic abnormalities, and +8 has been the most frequently reported karyotypic abnormality in most reports.[34, 35] Recently, 3 cases of aCML have been reported with t(4;22)(q12;q11), a translocation that fuses the platelet derived growth factor alpha receptor gene (PDGFalphaR) with BCR.[36, 37] This fusion leads to constitutive activation of the PDGF receptor. In addition, translocations involving PDGFRbeta have been reported. In one case, ETV6 was the partner gene, whereas in the other case reported to date, H4/D10S170 on chromosome band 10q21 was involved.[38, 39] Besides these chromosomal abnormalities, mutations of RAS have been reported in nearly 30% of cases of aCML that have been studied.[8]

have microcytosis. Platelet counts are decreased in at least 75% of the patients, and at times the thrombocytopenia is severe.[40, 42, 45]

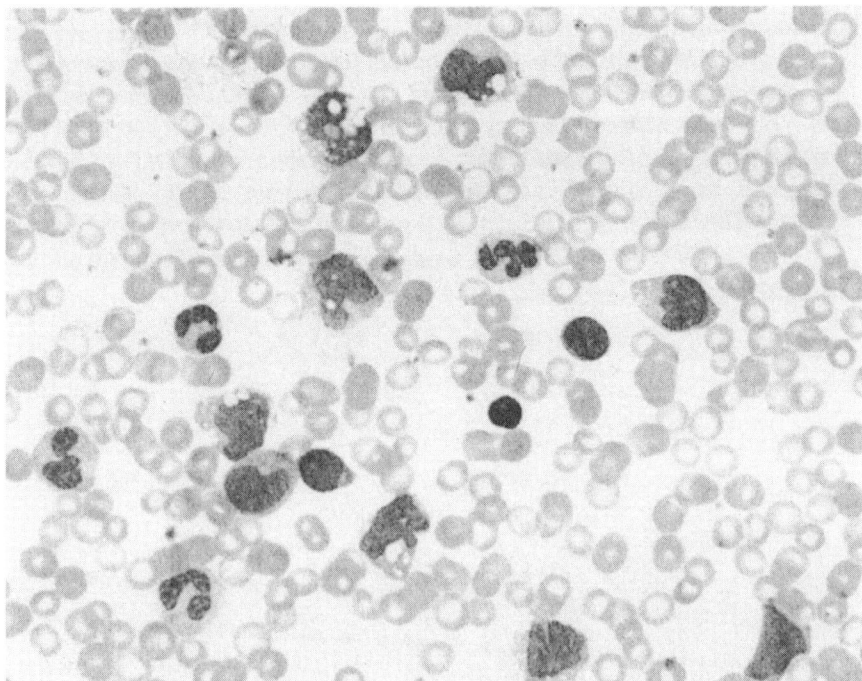

Figure 2-2. Peripheral blood smear from one-year-old boy with JMML. There are increased numbers of neutrophils and neutrophil precursors as well as of monocytes.

Most patients with JMML have hemoglobin F (Hb F) levels that are increased for their age. However, some authors have reported that patients with monosomy 7 and JMML are more likely to have normal or only modestly elevated HbF than do children with a normal karyotype or other cytogenetic abnormalities.[40]

Judging that a marrow specimen from a baby is hypercellular is not always easy; yet most investigators report that bone marrow biopy specimens and aspirates from patients with JMML are hypercellular or normocellular for the patient's age (Figure 2-3). In most cases, the M:E ratio is increased, but it may vary from less than 1:1 to >50:1.[40] Blasts and promonocytes usually account for fewer than 5% of the marrow cells, and by definition, for less than 20%. Auer rods are not seen. Usually, dysplasia is minimal, if present at all, but pseudo-Pelger-Huet neutrophils and neutrophils with cytoplasmic hypogranularity have been reported.[42] Erythroid precursors may show megaloblastic changes. Megakaryocytes are often reduced in number, but megakaryocytic dysplasia is not usual.

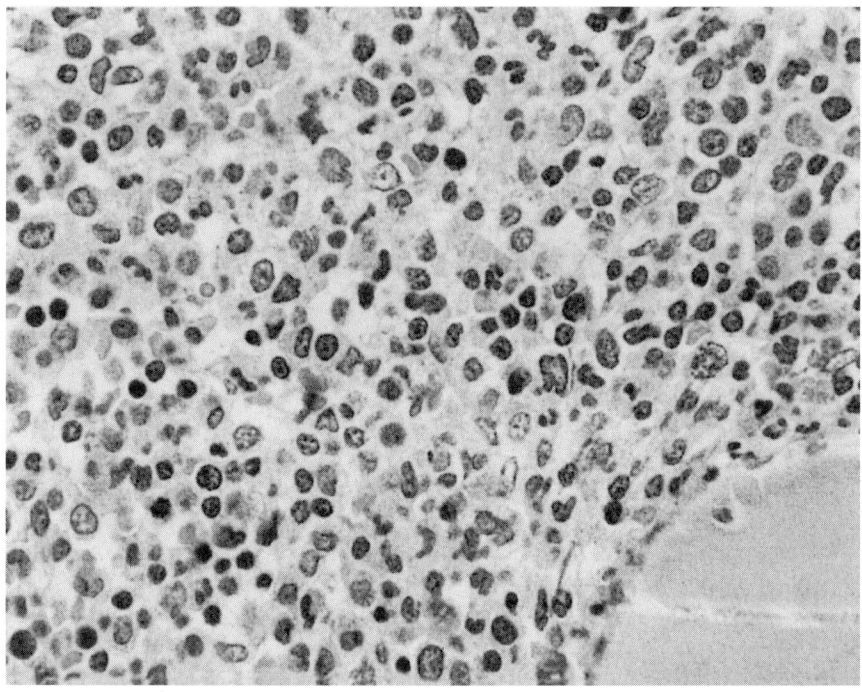

Figure 2-3. Bone marrow biopsy from patient with JMML. The marrow is hypercellular, and shows increased numbers of granulocytic and monocytic cells.

The hepatosplenomegaly observed clinically is due to leukemic infiltration. In the spleen, leukemic cells infiltrate the red pulp and compress and obliterate the white pulp. Liver biopsies often show both portal tract and sinusoidal infiltration. The skin is often infiltrated with myelomonocytic cells in the upper and lower dermis. Myelomonocytic infiltration of the lungs accounts for significant morbidity in JMML, and the cells spread from the peribronchial lymphatics into the alveolar septae.[46]

3.2.2.2   Cytogenetic and Genetic Findings

Normal karyotypes are reported in 40-70% of patients with JMML.[16, 40, 45] Monosomy 7 is noted in approximately 25% of patients, and about 10% are reported to have other cytogenetic abnormalities. Mutations in genes that encode for RAS, NF1, and SHP-2 have each been reported in about 30% of JMML patients; thus, overall, nearly 80-90% of patients will have one of these abnormalities.[6, 10, 11] These mutations are not specific for JMML and have been reported in AML, MDS, and other myeloproliferative diseases.

3.2.2.3   Other Laboratory Findings

More than one half of patients with JMML have polyclonal hypergammaglobulinemia of uncertain significance.[40, 42] Autoantibodies and a positive direct Coombs test have also been reported in up to 25% of cases.

As noted in the initial section on the pathogenesis as well as in Table 2-1, hypersensitivity of the myeloid progenitors to GM-CSF in in vitro studies is characteristic for JMML. This study should be performed in all cases, particularly if the diagnosis of JMML is not readily substantiated by other clinical and laboratory findings.

3.3   Differential Diagnosis of JMML

3.3.1   Infection

The clinical and morphologic findings of JMML can be imitated by a variety of infectious diseases, including viral diseases caused by EBV, CMV, and HHV-6.[16, 43, 47] However, the possibility that a patient with JMML may have a concomitant infection that further obscures the diagnosis must also be considered. Serologic investigations have shown that children with JMML have a similar prevalence of antibodies for CMV, EBV, and herpes virus type 1 as does a normal infant population.[44] The finding of a clonal chromosomal abnormality or other genetic defect, such as Nf1 mutation, would substantiate the neoplastic nature of the process in such cases.

3.3.2   Other Myeloid Diseases

Adult-type BCR/ABL+ CML is even less common in children than is JMML, particularly in those less than 5 years old. Nevertheless, cytogenetic and molecular studies should always be performed to exclude this possibility whenever the diagnosis of JMML is considered.

In contrast to JMML, "adult-type" MDS usually occurs in children above the age of 5 years. It lacks the features required for a diagnosis of JMML, is generally associated with leukopenia rather than leukocytosis, has more striking dysplasia that involves two or all three of the myeloid lineages, and has a lower frequency of hepatosplenomegaly than does JMML.[7, 40, 45] Children with MDS have also been reported to have a higher incidence of cytogenetic abnormalities than do those with JMML, and monosomy 7 as well as structural alterations of chromosomal 7 are particularly common. Thus, monosomy 7 can be seen in both childhood MDS and JMML, and the diagnosis depends on clinical, laboratory, and morphologic findings rather than on the karyotype alone.[41]

In some children with leukocytosis and monocytosis in the adolescent age range, the differental diagnosis of JMML vs. adult-type CMML may arise. There is little question that JMML shares many clinical and morphologic features with CMML. As noted previously, however, the consensus is that all leukemias of childhood, previously referred to as CMML, be included in the JMML category,[7] and that the diagnosis of CMML be made only in cases of childhood leukemia secondary to previous chemotherapy that otherwise meet the criteria for CMML[7]

The distinction between acute myeloid leukemia and juvenile myelomonocytic leukemia is based on the percentages of blasts in the blood and bone marrow. At the time of diagnosis, JMML has fewer than 20% blasts and promonocytes, whereas in acute leukemia, blasts and promonocytes account for 20% or more.[4] Still, at times it is difficult to decide whether a monocytic-lineage cell is a blast, a promonocyte, or a mature, reactive monocyte. A bone marrow biopsy may be particularly helpful in this regard, and the finding of sheets of blasts and immature cells points toward the diagnosis of AML.

3.4   Prognosis and Outcome of JMML

The prognosis of JMML is quite variable. Some patients have indolent disease with survival times in excess of 10 years, whereas in others the disease is very aggressive and the patients die within months of diagnosis. Unfortunately, the latter course is more common, and overall median survival times of only 1-4 years are commonly reported.[16, 40, 45] Factors that are reported to predict a worse outcome include age more than 2 years, platelet counts less than 100 x 10^9/L, and fetal hemoglobin >15%.[42] Patients who receive bone marrow transplantation are reported to have significantly better outcomes than do those who receive chemotherapy alone. In only 10-15% of patients with JMML transforms to overt acute leukemia. Most die due to organ infiltration by monocytic cells, infection, or hemorrhage.[16]

3.5   Chronic Myelomonocytic Leukemia (CMML)

If a single disorder could be considered as the prototype for the MDS/MPD category, it would be CMML. It is a clonal disorder of a bone marrow stem cell, and monocytosis is the major defining feature. Although absolute monocytosis is, by definition, always present, there is remarkable variation in the hematologic parameters. Some patients have prominent neutrophilia in addition to the monocytosis, whereas others have normal WBC counts or even leukopenia that is due to neutropenia (Figure 2-4). Some authorities have suggested that CMML should be divided into two diseases – one that has mainly myelodysplastic features and one that is more myeloproliferative in nature. The FAB group suggested that leukocytosis (WBC > 13 x 10^9/L) be the major criterion used for assigning a case to a myeloproliferative subcategory of CMML, whereas patients with lower WBC counts could be considered to have a myelodysplastic subtype.[48] Although it is likely that there are some pathogenetic differences between the myelodysplastic and the myeloproliferative types of CMML, several authors have presented data suggesting that the FAB proposal does not identify subgroups with unique clinical or biologic findings.[49, 50]

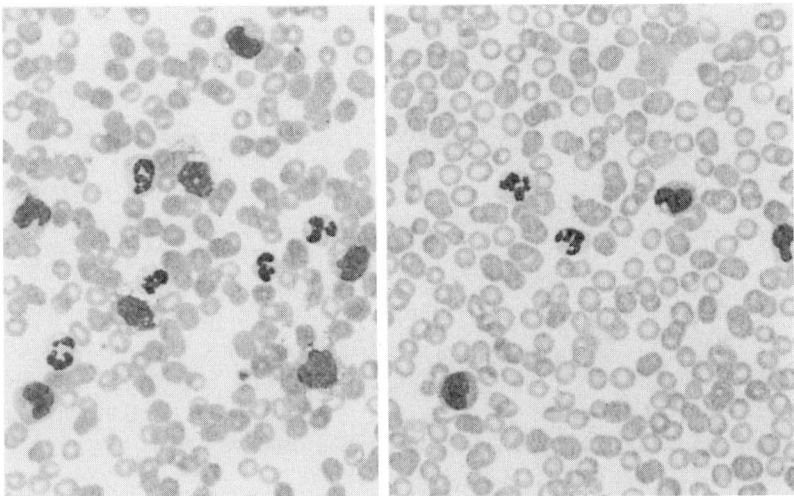

Figure 2-4. Composite photograph of blood smears from two different patients with CMML. This illustrates the heterogeneity of CMML, ranging from blood smears that show elevated WBC counts due to neutrophilia and monocytosis, to normal or even low WBC cell counts. In both patients illustrated, the number of monocytes exceeded 1,000 x 109/L.

3.6   Diagnosis of CMML

3.6.1   Clinical Findings

Most patients are 60-70 years old when they are first diagnosed to have CMML, but young adults have been reported as well.[24, 28, 49, 51, 52] In most series, men are affected 2-3 times more commonly than women. Symptoms most often include fever, infection, or hemorrhagic episodes in up to 30% of patients, and thrombotic complications in 10-15%.[28, 49, 51, 52] Up to 10% of patients have clinical manifestations of an autoimmune disease, such as vasculitic syndromes, arthritis, or even classical connective tissue diseases.[53] The incidence of any of these symptoms does not appear to be related to the magnitude of the WBC count.[49, 53]

Splenomegaly and hepatomegaly are found in 30-40% of patients, and are more common in those with leukocytosis. Lymphadenopathy is found in up to 15% of patients and skin involvement in 5-10%, and both are also more common in patients with high WBC counts.[28, 49]

3.6.2   Laboratory Findings

3.6.2.1   Hematologic and morphologic findings in blood, marrow, and extramedullary tissue

The criteria for the diagnosis of CMML are listed in Table 2-2. A review of the WBC counts commonly reported in patients with CMML underscores the variable manifestations of the disease. The counts range from 2.0 to nearly 500 x 10^9/L, with median values usually between $10 - 20$ x 10^9/L.[2, 24, 28, 49] Patients usually have modest thrombocytopenia, i.e., 80 to 100 x 10^9/L, but values from 1 to >700 x 10^9/L have been reported for platelet counts. Anemia is likewise usually mild, but hemoglobin values as low as 5 g/dL can occur.[2, 24, 28, 49]

Monocytosis is, by definition, present in all cases. When considered in absolute numbers, the range of monocytosis reported is also impressive, varying from 1 x 10^9/L to more than 200 x 10^9/L.[24, 28] (Figure 2-4) In the majority of patients, the monocyte count is below 5 x 10^9/L,[2, 28] but the percentage of monocytes is almost always >10% of the WBCs.[48] This is an important point to note because, in diseases with a markedly elevated WBC counts, only 1-2% monocytes in the leukocyte differential might result in an "absolute" monocytosis. The monocytes in the peripheral blood are generally mature in CMML, with unremarkable morphology, but they can exhibit abnormal granulation, unusual nuclear lobation, or finely dispersed nuclear chromatin.[54] Blasts and promonocytes may be present, but if their sum totals 10% or more of the WBCs, a diagnosis of CMML-2 should be made; if more than 20%, the diagnosis is AML rather than CMML, according to WHO recommendations.[4]

Table 2-2. Diagnostic criteria for CMML

1. Persistent peripheral blood monocytosis >1 x 10^9/L
2. No Philadelphia chromosome or *BCR/ABL* fusion gene
3. Less than 20% blasts in the blood or bone marrow
4. Dysplasia in one or more myeloid lineages. If myelodysplasia is absent or minimal, the diagnosis of CMML may still be made if the other requirements are present and:
    -an acquired, clonal cytogenetic abnormality is present in the marrow cells, or
    -the monocytosis has been persistent for at least 3 months <u>and</u>
    -all other causes of monocytosis have been excluded

Neutrophils may range from 0.3 to nearly 200 x 10^9/L, but are usually normal in number. Dysgranulopoiesis, including neutrophils with hypolobated or abnormally segmented nuclei or abnormal cytoplasmic granulation, is found in most cases.[52, 49] It is a commonly held belief that patients with higher WBC counts have less dyspoiesis than do those with lower counts, but some authors have reported that there is no significant relationship between the severity of dysplasia and the leukocyte count.[49] Immature neutrophils (promyelocytes, myelocytes) usually account for fewer than 10% of the WBCs. Mild basophilia is sometimes present, but basophils usually account for fewer than 2% of the WBCs. Eosinophilia is not uncommonly observed, and if persistently more than 1.5 X 10^9/L, a diagnosis of CMML with eosinophilia should be made.[4] Although a number of such cases are associated with translocations that involve PDGFRbeta on chromosome 5,[12-14] in most cases of CMML with eosinophilia a specific genetic defect has not yet been identified (Figure 2-5).

Bone marrow specimens are hypercellular in more than 75% of cases, but normocellular or even hypocellular specimens may be encountered.[2, 52] Granulocytes are often the most prominent bone marrow component, but an increase in erythroid precursors may be seen as well (Figure 2-6). Dysplastic features are usually present in one or both of these lineages.[49, 52] Monocytic proliferation is invariably present, but can be difficult to appreciate in the biopsy or even on bone marrow smears. Cytochemical studies that aid in the identification of monocytes, such as alpha naphthyl acetate esterase or alpha naphthyl butyrate esterase, used alone or in a combined stain with napthol ASD chloroacetate esterase, are recommended when a diagnosis of CMML is considered (Figure 2-7). Micromegakaryocytes and/or megakaryocytes with abnormally lobated nuclei are observed in more than 80% of cases.[24, 52] Substantial increases in marrow reticulin fibers are reported in nearly 30% of cases.[55] Lymphoid nodules are not uncommonly observed in the biopsy sections.[51]

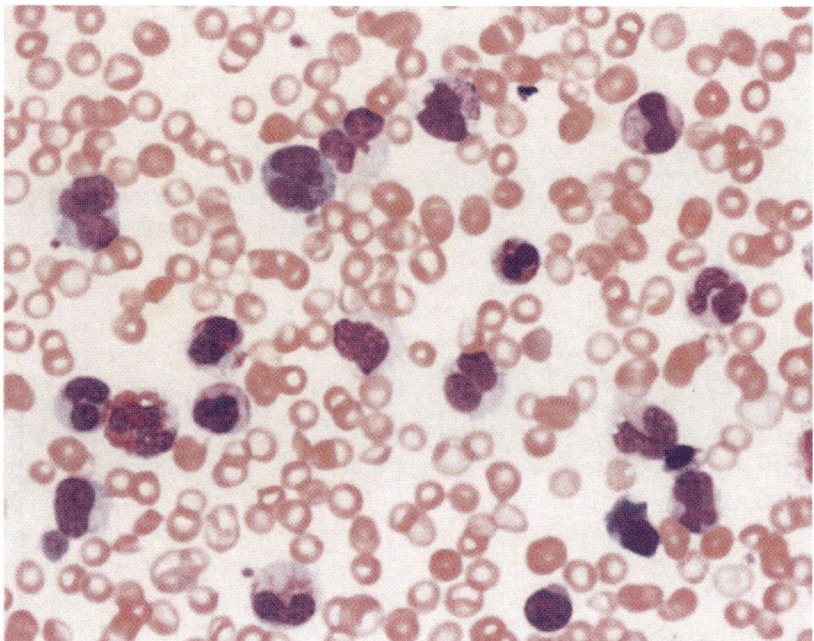

Figure 2-5. Patient with CMML associated with t(5;12)(q33;p13). This patient had significant eosinophilia in the peripheral blood as well as in the bone marrow specimen. Many of the eosinophils were somewhat degranulated.

The number of blasts and promonocytes should be carefully enumerated in both the blood and bone marrow. If their combined percentage is 5-19% in the blood, or 10-19% in the bone marrow, a diagnosis of CMML-2 should be made (Table 2-3). If Auer rods are noted, they also provide sufficient reason to include the patient in the CMML-2 category even if the blasts + promonocytes in the blood and bone marrow are less than 20%. Because patients who have increased numbers of blasts are reported to do poorly, patients who have CMML-2 would be expected to have a worse prognosis and a more rapid transformation to AML than do those with fewer blasts.[28, 52] (Figure 2-8) When the blast + promonocyte percentage is 20% or more, a diagnosis of overt acute leukemia should be made (see Table 2-3).

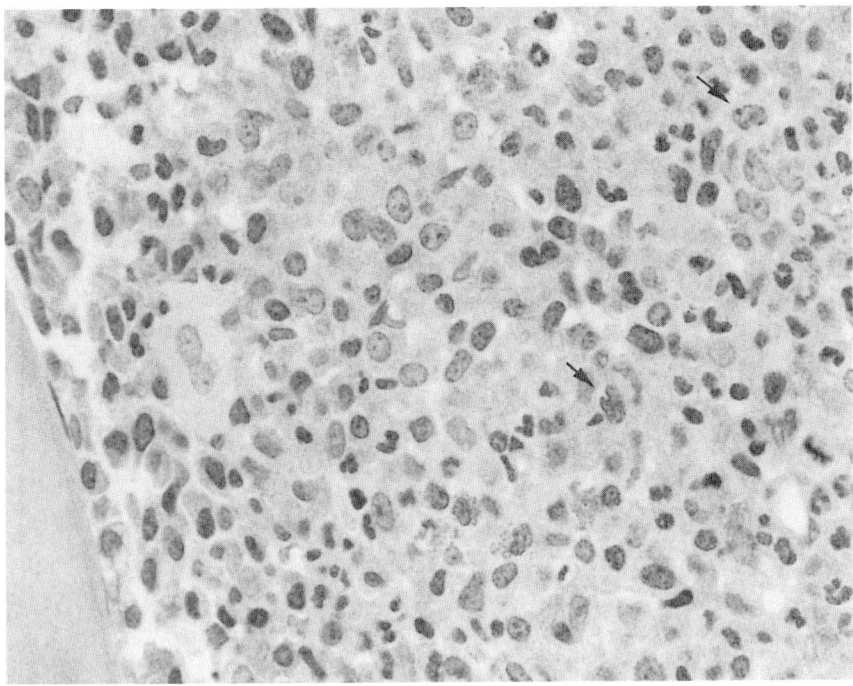

Figure 2-6. Bone marrow biopsy from patient with CMML. Frequently, the bone marrow biopsy specimen appears to show a very prominent granulocytic proliferation, and monocytes are frequently not easily appreciated. Monocytes often show folded or irregularly shaped nuclear contours (arrows).

Splenic enlargement is usually due to leukemic infiltration that is particularly prominent in the red pulp. Lymphadenopathy is seen in a minority of patients, but lymph nodes should always be biopsied, as this may indicate transformation to acute leukemia.

In rare patients with CMML, tumoral proliferations of plasmacytoid monocytes may be seen in the marrow, spleen, and/or lymph nodes.[56, 57] These cells have a round nucleus, finely dispersed nuclear chromatin, and a rim of eosinophilic or amphophilic cytoplasm. They express CD4, CD14, CD43, CD56, and CD68 and may exhibit CD2 and/or CD5 as well. Currently, the relationship between these cells and the leukemic myelomonocytic cells is not well understood.

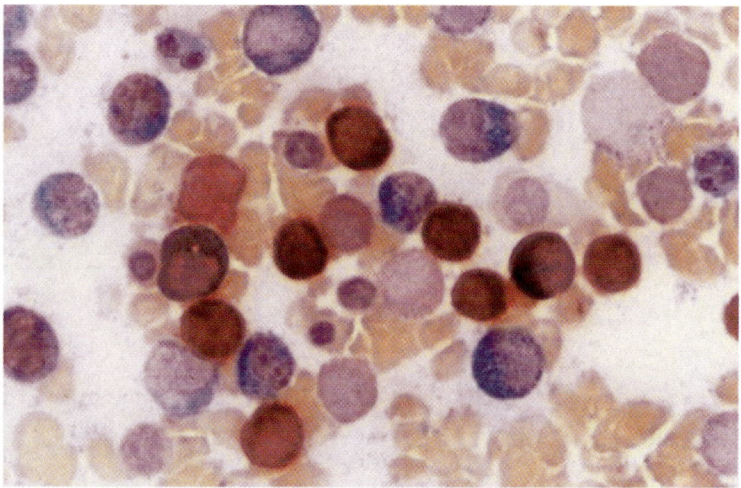

Figure 2-7. Combined esterase on aspirate smear of patient with CMML. Often, even in bone marrow aspirate smears, monocytes are not readily apparent. A non-specific esterase reaction (brown) is combined with Napthol ASD chloroacetate esterase (blue) and aids in detection of increased numbers of monocytes that demonstrate nonspecific esterase. Napthol ASD chloroacetate esterase will help to identify the neutrophil component. Rare cells may demonstrate both reaction products simultaneously.

Table 2-3. Diagnostic criteria for morphologic variants of CMML*

Diagnose CMML-1 when blasts <5% in blood, <10% in bone marrow

Diagnose CMML-2 when blasts 5-19% in blood, or 10-19% in marrow, or if Auer rods are present and blasts are <20% in blood or marrow

Diagnose CMML-1 or CMML-2 with eosinophilia when the criteria above are present and when the eosinophil coune in the peripheral blood is >1.5 x 10⁹/L

*In this classification of CMML, blasts include myeloblasts, monoblasts, and promonocytes.

3.6.2.2   Cytogenetic/Genetic Findings

No specific cytogenetic or genetic abnormalities have yet been identified in CMML. Abnormal karyotypes are reported in 20-40% of cases of CMML. Trisomy 8, -7, -5 plus –7, del(12p), del(20q), i(17), and complex karyotypes are the most commonly reported findings.[28, 29, 49] As noted in the pathogenesis section above, most of the patients with leukemic cells that exhibit t(5;12)(q33;p13) have been reported to have CMML with eosinophilia.[12-14] Although important as a model for leukemogenesis, this translocation, as well as others involving the PDGFRbeta on chromosome 5, are uncommon. Abnormalities involving MLL at 11q23 are also unusual in CMML, and, if present, suggest a diagnosis of AML rather than CMML.

Point mutations of N-ras or K-ras genes reportedly occur in 20-40% of patients.[9, 28]

3.6.2.3 Other Laboratory Findings

Serum lysozyme levels are usually elevated and parallel the degree of monocytosis in the blood.[51, 52, 58] Polyclonal hypergamaglobulinemia has been reported in 50-60% of patients, and rarely, monoclonal proteins may even be detected.[58, 59] A positive Coomb's test when there is no prior transfusion history has been reported in almost 20% of patients evaluated in one study.[59]

3.7 Differential Diagnosis of CMML

3.7.1 Ph+, BCR/ABL+ CML

The distinction between BCR/ABL+ CML and CMML is usually made on the basis of morphology combined with cytogenetics and molecular genetic studies. The BCR/ABL fusion gene is always present in CML and never present in CMML. Occasional cases of CML with a breakpoint in the minor BCR region that leads to a p190 protein may demonstrate monocytosis and resemble CMML, however. Therefore, cytogenetic and genetic testing for the BCR/ABL fusion gene is strongly recommended whenever a diagnosis of CMML is considered. The findings in the peripheral blood of patients with CMML usually differ from those in CML in that there are fewer basophils and fewer immature granulocytes in CMML, whereas monocytes >3% and granulocytic dysplasia are very uncommon in the chronic phase of CML. However, there may be monocytosis in the blood of BCR/ABL + CML after certain types of therapy and granulocytic dysplasia may be seen at the time of transformation of CML to more aggressive phases.[4] Furthermore, the bone marrow biopsy in CMML often shows prominent granulocytic proliferation, and the marrow monocytosis may not be appreciated without special stains. Thus, at times, morphologic inspection of the blood and marrow alone may not be entirely conclusive. Genetic studies are essential in all cases.

3.7.2 Atypical CML (aCML)

aCML is discussed in detail below. Briefly, it is distinguished from CMML mainly based on the percentage of monocytes in the peripheral blood. Rarely does the monocyte percentage exceed 3-4% in aCML, and according to the FAB and WHO guidelines, it should be less than 10% (see Table 2-4). In addition, granulocytic dysplasia is often more severe in aCML than in CMML.[48] Both diseases lack a Ph chromosome or BCR/ABL fusion gene.

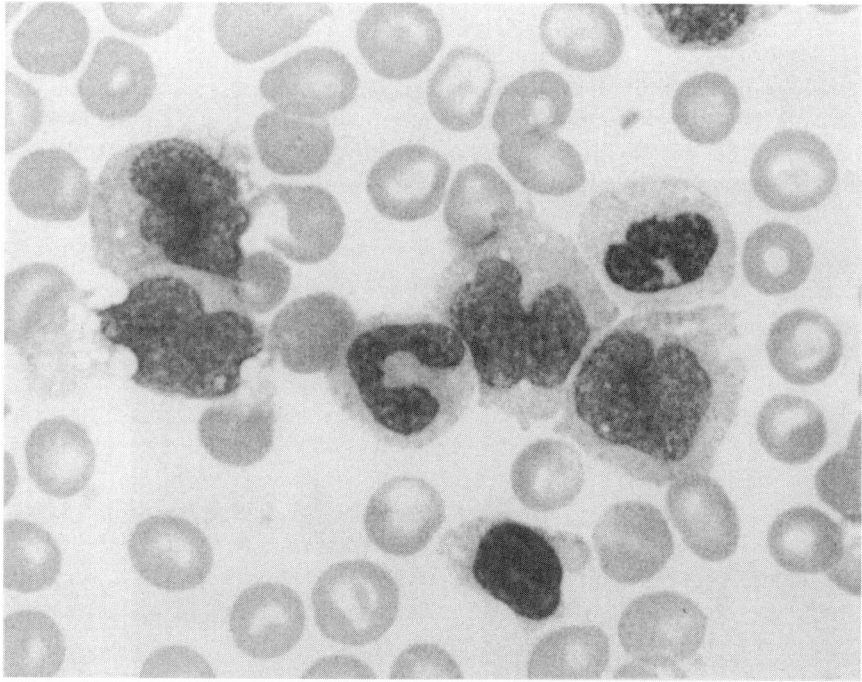

Figure 2-8. This slide illustrates increased numbers of immature monocytes in a patient with CMML-2. The finding of increased number of immature monocytic cells in the blood, including promonocytes and blasts (see Figure 2-9) should always prompt a bone marrow evaluation, because often the marrow will show more immaturity. If promonocytes and blasts account for 5-19% of the white blood cells in the blood, a diagnosis of CMML-2 should be made.

Table 2-4. Diagnostic criteria for aCML

1. Peripheral blood leukocytosis due to increased numbers of mature and immature neutrophils
2. Prominent dysgranulopoiesis
3. No Ph chromosome or *BCR/ABL* fusion gene
4. No or minimal absolute basophilia; basophils <2% of WBCs
5. No or minimal absolute monocytosis; monocytes <10% of WBCs
6. Hypercellular bone marrow with granulocytic proliferation and dysplasi, with or without dysplasia in the erythroid and megakaryocytic lineages
7. Fewer than 20% blasts in the bone marrow

3.7.3   Acute Myelomonocytic and Acute Monocytic Leukemia

Acute leukemia must always be considered in the differential diagnosis of CMML, particularly of CMML-2. A bone marrow aspirate and biopsy are particularly crucial for distinguishing between these entities, because immature monocytes and blasts are often more prominent in the bone marrow than in the blood in each of these diseases. Furthermore, differentiating among monocytes, promonocytes, and monocytic blasts is sometimes very difficult. In CMML, most of the monocytes are mature or have only mildly dispersed nuclear chromatin and no or inconspicuous nucleoli. In contrast, very finely dispersed nuclear chromatin, delicate nuclear folding or creasing, and prominent nucleoli are more in keeping with promonocytes or blasts (the promonocyte is considered as a "blast equivalent" in the WHO classification) (Figure 2-9). Thinly cut sections of the bone marrow biopsy specimens may be particularly helpful for making a distinction between AML and CMML, because it may be easier to appreciate the immaturity of the monocytic cells, as well as to appreciate how much or little granulocytic maturation is present.

3.8   Progression and Prognosis of CMML

In view of the variable clinical, morphologic, and biologic properties of CMML, it is not surprising that survival times for affected patients also vary widely. Although median survival times of 20-40 months are reported in most series, the range of survival for individual patients varies from 1 to more than 120 months.[2, 28, 49] Adverse prognostic factors have been reported to include thrombocytopenia (< 100 x 10^9/L), anemia <12 g/dL, immature granulocytes in the blood, serum LDH > 700 U/L, and bone marrow blasts >10%.[28, 49, 51, 52] Transformation of CMML to AML does occur, but only in 20-30% of patients. More deaths result from the complications of the disease, such as infection, without evidence of transformation.[28, 29, 49]

3.9   Atypical Chronic Myeloid Leukemia (aCML)

It could be argued that there is no myeloid disease that has a more inappropriate name than does aCML. To most physicians and students, "atypical chronic myeloid leukemia" has the connotation that the disease is merely an atypical form of chronic myelogenous leukemia. However, our current understanding of aCML and of the entity classically referred to as "CML" suggests that there are many differences between these two disorders.[4, 48, 60] Importantly, aCML does not have a Ph chromosome or BCR/ABL fusion gene. Furthermore, although aCML does have myeloproliferative aspects, including an elevated WBC count and splenomegaly, it is characterized by remarkable granulocytic and often multilineage dysplasia, and, in most of the series reported to date, an aggressive clinical course.[34, 35, 60] Because of its myeloproliferative and myelodysplastic features, it is appropriate to place aCML in the broad category of MDS/MPD. It is to be hoped that the inclusion of this disease as a distinct entity in the WHO classification will allow more cases to be recognized and more completely investigated.

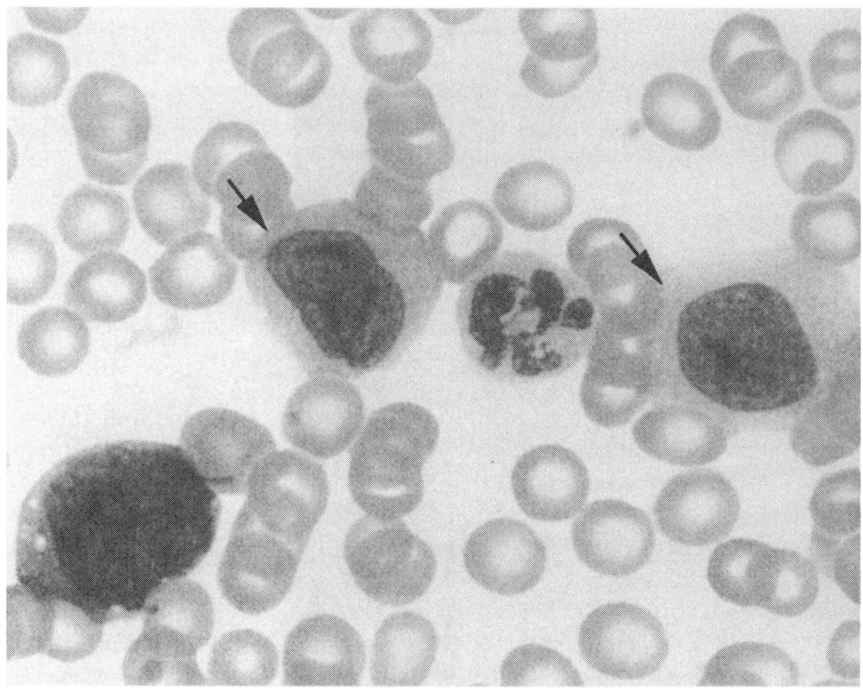

Figure 2-9. The peripheral blood smear from a patient with a diagnosis of CMML-2 progressing to AMML. This photograph illustrates 1 blast and 2 promonocytes (arrows) as well a dysplastic neutrophil. Often the distinction between CMML and AMoL or AMML is quite difficult. In the WHO classification, the promonocytes are considered as "blast" equivalents.

3.10 Diagnosis of aCML

3.10.1 Clinical Findings

Most of the cases reported to date have occurred in older patients, usually in the seventh or eighth decade of life, but younger patients may be affected as well.[34-36] The male to female ratio varies from 1:1 to 2.5:1. In the few cases reported to date, symptoms related to anemia or thrombocytopenia have predominated. Splenomegaly is often prominent, and the chief complaint may be related to a significantly increased spleen size. However, some patients have been reported who initially had laboratory and bone marrow findings that were considered typical for "refractory anemia," and who, after a period of 1-9 years, developed findings typical of aCML and had a poor survival thereafter.[61]

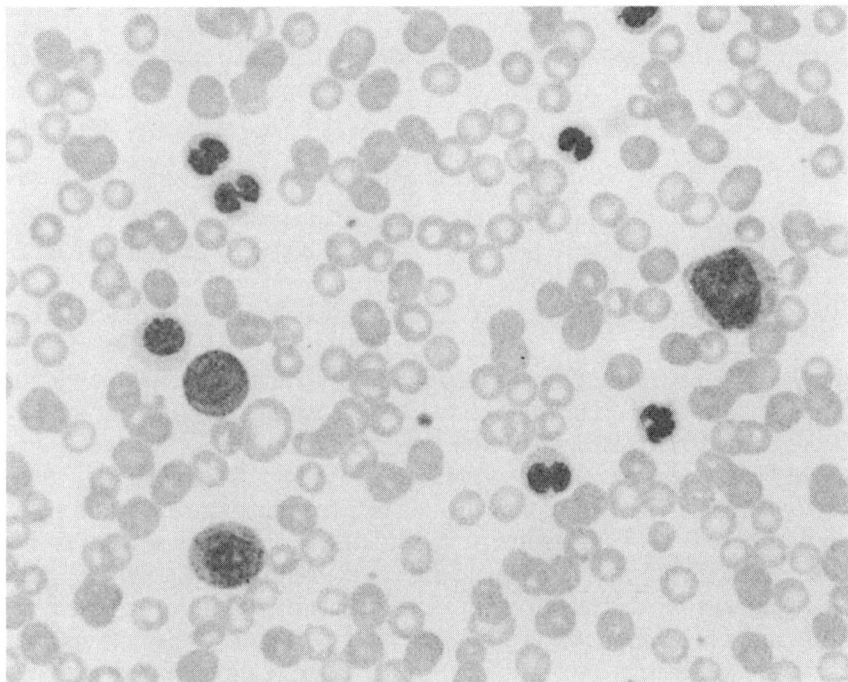

Figure 2-10. Peripheral blood smear from a patient with aCML. This patient has an elevated white cell count, with immature neutrophils and with dysplastic, Pelger-Huet-like nuclei. Even occasional blasts are present. Note the thrombocytopenia.

3.10.2   Laboratory Findings

3.10.2.1   Hematologic and morphologic findings in blood, marrow, and extramedullary tissues

In the peripheral blood there is always leukocytosis (Table 2-4), but the median values reported range from 35-96 x 10^9/L, although individual cases have been reported with WBC counts in excess of 300 x 10^9/L.[34, 35, 60] Thrombocytopenia is often present and may be severe, but thrombocytosis can occur as well. Anemia is usually present.

The peripheral blood smear is most remarkable for showing pronounced dysgranulopoiesis. Neutrophils, many of which have hypogranular cytoplasm or abnormally lobated nuclei, are usually the predominant cells (Figure 2-10). Immature neutrophils account for 10-20% or more of the WBCs, but the percentage of blasts is usually less than 5% and always less than 20%.[4,34] In most cases, basophils account for < 2% of the WBCs.[48, 60] It is important to enumerate monocytes carefully, because they are a key feature in distinguishing aCML from CMML. In aCML, there may be slight absolute monocytosis, but monocytes usually comprise fewer than 3% and always less than 10% of the white cells.[48, 60] Evidence of dyserythropoiesis, such as macro-ovalocytosis, is commonly observed in the blood smear.

The bone marrow biopsy specimen is hypercellular and shows prominent granulocytic proliferation resembling that in a myeloproliferative disease. Erythropoiesis has been reported by some to be more prominent than in BCR/ABL+ CML,[2, 48] whereas others have reported erythroid hypoplasia.[34] Blasts may be modestly increased in number, but should always be less than 20% of the marrow cells. As in the peripheral blood smear, granulocytic dysplasia is marked and can be seen in the aspirate smears and often in the biopsy specimen as well. Megakaryocytes are variable in number, but may be decreased, increased, or normal. In almost all cases, however, some degree of megakaryocytic dysplasia is present.[34, 35] (Figure 2-11) Dyserythropoiesis is also commonly found. The number of reticulin fibers are increased in some patients at the time of diagnosis, and is not uncommonly increased during the course of the disease.

Splenomegaly and hepatomegaly are frequently observed, but there are no studies that detail the histologic findings in these organs in aCML. However, the pattern of involvement would be expected to be similar to that observed in other myeloid diseases, i.e., mainly red pulp involvement of the spleen and a mixed sinus and periportal infiltrate in the liver.

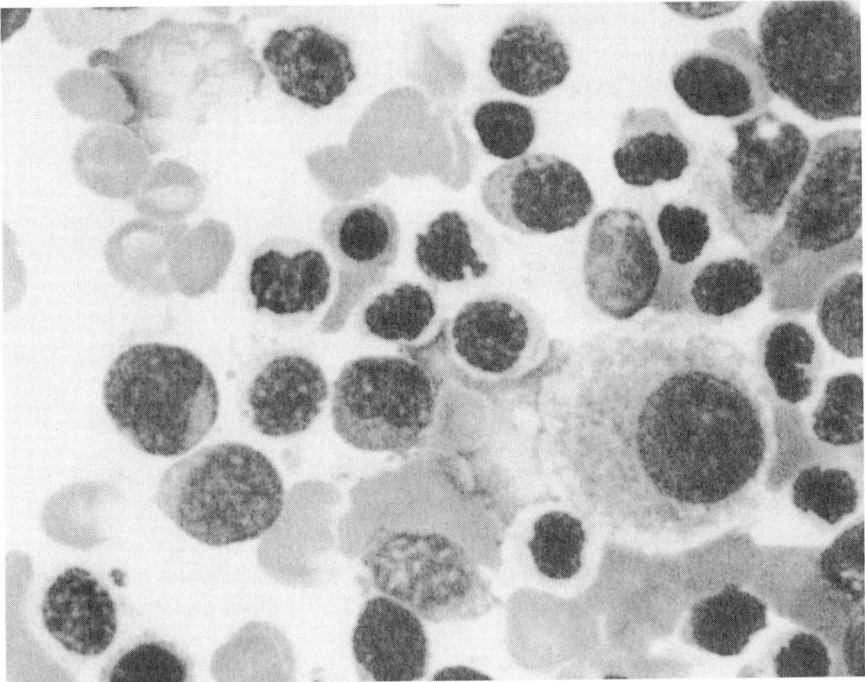

Figure 2-11. The bone marrow aspirate smear from the same patient illustrated in Figure 2-10 demonstrates not only dyspoietic neutrophils, but also a hypolobated, dysplastic megakaryocytes.

3.10.2.2 Cytogenetics/genetics

The majority of patients with aCML have chromosome abnormalities. As noted previously, +8 is the most common cytogenetic abnormality reported, but deletions involving chromosome arms 12q, 12p, 20q, 17p and 13q are other abnormalities that can be seen.[34, 35] The recent reports of t(4;11)(q12;q11) in aCML are particularly exciting because they have the potential to further our understanding of this disease process. On the other hand, details of the clinical and morphologic findings have not been described for cases with this abnormality reported to date, and whether they meet the diagnostic criteria for aCML is not clear.[36, 37]

3.11   Differential Diagnosis of aCML

3.11.1   Chronic Myelomonocytic Leukemia

The differences between CMML and aCML have already been described above in the discussion of the differential diagnosis of CMML. Differences in the reported median survival times of CMML and aCML argue that they are biologically separate entities, but in practice the distinction between them is somewhat arbitrary and at times cannot be made with any degree of confidence. A meaningful discussion of the differences between these two disorders awaits a further understanding of their pathogenesis.

3.11.2   Syndrome of Abnormal Chromatin Clumping

A small number of patients have been reported to have remarkably exaggerated clumping of the nuclear chromatin of neutrophils in the setting of a myeloproliferative disorder.[62-64] Most patients have leukocytosis due to immature and mature neutrophils, with such marked clumping of chromatin that the nucleus appears fragmented and hypolobated. There is often severe anemia and thrombocytopenia. The marrow is hypercellular, and dysplastic changes can be seen in the erythroid precursors and the megakaryocytes. Although neutrophils with such abnormal chromatin condensation can be seen in cases of MDS as a manifestation of marked apoptosis, the association of this finding with an elevated WBC count and other myeloproliferative features is what makes the syndrome of abnormal chromatin clumping unique. Overall, however, the clinical and morphologic features overlap those of aCML, so that, in the WHO classification, the syndrome of abnormal chromatin clumping is considered to be a variant of aCML.[4]

3.12   Myelodysplastic/myeloproliferative Disease, Unclassifiable (MDS/MPD, U)

It is apparent from the criteria for the diagnosis of MDS/MPD,U that the authors of the WHO Classification were concerned that this category might become a repository for cases with insufficient clinical or laboratory data, or inadequate blood or marrow specimens to allow one to decide whether they were MDS or CMPD.[65] (Table 2-5) Such concern, of course, is appropriate for any "unclassifiable" category of disease. On the other hand, there are some patients who initially have features that support a diagnosis of MDS and of MPD, but that do not meet the criteria for the other entities included in the MDS/MPD category. Such cases should prompt careful review, with attention to the details to make certain that a better-defined classification cannot be made that will allow specific and appropriate therapy for the patient. Still, even the most meticulous pathologist and hematologist will encounter occasional patients with diseases that seem to defy accurate classification. In such cases, the use of the term "unclassifiable" is justified.

Table 2-5. Myelodysplastic /Myeloproliferative Disease, Unclassifiable

Clinical, laboratory and morphologic features of one of the categories of MDS and fewer than 20% blasts in blood an marrow, and

-Prominent myeloproliferative features (e.g. platelet count $\geq$ 600 x 10^9/L associated with megakaryocytic proliferation, or WBC count $\geq$ 13.0 x 10^9/L) with or without splenomegaly, and

-No preceding history of an underlying CMPD or of MDS, no history of recent cytotoxic or growth factory therapy that could explain the myelodysplastic or myeloproliferative features, and no Ph chromosome or BCR/ABL fusion gene, del (5q), t(3;3)(q21;q26) or inv(3)(q21q26)

Or the patient has mixed myeloproliferative and myelodysplastic features and cannot be assigned to any other category of MDS, CMPD, or MDS/CMPD

REFERENCES

1. Bennett J.M., Catovsky D., Daniel M.T., et al. Proposals for the classification of the myelodysplastic syndromes. Br J Haematol 1982;51:189-199.
2. Michaux J.L., Martiat P. Chronic myelomonocytic leukaemia (CMML) - a myelodysplastic or myeloproliferative syndrome? Leuk Lymph 1993;9:35-41.
3. Bain B.J. The relationship between the myelodysplastic syndromes and the myeloproliferative disorders. Leuk Lymphoma 1999;34:443-449.
4. Jaffe E.S., Harris N.L., Stein H., Vardiman J.W. (eds): World Health Organization Classification of Tumours. Pathology and Genetics of Tumours of Haematopoietic and Lymphoid Tissues. Lyon: IARC Press, 2001.
5. Neuwirtová R., Mociková K., Musilová J., et al. Mixed myelodysplastic and myeloproliferative syndromes. Leuk Res 1996; 20:717-726.
6. Emanuel P.D., Shannon K.M., Castleberry R.P. Juvenile myelomonocytic leukemia: molecular understanding and prospects for therapy. Mol Med Today 1996;2:468-475.
7. Hasle H., Niemeyer C.M., Chessells J.M., et al. A pediatric approach to the WHO classification of myelodysplastic and myeloproliferative disease. Leukemia 2003;17:277-282.
8. Cogswell P.C., Morgan R., Dunn M., et al. Mutations of the Ras protooncogenes in chronic myelogenous leukemia: a high frequency of Ras mutations in bcr/abl rearrangement-negative chronic myelogenous leukemia. Blood 1989;74:2629-2633.
9. Hirsch-Ginsberg C., LeMaistre A.C., Kantarjian H., et al. RAS mutations are rare events in Philadelphia chromosome-negative/bcr gene rearrangement-negative chronic myelogenous leukemia, but are prevalent in chronic myelomonocytic leukemia. Blood 1990;76:1214-1219.

10. Side L.E., Emanuel P.D., Taylor B., et al. Mutations of the NF1 gene in children with juvenile myelomonocytic leukemia without clinical evidence of neurofibromatosis, type 1. Blood 1998;92:267-272.

11. Tartaglia M., Niemeyer C.M., Fragele A., et al. Somatic mutations in PTPN11 in juvenile myelomonocytic leukemia, myelodysplastic syndromes and acute myeloid leukemia. Nat Genet 2003;34:148-150.

12. Golub T.R., Barker G.F., Lovett M., et al. Fusion of PDGF receptor beta to a novel ets-like gene, tel, in chronic myelomonocytic leukemia with t(5;12) chromosomal translocation. Cell 1994;77:307-316.

13. Carroll M., Tomasson M.H., Barker G.F., et al. The TEL/platelet-derived growth factor beta receptor (PDGFbetaR) fusion in chronic myelomonocytic leukemia is a transforming protein that self-associates and activates PDGFbeta R kinase-dependent signaling pathways. Proc Natl Acad Sci USA 1996;93:145-150.

14. Tomasson M.H., Williams I.R., Hasserjian R., et al. TEL/PDGFbetaR induces hematologic malignancies in mice that respond to a specific tyrosine kinase inhibitor. Blood 1999;93:1707-1714.

15. Kelly L., Clark .J, Gilliland D.G. Comprehensive genetic analysis of leukemia: clinical and therapeutic implications. Cur Opinion Oncol 2002;14:10-18.

16. Emanuel P.D. Myelodysplasia and myeloproliferative disorders in children: an update. Review. Br J Haematol 1999;103:852-863.

17. Suda T., Miura Y., Mizoguchi H., et al. Characterization of hematopoietic precursor cells in juvenile-type chronic myelocytic leukemia. Leuk Res 1982;6:43-53.

18. Emanuel P.D., Bates L.J., Castleberry R.P., et al. Selective hypersensitivity to granulocyte-macrophage colony-stimulating factor by juvenile chronic myeloid leukemia hematopoietic progenitors. Blood 1991;77:925-929.

19. Busque L., Gilliland D.G., Prachal J.T., et al. Clonality in juvenile chronic myelomonocytic leukemia. Blood 1995;85:21-30.

20. Freeburn R.W., Gale R.E., Wagner H.M., Linch D.C. Analysis of the coding sequence for the GM-CSF receptor alpha and beta chains in patients with juvenile chronic myeloid leukemia (JCML). Exp Hematol 1997;25:306-311.

21. Miyauchi J., Asada M., Sasaki M., et al. Mutations of the N-ras gene in juvenile chronic myelogenous leukemia. Blood 1994;83:2248-2254.

22. Flotho C., Valcamonica S., Mach-Pascual S., et al. RAS mutations and clonality analysis in children with juvenile myelomonocytic leukemia (JMML). Leukemia 1999;13:32-37.

23. Side L., Taylor B., Cayouette M., et al. Homozygous inactivation of the NF1 gene in bone marrow cells from children with neurofibromatosis type 1 and malignant myeloid disorders. N Eng J Med 1997;336:1713-1720.

24. Martiat P., Michaux J.L., Rodhain J. for the Groupe Français de Cytogénétique Hématologique. Philadelphia-negative (Ph-) chronic myeloid leukemia (CML): comparison with Ph+ CML and chronic myelomonocytic leukemia. Blood 1991;78:205-211.

25. Emanuel P.D., Zhu S.W., Bates L.J., Zuckerman K.S. Hypersensitivity to hemopoietic growth factors in chronic myelomonocytic leukemia. Blood 1991;78(Suppl.1), 567a .

26. Cambier N., Baruchei A., Schlageter M.H., et al. Chronic myelomonocytic leukemia: from biology to therapy. Hematology and Cell Therapy 1997;39:41-48.

27. Ramshaw H.S., Bardy P.G., Lee M.A., et al. Chronic myelomonocytic leukemia requires granulocyte-macrophage colony-stimulation factor for growth in vitro and in vivo. Exp Hematol 2002;30:1124-1131.

28. Onida F., Kantarjian H.M., Smith T.L., et al. Prognostic factors and scoring systems in chronic myelomonocytic leukemia: a retrospective analysis of 213 patients. Blood 2002;99:840-849.

29. Groupe Francais de Cytogenetique Hematologique. Chronic myelomonocytic leukemia: Single entity or heterogeneous disorder? A prospective multicenter study of 100 patients. Cancer Genet Cytogenet 1991;55:57-65.

30. Toyama K., Ohyashiki K., Yoshida Y.. Clinical implications of chromosomal abnormalities in 401 patients with myelodysplastic syndromes: a multicentric study in Japan. Leukemia 1993;7:499-508.

31. Ross T.S., Bernard O.A., Berger R., Gilliland D.G. Fusion of Huntingtin interacting protein 1 to platelet derived growth factor beta receptor (PDGFbetareceptor) in chronic myelomonocytic leukemia with t(5;7)(q33;q11.2). Blood 1998;91:4419-4426.

32. Magnusson M.K., Meade K.E., Nakamura R., et al. Activity of STI571 in chronic myelomonocytic leukemia with a platelet-derived growth factor beta receptor fusion oncogene. Blood 2002;100:1088-1091.

33. Wilbanks A.M., Mahajan S., Frank D.A., et al. TEL/PDGFbetaR fusion protein activates STAT1 and STAT5: a common mechanism for transformation by tyrosine kinase fusion proteins. Exp Hematol 2000;28:584-593.

34. Hernandez J.M., del Canizo M.C., Cuneo A., et al. Clinical, hematological and cytogenetic characteristics of atypical chronic myeloid leukemia. Ann Oncol 2000;11:441-444.

35. Shukralla N., Finiewicz K., Roulston D., et al. Is atypical chronic myeloid leukemia a high white count myelodysplastic disorder? Mod Pathol 1997;10:134a.

36. Baxter E.J., Hochhaus A., Bolufer P., et al. The t(4;22)(q12;q11) in atypical chronic myeloid leukemia fuses BCR to PDGFRalpha. Human Mol Genet 2002;11:1391-1397.

37. Trempat P., Villalva C., Laurent G., et al. Chronic myeloproliferative disorders with rearrangement of the platelet-derived growth factor alpha receptor: a new clinical target for STI571/Glivec. Oncogene 2003;22:5702-5706.

38. Siena S., Sammarelli G., Grimoldi M.G., et al. New reciprocal translocation t(5;10)q33;q22) associated with atypical chronic myeloid leukemia. Haematologica 1999;84:369-372.

39. Aurich J., Duchayne E., Huguet-Rigal F., et al. Clinical, morphological, cytogenetic and molecular aspects of a series of Ph-negative chronic myeloid leukemias. Hematol Cel Ther 1998;40:149-158.

40. Niemeyer C.M., Arico M., Biondi A., et al. Chronic myelomonocytic leukemia in childhood: A retrospective analysis of 110 cases. Blood 1997;89:3534-3543.

41. Hasle H., Arico M., Biondi A., et al. Myelodysplastic syndrome, juvenile myelomonocytic leukemia, and acute myeloid leukemia associated with complete or partial monosomy 7. Leukemia 1999;13:376-385.

42. Arico M., Biondi A., Pui C.H. Juvenile myelomonocytic leukemia. Blood 1997;90:479-488.

43. Pinkel D. Differentiating juvenile myelomonocytic leukemia from infectious disease. Blood 1998;91:365-367.

44. Niemeyer C.M., Fenu S., Hasle H., et al. Response (letter); Differentiating juvenile myelomonocytic leukemia from infectious disease. Blood 1998;91:365-367.

45. Luna-Fineman S., Shannon K.M., Atwater S.K., et al. Myelodysplastic and myeloproliferative disorders of childhood: A study of 167 patients. Blood 1999;93:459-466.

46. Hess J.L., Zutter M.M., Castleberry R.P., Emanuel P.D.. Juvenile chronic myelogenous leukemia. Am J Clin Pathol 1996;105:238-248.
47. Herrod H., Dow L., Sullivan J. Persistent Epstein-Barr virus infection mimicking juvenile chronic myelogenous leukemia: Immunologic and hematologic studies. Blood 1983;61:1098-1105.
48. Bennett J.M., Catovsky D., Daniel M.T., et al. The chronic myeloid leukaemias: guidelines for distinguishing chronic granulocytic, atypical chronic myeloid, and chronic myelomonocytic leukaemia: proposals by the French-American-British Cooperative Leukaemia Group. Br J Haematol 1994;87:746-754.
49. Germing U., Gattermann N., Minning H., et al. Problems in the classification of CMML – dysplastic versus proliferative type. Leuk Res 1998;22:871-878.
50. Voglová J., Chrobák L., Neuwirtová R., et al. Myelodysplastic and myeloproliferative type of chronic myelomonocytic leukemia-distinct subgroups or two stages of the same disease? Leuk Res 2001;25:493-499.
51. Fenaux P., Beuscart R., Lai J.L., et al. Prognostic factors in adult chronic myelomonocytic leukemia: an analysis of 107 cases. J Clin Oncol 1988;6:1417-1424.
52. Storniolo A.M., Moloney W.C., Rosenthal D.S., et al. Chronic myelomonocytic leukemia. Leukemia 1990;4:766-770.
53. Saif M.W., Hopkins J.L., Gore S.D. Autoimmune phenomena in patients with myelodysplastic syndromes and chronic myelomonocytic leukemia. Leuk Lymph 2002;43:2083-2092.
54. Kouides P.A., Bennett J.M. Morphology and classification of the myelodysplastic syndromes and their pathologic variants. Semin Hematol 1996;33:95-110.
55. Maschek H., Georgii A., Kaloutsi V., et al. Myelofibrosis in primary myelodysplastic syndromes: a retrospective study of 352 patients. Eur J Haematol 1992;48:208-214.
56. Baddoura F.K., Hanson C., Chan W.C. Plasmacytoid monocyte proliferation associated with myeloproliferative disorders. Cancer 1992;69:1457-1467.
57. Harris N.L., Demirjian Z. Plasmacytoid T-zone cell proliferation in a patient with chronic myelomonocytic leukemia. Histologic and immunohistologic characterization. Am J Surg Pathol 1991;15:87-95.
58. Fenaux P., Jouet J.P., Zandecki M., et al. Chronic and subacute myelomonocytic leukaemia in the adult: a report of 60 cases with special reference to prognostic factors. Br J Haematol 1987;65:101-106.
59. Solal-Celigny P., Desaint B., Herrera A., et al. Chronic myelomonocytic leukemia according to the FAB classification: analysis of 35 cases. Blood 1984;63:634-638.
60. Shepherd P.C.A., Ganesan T.S., Galton D.A.G. Haematological classification of the chronic myeloid leukaemias. Bailliere's Clinical Haematology 1987;1:887-906.
61. Oscier D.G. Atypical chronic myeloid leukaemia, a distinct clinical entity related to the myelodysplastic syndrome? Br J Haematol 1996;92:582-586.
62. Felman P., Bryon P.A., Gentilhomme O., et al. The syndrome of abnormal chromatin clumping in leucocytes: a myelodysplastic disorder with proliferative features? Br J Haematol 1988;70:49-54.
63. Invernizzi R., Custodi P., De Fazio P., et al. The syndrome of abnormal chromatin clumping in leucocytes: clinical and biological study of a case. Haematologica 1990;75:532-536.
64. Brizard A., Huret J.L., Lamotte J.I., et al. Three cases of myelodysplastic-myeloproliferative disorder with abnormal chromatin clumping in granulocytes. Correspondence. Br J Haematol 1989;72:294-295.

65. Bain B., Vardiman J.W., Imbert M., Pierre R. Myelodysplastic/myeloproliferative disease, unclassifiable, in Jaffe ES, Harris NL, Stein H, Vardiman JW (Eds): World Health Organization Classification of Tumours. Pathology and Genetics of Tumours of Haematopoietic and Lymphoid Tissues. Lyon: IARC Press, 2001.

Chapter 3

RELEVANCE OF PATHOLOGIC CLASSIFICATIONS AND DIAGNOSIS OF ACUTE MYELOID LEUKEMIA TO CLINICAL TRIALS AND CLINICAL PRACTICE

Martin S. Tallman
Northwestern University Feinberg School of Medicine, and Robert H. Lurie Comprehensive Cancer Center, Chicago, Illinois

1. INTRODUCTION

Major progress has occurred during the past 40 years in our understanding of both the biology of acute myeloid leukemia (AML) as well as of therapy and prognosis. The foundation of such progress lies in the recognition that AML represents a heterogeneous group of diseases. The number of subtypes of AML has expanded since the original description of the FAB classification in 1976 which is based primarily on morphology.[1,2] It is now well recognized that subtypes of AML have different cytogenetic and molecular genetic features, cell surface antigen expression, clinical manifestations, treatments and prognoses.

In general, the treatment of younger adults with AML has improved during the last 40 years.[3,4] Such progress is attributable to both changes in supportive care as well as increased intensity of post remission therapy.[4] However, both large cooperative group and single institution studies confirm that similar progress has not occurred in older adults.[5-7] Differences in outcome relate in part to the age of the patient. However, other factors, including the presence of an antecedent hematologic disorder, cytogenetic abnormalities, and molecular findings such as surface antigen expression, and multidrug resistance markers, contribute to prognosis. This chapter will focus on several specific subtypes of AML which reflect the importance of evolving changes in the pathologic classification of AML in the development of new therapies which have influenced prognoses.

2.   CLASSIFICATIONS

2.1   French-American-British Classification

Although the French-American-British (FAB) classification remains a useful common language among hematopathologists, clinical investigators, and clinicians, important new insights into the biology of AML have limited its utility and provided a foundation for new classifications.[1,8,9] The FAB classification is based solely on the morphology of the leukemic cells and basic cytochemical stains. Subsequent to the initial publication describing the FAB classification, several additional subtypes of AML were defined including undifferentiated AML (FAB M0) and acute megakaryocytic leukemia (FAB M7) which rely on immunophenotyping to establish a definitive diagnosis.[10,11] Head has proposed a classification which separates AML into those which arise de novo and those which evolve from prior myelodysplastic syndromes.[8] The latter group is recognized by resistant leukemia, specific cytogenetic abnormalities, often similar to those found in patients with myelodysplastic syndromes, early relapse and evidence of dysplastic morphologic features.

Table 3-1. WHO Classification of Acute Myeloid Leukemia (adapted from Brunning[9])

AML with recurrent genetic abnormalities
-AML with t(8;21); (*AML1/ETO*)
-AML with abnormal bone marrow eosinophils, inv (16)(p13q22) or t(16;16)(p13;q22); (*CBFβ*/MYH11)
-Acute promyelocytic leukemia with t(15;17)(q22;q12)(*PML/RARα*) and variants
-AML with 11q23 (*MLL*) abnormalities
AML with multilineage dysplasia (dysplasia involving >50% of all cell lineages)
-Following a myelodysplastic syndrome or myelodysplastic syndrome/myeloproliferative disorder
-Without antecedent myelodysplastic syndrome
Acute myeloid leukemia and myelodysplastic syndromes, therapy-related
-Alkylating agent-related
-Topoisomerase type II inhibitor-related (some may be lymphoid)
-Other types
Acute myeloid leukemia not otherwise categorized
-Classification analogous to FAB MO through M7
-Acute basophilic leukemia
-Acute panmyelosis with myelofibrosis
-Myeloid sarcoma

2.2   World Health Organization Classifications

More recently, the World Health Organization (WHO) classification has been described which takes into account specific nonrandom cytogenetic abnormalities, molecular genetic changes, the identification of an antecedent hematologic disorder (secondary AML) evolving after exposure to prior chemotherapy for another malignancy, and the presence of antigen expression on leukemic cells.[9,12] (Table 3-1) Among the most important changes proposed in the WHO classification is a reduction in the percentage of blasts in the bone marrow sufficient to establish a diagnosis of AML. The new WHO classification establishes 20% as the threshold to make a diagnosis of AML. In addition, it has been proposed that patients with t(8;21)(q22;q22), inv(16)(p13q22), t(16;16)(p13;q22) and t(15;17)(q22;q22) should be considered to have AML regardless of the blast percentage or the marrow.[12] The previous classification of the myelodysplastic syndrome (MDS), refractory anemia with excess blasts in transformation (RAEBIT) has been eliminated. Such a change appears justified since patients with RAEBIT have a similar outcome as those with AML when treated with similar intensive antileukemic chemotherapy.[13] The importance of determining cytogenetic abnormalities as well as molecular genetic abnormalities is emphasized, since cytogenetic abnormalities represent the most important prognostic factor in AML. These include the identification of fusion transcripts associated with core binding factor leukemias and the fusion transcript pathognomonic of acute promyelocytic leukemia (APL). Definitions for diagnosis and response, previously established by a National Cancer Institute-sponsored workshop,[14] recently have been revisited.[15] The importance in classifying patients with AML by cytogenetic risk group as well as primary or secondary AML is emphasized, particularly when determining eligibility for participation in large clinical trials so that uniform comparisons of outcome with various treatments can be made. It has been recommended that contemporary clinical trials for patients with AML include patients with what was previously identified as RAEBIT.[14,15] In addition, new categories of response have been proposed, including early treatment assessment at 7-10 days, morphologic leukemia-free state where persistent phenotype abnormalities by flow cytometry is viewed as evidence of persistent disease, morphologic CR with incomplete blood count recovery, cytogenetic CR requiring a normal karyotype, molecular CR for specific subtypes of AML (APL) where the prognostic significance of a molecular CR has been firmly established and partial remission which is particularly applicable for phase I and II clinical trials which evaluate the safety and efficacy of novel agents or strategies.

3.   CORE BINDING FACTOR LEUKEMIAS

Core binding factor leukemias represent subgroups of AML which have rearrangements involving gene encoding for the core binding factor (CBF) alpha-2 (AML1, RUNX1) and the beta subunits, and include FAB M2 AMLs with t(8;21)(q22;q22), inv(16)(p13q22), and t(16;16)(p13;q22).[16-20] Such specific cytogenetic changes lead to the generation of fusion genes which include AML1-ETO and CBF-MYH11, respectively. Such patients have cytogenetic abnormalities which are included among the favorable-risk cytogenetic classifications.[21,22] (Table 3-2) These patients appear to have an improved prognosis compared to many patients with other cytogenetic subtypes of AML and those with a normal karyotype when given consolidation with intensive post remission chemotherapy, which often includes high-dose cytarabine.

Table 3-2. Cytogenetic Risk Groups for Acute Myeloid Leukemia (from Slovak et al[21])

Favorable	Inv(16)/t(16;16)/del(16); t(15;17) without secondary aberrations; t(8;21) lacking del(9) or complex karyotype
Standard	Normal or +8, +6, -y, del(12p)
Unfavorable	del(5q)/-5, -7/del(7q), abn 3q, 9q, 11q, 20q, 21q, 17p, del(9q), t(6;9), t(9;22), complex karyotypes with ≥ 3 unrelated abn

3.1   t(8;21)(q22;q22) Translocation

Patients with FAB M2 morphology and the t(8;21)(q22;q22) translocation have a distinct cytogenetic and clinical subtype of AML. This specific cytogenetic abnormality is seen in approximately 40% of patients with AML who have the FAB M2 subtype. This specific balanced reciprocal translocation, leads to the formation of the AML1-ETO fusion transcript.[16-18] The AML1 gene forms a heterodimeric complex with CBFβ which appears to regulate the transcription of target genes while adding to the DNA sequence TGT/cGGT. AML1 interacts with target genes through its activation domain with the multifunctional transcription coactivators p300 and CBP which activate transcription by acetylating chromatin. While the majority of patients have a balanced reciprocal translocation, this specific cytogenetic abnormality is frequently accompanied by additional cytogenetic chromosome abnormalities such as loss of a sex chromosome and deletion of the long arm of chromosome 9.[19,20]

The majority of patients with the t(8;21)(q22;q22) have leukemic cells which express HLA-DR CD34, CD33, CD13, CD19 and less frequently, CD56.[23,24] This is a relatively distinct immunophenotype with expression of both myeloid and stem cell antigens. There is a subgroup of patients that express the antigen CD56, which identifies the neural cell adhesion molecule, associated with the development of extramedullary disease.[25] [26] Such expression of CD56 in this subgroup of patients has been associated with significantly inferior complete remission (CR) duration and overall survival (OS) compared to other patients with this translocation who do not express the CD56 antigen.[27] Several reports also suggest an inferior outcome among patients with APL who express CD56 (discussed below).

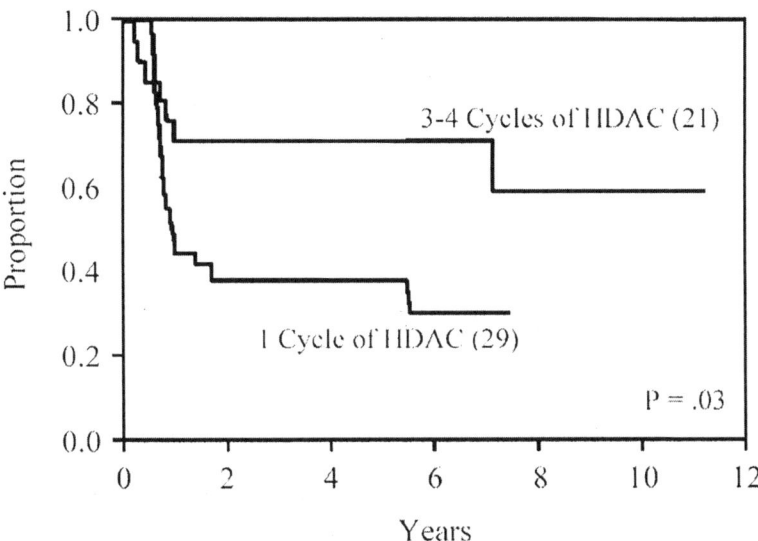

Figure 3-1. Disease-free survival for patients with t(8;21)(q22;q22) (from Byrd[31])

Patients with FAB M2 morphology who have the t(8;21)(q22;q22) constitute a subgroup of patients with favorable-risk cytogenetics.[28] Such patients appear to have a significantly more favorable outcome than those with other subtypes of AML including those patients with normal karyotypes, when similarly treated with intensive postremission chemotherapy.[29,30] It has been suggested that such patients fare particularly well if given intensive consolidation chemotherapy with multiple cycles of high-dose cytarabine (HDAC).[31,32] (Figure 3-1) Whether patients definitely need what is considered high-dose cytarabine at 2-3 gm/m2 per dose, is not clear, since there are data from the Medical Research Council (MRC) in the United Kingdom which suggest that patients do equally well with lower doses of cytarabine at the 1 gm/m2 per dose.[28] However, even within this relatively favorable subtype of AML, the prognosis varies depending on antigen expression as discussed above and presenting white blood cell count.[33] The identification of this particular subtype of AML represents an example of the importance of correlating morphology, immunophenotyping, and cytogenetics to guide therapy.

3.2   inv(16)(p13q22) and t(16;16)(p13;q22) Cytogenetic Abnormalities

A second subtype of AML which is considered a core binding factor leukemia, are those associated with either inv(16)(p13q22) or t(16;16)(p13;q22) which result in the formation of the CBFβ-MYH11 fusion transcript.[34-38] Patients with such cytogenetic abnormalities have often bone marrows with an increased number of abnormal-appearing eosinophils. Some patients may have cryptic translocations not identifiable by routine karyotyping of metaphase cells, but all patients with this subtype will have the fusion transcript detected. Patients who have evidence of a trisomy 22, a common additional cytogenetic abnormality in patients with inv(16), should be carefully screened for cryptic translocations involving chromosome 16 or inversion, or inv(16) and the fusion transcript should be carefully searched for. This may be particularly important because this finding of inv(16) with trisomy 22 has been associated in some, but not all reports, with central nervous system involvement.[39-42] Overall, the subtype of M4 with abnormal eosinophilia occurs in approximately 5% of adults with AML. The cells have a myelomonocytic morphologic appearance. In up to 30% of the marrow cells may have morphologically and histochemically abnormal eosinophils, or eosinophilic precursors.

Although these specific abnormalities of chromosome 16 as detailed above are associated with FAB M4 morphology with abnormal-appearing eosinophils, the expression of the CBFβ/MYH11 can be associated with other morphologic subtypes, including M1, M2, and M5 with or without eosinophilia.[43]

Similar to the case of patients with the t(8;21)(q22;q22) abnormality, there are data to suggest that patients with inv(16)(p13q22) and t(16;16)(p13q22) have leukemic cells which also are particularly sensitive to multiple cycles of intensive post remission chemotherapy, often with high-dose cytarabine. Both single institution and cooperative group studies show that with intensive post remission consolidation chemotherapy, the long-term event-free survival ranges between approximately 55-70%.[28,44,45] (Figure 3-2) There are other cytogenetic abnormalities, usually translocations, which are also CBF leukemias. (Table 3-3)

Overall Survival of Patients with Cytogenetic Abnormalities

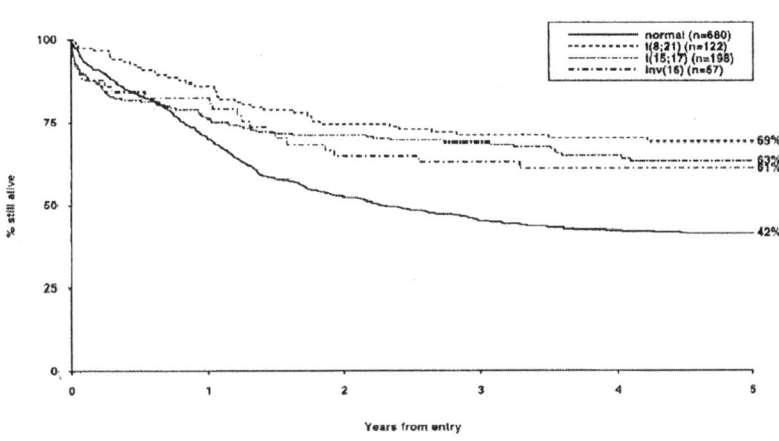

Figure 3-2. Overall survival of patients with cytogenetic abnormalities (from Grimwade[28])

Table 3-3. Core Binding Factor Leukemias

Translocation	Genes Involved
t(8;21)	AML1-ETO
t(3;21)	AML1-EAP, MDS1, EVI1
t(12;21)	TEL(ETV6)
inv(16), t(16;16)	CBFβ-MYH11

3.3   Quantitation of Minimal Residual Disease by Real-time Reverse Transcriptase Polymerase Chain Reaction (PCR)

Molecular techniques to amplify and detect DNA and RNA from leukemic cell s now permit the identification of minimal amounts of leukemia in blood and bone marrow.[46] The presence of fusion transcripts in patients with CBF leukemias not only is important in establishing the correct diagnosis, but also facilitates the identification of those patients in apparent CR with minimal residual disease (MRD).[47] Recent studies have suggested one important difference between patients with the t(8;21)(q22;q22) and patients with either inv(16)(p13q22) and t(16;16)(p13q22) is that patients with the former subtype may have persistence of the molecular fusion transcript and yet enjoy long-term disease free survival.[48] Interestingly enough, the AML1/ETO transcript has been detected in non-leukemic stem cells.[49] Perhaps the most progress in the detection of minimal residual disease by molecular techniques has been realized in patients with APL. The quantitation of minimal residual disease by real-time reverse transcriptase polymerase chain reaction (RT-PCR) can be useful to identify a threshold below which relapse is uncommon, in patients with APL.[50]

3.4   Identification of Minimal Residual Diseases by Immunophenotyping

The identification of minimal residual disease by detecting aberrant phenotypes by multiparametric flow cytometry in patients in morphologic CR has emerged as a potentially useful strategy.[51,52] Such techniques appear sensitive and quantification of the number of residual cells with the leukemic phenotype has been used to classify patients into risk categories with different risks of relapse. (Figure 3-3) High-risk patients may be candidates for alternative novel treatment strategies.

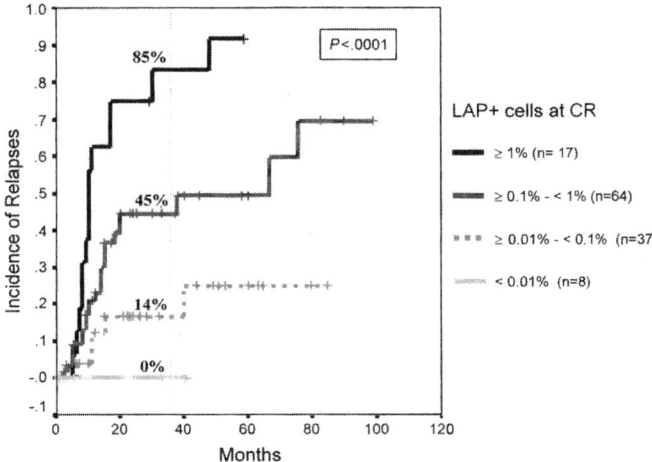

Figure 3-3. Relapse rates in the 4 AML risk categories according to number of leukemia-associated-phenotype (LAP) cells in the first bone marrow in morphologic complete remission (from San Miguel[51]).

4.   ACUTE PROMYELOCYTIC LEUKEMIA

Acute promyelocytic leukemia (APL) represents another distinct subtype of AML. The disease is associated with a specific balanced reciprocal translocation, t(15;17)(q22;q21).[53] This specific chromosomal translocation results in a fusion transcript, the PML-RARα chimeric gene. Recent studies have contributed to an understanding of the molecular pathogenesis of APL. As a result of the fusion of retinoic acid receptor alpha gene to the PML gene, there is increased affinity for the nuclear co-repressor protein complex.[54] The formation of this protein complex in turn attracts histone deacetylase which alters chromatin confirmation and inhibits transcription. The leukemic promyelocytes undergo differentiation with exposure to the natural vitamin A derivative all-trans retinoic acid (ATRA). Retinoic acid induces release of the nuclear co-repressor complex and histone deacetylase which leads to normal chromatin confirmation and normal transcription. Not only does this model provide a plausible mechanism for leukemogenesis, but it also provides the rationale for exploring histone deacetylase inhibitors.[55-57]

The morphologic appearance of leukemic promyelocytes is quite characteristic. In approximately 85% of patients, these cells have heavy, numerous, and often bizarre appearing primary azurophilic granules which can often obscure a bilobed or reniform nuclear contour.[58] Collections of Auer rods can be seen. Several variants which morphologically can appear virtually indistinguishable from classical APL have been described. The identification of these variants is important because the most common, which is associated with the formation of the PLZF-RARα fusion transcript, is not sensitive to the differentiating effects of ATRA.[59] Recently, a variety of specific genetic patterns have been identified in patients with APL undergoing differentiation therapy with ATRA whereby a variety of genes have been shown to be upregulated within 24-48 hours after ATRA exposure.[60] In addition, a variety of genes are downregulated and suppressed within 8 hours.

The leukemic promyelocytes have a distinctive immunophenotype which include the lack of or low expression of HLA-DR and CD34, expression of CD13, CD33, and CD9.[61-64] The leukemic promyelocytes have a peculiar sensitivity to the cytotoxic effects of anthracyclines.[65] This has been thought to be, in part, related to absence of expression of the multidrug resistance mediator P-glycoprotein.[66,67] Expression of CD2 has been associated with the microgranular variant or with the short (bcr3) PML-RARα transfusion transcript subtype.[68,69] Recently, ATRA has been shown to induce the expression of CD52 on the leukemic cells of patients with APL during differentiation.[70] Expression of CD56 has been associated with a poor outcome in APL.[71,72] Immunophenotype alone is insufficient to establish a diagnosis of APL since, for example, a similar immunophenotype can be observed in patients with natural killer AML which may resemble APL morphologically.[73,74] Correlation with cytogenetics and molecular genetics may be critical to distinguish these 2 subtypes of AML which have different treatment.

Clinically, patients with APL have a high incidence of bleeding due to a complex coagulopathy manifested by disseminated intravascular coagulation, hyperfibrinolysis, or both, and in some cases, direct proteolysis.[75-80] Historically, hemorrhage, often intracerebral, has been the major cause of early death.[75,80,81] All-trans retinoic acid appears to reduce clinical bleeding and biochemical parameters of the coagulopathy return to normal.[77-79] However, the impact on early mortality is less clear. Although mortality has declined in some studies, it has not in others.[77,81-83]

Before 1986, APL was treated as all other subtypes of AML with intensive cytotoxic chemotherapy. With the introduction of ATRA in 1987 as a differentiating agent, and arsenic trioxide in 1992 as a inducer of both differentiation and apoptosis, dramatic improvement has occurred in the outcome for both patients with de novo, as well as relapsed APL.[53,81,84]

Therapy for patients with APL differs from all other subtypes in 3 ways. Firstly, ATRA is now included in the treatment of all patients in induction. It has become routine to combine ATRA with anthracycline-based chemotherapy, both because of potential synergism which appears to prevent relapse, as well as the apparent ability of the combination to diminish the most important side effect of ATRA therapy, namely the retinoic acid syndrome.[82,85-87] Secondly, chemotherapy strategies appear to rely more on anthracyclines, than the combination of anthracyclines plus cytarabine.[65] While it has not been conclusively established, it appears that induction and consolidation therapy can be accomplished successfully without cytarabine.[88-90] Thirdly, maintenance therapy, a strategy not generally beneficial in other subtypes of AML, appears to play a role in patients with APL.[82,83,88,89] The mechanism by which maintenance therapy appears to be effective has not been established. An antiangiogenic mechanism of action for low-dose cytotoxic maintenance chemotherapy has been proposed whereby cytotoxic chemotherapy may have a preferential effect on newly formed endothelial cells.[91] Interestingly enough, increased angiogenesis and vascular endothelial growth factor production has been shown to be increased in patients with APL, and such processes appear to be inhibited by ATRA.[92] Recent data from the Italian Cooperative Group, GIMEMA, suggest that patients who are in a molecular CR following intensive consolidation may not benefit from maintenance therapy.[93] In the GIMEMA protocol for APL, consolidation is more intensive than in other cooperative group protocols and this fact may account for the lack of benefit of maintenance recently reported.

With current strategies,[82,88,89] now 70-80% of patients with APL can be expected to be cured of their disease.[81,87,94,95] (Figure 3-4) This dramatic improvement has occurred primarily because of the introduction of ATRA in induction and as maintenance therapy. This represents a paradigm for the identification of molecularly targeted therapy and represents the only clinically meaningful example of differentiation therapy. Quantitative real time RT-PCR for the PML-RARα fusion transcript in patients with APL can be useful not only to establish the diagnosis, but also to follow patients in apparent molecular CR.[87,96] Thresholds can be identified which can predict patients at high risk of relapse.[50] (Figure 3-5) Such a strategy will useful to identify those patients in apparent CR who may benefit from additional therapy such as arsenic trioxide (ATO) or targeted antibody therapy with gemtuzumab ozogamicin.[97]

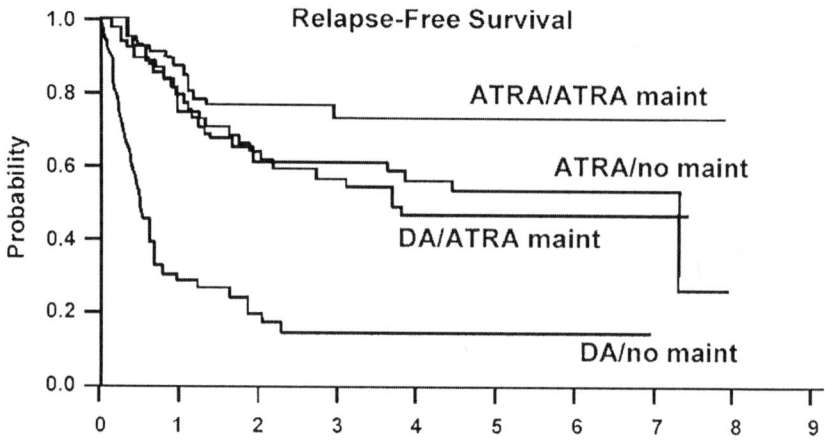

Figure 3-4. North American intergroup protocol for acute promyelocytic leukemia, median follow-up 6 years (from Tallman[95])

For the small percentage of patients with APL who do relapse, arsenic trioxide (ATO) has emerged as the treatment of choice for patients with relapsed or refractory disease. Investigators from China initially reported that ATO induces complete remission in the majority of such patients.[98] Subsequently, studies in the United States and elsewhere have confirmed these initial observations.[99-101] Most importantly, recent studies have suggested that approximately 50% of patients receive a molecular CR after one cycle of ATO, and approximately 80% of patients do so after two 5-week cycles.[100] Many patients enjoy a prolonged disease-free survival after ATO treatment to induce second CR followed by additional courses of ATO as consolidation and maintenance.[100] Potential toxicity of ATO therapy include prolongation of the QTc interval and the APL differentiation syndrome, a cardiorespiratory distress syndrome reminiscent of the retinoic acid syndrome, and similarly, very responsive to dexamethasone. Patients who achieve a second CR with ATO may do well with maintenance arsenic therapy for four cycles. However, some will relapse, and an attractive alternative appears to be high-dose chemotherapy with autologous hematopoietic stem cell transplantation, if one can harvest and reinfuse molecularly negative cells.[102] For those patients who remain persistently molecularly positive, allogeneic hematopoietic stem cell transplantation offers the benefit of a potentially potent graft-vs-leukemia effect, and may be useful for patients with advanced disease.[103]

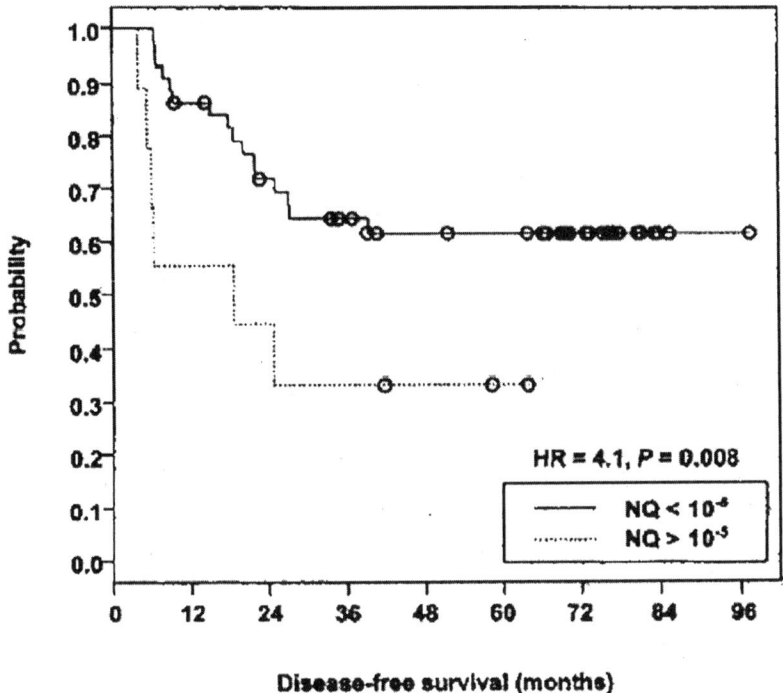

Figure 3-5. Kaplan-Meier analysis comparing disease-free survival of patients with PML-RARα normalized quotient (NQ) exceeding 10^{-5} vs. patients with NQ below 10^{-5} (from Gallagher[50])

5.   TARGETING CD33-POSITIVE ACUTE MYELOID LEUKEMIA

The CD33 antigen is a transmembrane protein expressed on the leukemic cells for the majority of patients with AML.[104] This antigen is not expressed on non-hematopoietic cells. These observations make it an appealing target for antibody therapy.[105,106] Gemtuzumab ozogamicin is an immunoconjugate of a humanized anti-CD33 monoclonal antibody chemically linked to a semisynthetic derivative of a very potent cytotoxic antitumor antibiotic, calicheamicin.[107] (Figure 3-6) A phase I dose-escalation trial in 40 patients with relapsed or refractory AML showed that leukemia was eliminated from the blood and marrow in 8 (20%) patients.[108] Subsequently, three multicenter phase II trials were conducted in 142 patients in first relapse with a relatively long first remission duration (median approximately 11 months) and no antecedent hematologic disorder.[109] Complete remission, but with incomplete recovery of platelet count to ≥ 100,000, was obtained in 30% of patients. Non-hematologic toxicities were modest and included grade 3 or 4 hyperbilirubinemia in 23%, elevated hepatic transaminases in 17%, and infections in 28%. An hepatic veno-occlusive disease-like syndrome has been reported in a small percentage of patients.[110-112] This agent represents a novel delivery technique with modest toxicity. The phase II trials were encouraging, and despite the relatively favorable population of patients, that gemtuzumab ozogamicin has been incorporated into chemotherapy programs for induction with excellent CR rates of 86% after 1 cycle.[113,114]

6.   SUMMARY

Many new insights into the diagnosis, pathogenesis, clinical manifestation, treatment and prognosis of patients with AML reflect the heterogeneity of the disease. The initial descriptions of the various subtypes of AML, established by the FAB classification, were based on morphology and cytochemical stains. Although morphology remains the foundation for the diagnosis, additional diagnostic studies including immunophenotyping, cytogenetic evaluation, and molecular genetic studies have become critical, and in some specific cases, mandatory, complementary tools. Several specific subtypes of AML are now treated with directed or targeted therapy. Acute promyelocytic leukemia is currently the only example of a subtype of AML to which specific therapy targeted to a molecular genetic abnormality is available and this subtype now is highly curable. Future studies will address newly identified prognostic factors and gene mutations such as FLT3, [115-122] Wilm's tumor (WTI),[123,124] and CEBPA[125] which will enable the further pathologic classification of patients with AML. Finally, microarray analysis will likely identify genes critically involved in the pathogenesis of specific pathologic subtypes.[125]

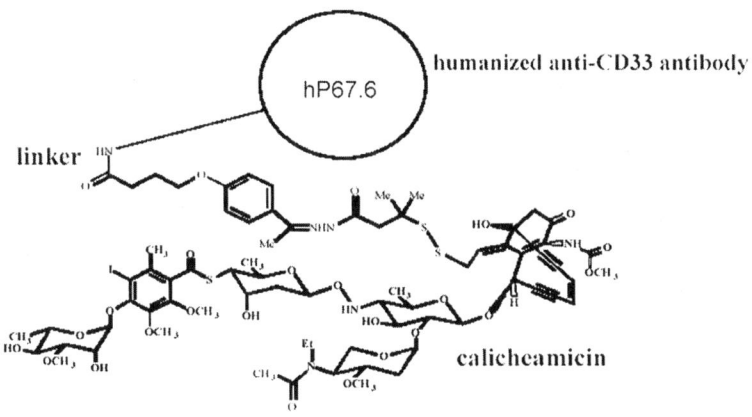

Figure 3-6. Structure of gemtuzumab ozogamicin

REFERENCES

1. Bennett J. Proposals for the Classification of the Acute Leukemias. Br J Haematol 1976; 33:451-458.
2. Head D, Savage R, Cerezo L, et al: Reproducibility of the French-American-British Classification of Acute Leukemia: The Southwest Oncology Group Experience. Am J Hematol 1985; 18:47-57.
3. Burnett A. Introduction: Modern management of acute myeloid leukemia. Seminars in Hematology 2001; 38:1-2.
4. Bennett J, Young M, Andersen J, et al. Long-term survival in acute myeloid leukemia: the Eastern Cooperative Oncology Group experience. Cancer 1997; 80:2205-2209.
5. Rowe J. Treatment of acute myelogenous leukemia in older adults. Leukemia 2000; 14:480-487.
6. McMullin M, Mackenzie G. Survival from acute myeloid leukaemia in patients over 55 years of age in Northern Ireland: a discrete population. Hematology 2001; 6:103-110.
7. Dalley C, Rohatiner A, Bradburn M, et al. Acute myelogenous leukaemia in patients 60 years and older: A retrospective analysis from St. Bartholomew's Hospital 1969-1999. Hematology 2001; 6:163-75.
8. Head D. Revised classification of acute myeloid leukemia. Leukemia 1996; 10:1826-1831.
9. Brunning RD, Matutes E, Harris NL, et al. Acute myeloid leukemia. in: Jaffe ES, Harris NL, Stein H, Vardiman JW eds: World Health Organization Classification of

Tunours. Tumours of Haematopoietic and Lymphoid Tissues. London, IARC Press, 2001: pp 75-107.

10. Bennett J, Catovsky D, Daniel M, et al. Proposal for the recognition of minimally differentiated acute myeloid leukemia (AML-M0). Br J Haematol 1991; 78:325-329.

11. Matsuo T, Bennett J. Acute leukemia of megakaryocyte lineage (M7). Cancer Genet Cytogenet 1988; 34:1-3.

12. Vardiman J, Harris N, Brunning R. The World Health Organization (WHO) classification of the myeloid neoplasms. Blood 2002; 100:2292-2302.

13. Estey E, Thall P, Beran M, et al. Effect of diagnosis (RAEB, RAEB-t or AML) on outcome of AML-type chemotherapy. Blood 1997; 90:2969-2977.

14. Cheson B, Cassileth P, Head D, et al. Report of the National Cancer Institute-sponsored workshop on definitions of diagnosis and response in acute myeloid leukemia. J Clin Oncol 1990; 8:813-819.

15. Cheson B, Bennett J, Kopecky K, et al. Recommendations of the international working group to standardize response criteria and treatment outcomes for therapeutic trials in acute myeloid leukemia. J Clin Oncol 2003; 21:4642-4649.

16. Shimada H, Ichikawa H, Nakamura S, et al. Analysis of genes under the downstream control of the t(8;21) fusion protein AML1-MTG8: overexpression of the TIS11b (ERF-1, cMG1) gene induces myeloid cell proliferation in response to G-CSF. Blood 2000; 96:655-662.

17. Wang J, Wang M, Johnson M. Transformation properties of the ETO gene, fusion partner in t(8;21) leukemias. Cancer Res 1997; 57:2951-2955.

18. Shimada H, Ichikawa H, Ohki M. Potential involvement of the AML1-MTG8 fusion protein in the granulocytic maturation characteristic of the t(8;21) acute myelogenous leukemia revealed by microarray analysis. Leukemia 2002; 16:874-885.

19. Nishii K, Usui E, Katayama N, et al. Characteristics of t(8;21) acute myeloid leukemia (AML) with additional chromosomal abnormality: concomitant trisomy 4 may constitute a distinctive subtype of t(8;21) AML. Leukemia 2003; 17:731-737.

20. Nucifora G, Rowley J. AML1 and the 8;21 and 3;21 translocations in acute and chronic myeloid leukemia. 1995; Blood 86:1-14.

21. Slovak M, Kopecky K, Cassileth P. Karyotypic analysis predicts outcome of preremission and postremission therapy in adult acute myeloid leukemia: a Southwest Oncology Group/Eastern Cooperative Oncology Group study. Blood 2000; 96:4075-4083.

22. Dastugue N, Payen C, Lafage-Pochitaloff M, et al. Prognostic significance of karyotype in de novo acute myeloid leukemia. Leukemia 1995; 9:1411-1498.

23. Porwit-MacDonald A, Janossy G, Ivory K, et al. Leukemia-associated changes identified by quantitative flow cytometry. IV. CD34 overexpression in acute myelogenous leukemia M2 with t(8;21). Blood 1996; 87:1162-1169.

24. Baer M, Stewart C, Lawrence D, et al. Expression of the neural cell adhesion molecule CD56 is associated with short remission duration and survival in acute myeloid leukemia with t(8;21)(q22;q22). Blood 1997; 90:1643-1648.

25. Byrd J, Weiss R, Arthur D, et al. Extramedullary leukemia adversely affects hematologic complete remission rate and overall survival in patients with t(8;21)(q22;q22): results from Cancer and Leukemia Group B 8461. J Clin Oncol 1997; 15:466-475.

26. Byrd J, Edenfield W, Shields D, et al. Extramedullary myeloid tumors in acute nonlymphocytic leukemia: a clinical review. J of Clin Oncol 1995; 13:1800-1816.

27. Raspadori D, Damiani D, Lenoci M, et al. CD56 antigenic expression in acute myeloid leuiemia identifies patients with poor clinical prognosis. Leukemia 2001; 15:1161-1164.

28. Grimwade D, Walker H, Oliver F, et al. The importance of diagnostic cytogenetics on outcome in AML: analysis of 1,612 patients entered into the MRC AML 10 trial. The Medical Research Council Adult and Children's Leukaemia Working Parties. Blood 1998; 92:2322-2333.

29. Byrd J, Mrozek K, Dodge R, et al. Pretreatment cytogenetic abnormalities are predictive of induction success, cumulative incidence of relapse, and overall survival in adult patients with de novo acute myeloid leukemia: results from Cancer and Leukemia Group B (CALGB 8461). Blood 2002; 100:4325-4336.

30. Bloomfield C, Lawrence D, Byrd J, et al. Frequency of prolonged remission duration after high-dose cytarabine intensification in acute myeloid leukemia varies by cytogenetic subtype. Cancer Res 1998; 58:4173-4179.

31. Byrd J, Dodge R, Carroll A, et al. Patients with t(8;21)(q22;q22) and acute myeloid leukemia have superior failure-free and overall survival when repetitive cycles of high-dose cytarabine are administered. J Clin Oncol 1999; 17(12):3767-75.

32. Palmieri S, Sebastio L, Mele G, et al. High-dose cytarabine as consolidation treatment for patients with acute myeloid leukemia with t(8;21). Leuk Res 2002; 26:539-543.

33. Nguyen S, Leblanc T, Fenaux P, et al. A white blood cell index as a main prognostic factor in t(8;21) acute myeloid leukemia (AML): a survey of 161 cases from the French AML Intergroup. Blood 2002; 99:3517-3523.

34. Liu P, Tarle S, Hajra A, et al. Fusion between transcription factor CBFbeta/PEBP2beta and a myosin heavy chain in acute myeloid leukemia. Science 1993; 261:1041-1044.

35. Shurtleff S, Meyers S, Hiebert S, et al. Heterogeneity in CBFB/MYH11 fusion messages encoded by the inv(16)(p13;q22) and the t(16;16)(p13;q22) in acute myelogenous leukemia. Blood 1995; 85:3695-3703.

36. Costello R, Sainty D, Lecine P, et al. Detection of CBFbeta/MYH11 fusion transcripts in acute myeloid leukemia: heterogeneity of cytological and molecular characteristics. Leukemia 1997; 11:644-650.

37. Langabeer S, Walker H, Gale R, et al. Frequency of CBFbeta/MYH11 fusion transcripts in patients entered into the UK MRC AML trials. Br J Haematol 1997; 96:736-739.

38. Poirel H, Radford-Weiss I, Rack K, et al. Detection of the chromosome 16 CBFbeta-MYH11 fusion transcript in myelomonocytic leukemias. Blood 1995; 85:1313-1322.

39. Ohyashi K, Oyashi J, Iwabuchi A, et al. Central nervous system involvement in acute nonlymphocytic leukemia with inv(16)(p13q22). Leukemia 1988; 2:398-399.

40. Holmes R, Keating M, Cork A, et al. A unique pattern of central nervous system leukemia in acute myelomonocytic leukemia associated with inv(16)(p13q22). Blood 1985; 65:1071-1078.

41. Dechary D, Bernard P, Lacome F, et al. Acute myeloid leukemia with hypereosinophilia and chromosome 16 anomaly. Cancer Genet Cytogenet 1986; 20:241-246.

42. Larson R, Williams S, Le Beau M, et al. Acute myelomonocytic leukemia with hypereosinophilia and inv(16) or t(16;16) has a favorable prognosis. Blood 1986; 68:1242-1249.

43. Monahan B, Rector J, Liu P, et al. Clinical aspects of expression of inversion 16 chromosomal fusion trancript CBFB/MYH11 in acute myelogenous leukemia subtype M1 with abnormal bone marrow eosiniphilia. Leukemia 1996; 10:1653-1675.

44. Razzouk B, Raimondi S, Srivastava D, et al. Impact of treatment on the outcome of acute meyloid leukemia with inversion 16: a single institution's experience. Leukemia 2001; 15:1326-1330.

45. Buonamici S, Ottaviani E, Testoni N, et al. Real-time quantitation of minimal residual disease in inv(16)-positive acute myeloid leukemia may indicate risk for clinical relapse and may identify patients in a curable state. Blood 2002; 99:443-449.

46. Jaeger V, Kainz B. Monitoring minimal residual disease in AML: the right time for real time. Ann Hematol 2003; 82:139-147.

47. Krauter J, Gorlich K, Ottmann O, et al. Prognostic value of minimal residual disease quantification by real-time reverse trascriptase polymerase chain reaction in patients with core binding factor leukemias. J Clin Oncol 2003; 21:4413-4422.

48. Varella-Garcia M, Hogan C, Odom L, et al. Minimal residual disease (MRD) in remission t (8;21) AML and in vivo differentiation detected by FISH and CD34+ cell sorting. Leukemia 2001; 15:1408-1414.

49. Miyamoto T, Weissman I, Akashi K, et al. AML1/ETO-expressing nonleukemic stem cells in acute myelogenous leukemia with 8;21 translocation. Proc Natl Acad Sci USA 2000; 97:7521-7526.

50. Gallagher R, Yeap B, Bi W. Quantitative real-time RT-PCR analysis of PML-RARalpha mRNA in acute promyelocytic leukemia: assessment of prognostic significance in adult patients from intergroup protocol 0129. Blood 2003; 101:2521-2528.

51. San Miguel J, Vidriales M, Lopez-Berges C, et al. Early immunophenotypical evaluation of minimal residual disease in acute myeloid leukemia identifies different patient risk groups and may contribute to postinduction treatment stratification. Blood 2001; 98:1746-1751.

52. San Miguel J, Martinez A, Macedo A, et al. Immunophenotyping investigation of minimal residual disease is a useful approach for predicting relapse in acute myeloid leukemia patients. Blood 1997; 90:2455-2470.

53. Grignani F, Fagioli M, Alcalay M, et al. Acute promyelocytic leukemia: from genetics to treatment. Blood 1994; 83:10-25.

54. Grignani F, De Matteis S, Nervi C, et al. Fusion proteins of the retinoic acid receptor-alpha recruit histone deacetylase in promyelocytic leukemia. Nature 1998; 391:815-818.

55. Gottlicher M, Minucci S, Zhu P, et al. Valproic acid defines a novel class of HDAC inhibitors inducing differentiation of transformed cells. Embo J 2001; 20:6969-6978.

56. Maeda T, Towatori M, Kosugi H, et al. Up-regulation of costimulatory/adhesion molecules by histone deacetylase inhibitors in acute myeloid leukemia cells. Blood 2000; 96:3847-3856.

57. Kitamura K, Hoshi S, Koike M, et al. Histone deacetylase inhibitor but not arsenic trioxide differentiates acute promyelocytic leukaemia cells with t(11;17) in combination with all-trans retinoic acid. Br J Haematol 2000; 108:696-702.

58. O'Connor S, Evans P, Morgan G, et al. Diagnostic approaches to acute promyelocytic leukaemia. Leuk Lymphoma 1999; 33:53-63.

59. Sainty D, Liso V, Cantu-Rajnoldi A, et al. A new morphologic classification system for acute promyeloctyic leuekmia distinguishes cases with underlying PLZF/RARA gene rearrangements. Blood 2000; 96:1287-1296.

60. Liu T-X, Zhang J-W, Tao J, et al. Gene expression networks underlying retinoic acid-induced differentiation of acute promyelocytic leukemia cells. Blood 2000; 96:1496-1504.

61. Lo Coco F, Avvisati G, Diverio D, et al. Rearrangements of the RARalpha gene in acute promyelocytic leukemia: correlations with morphology and immunophenotype. Br J Haematol 1991; 78:494-499.

62. Erber W, Asbahr H, Rule S, et al. Unique immunophenotype of acute promyelocytic leukemia as defined by CD9 and CD68 antibodies. Br J Haematol 1994; 88:101-104.

63. Paietta E, Andersen J, Gallagher R, et al. The immunophenotype of acute promyelocytic leukemia (APL): an ECOG study. Leukemia 1994; 7:1108-1112.

64. Guglielmi C, Martelli M, Diverio D, et al. Clinical and biological relevance of immunophenotype in acute promyelocytic leukemia. Br J Haematol 1998; 102:1035-1041.

65. Bernard J, Weil M, Boiron M, et al. Acute promyelocytic leukemia: results of treatment by daunorubicin. Blood 1973; 41:489-496.

66. Paietta E, Andersen J, Racevskis J, et al. Significantly lower P-glycoprotein expression in acute promyelocytic leukemia than in other types of acute myeloid leukemia: immunological, molecular and functional analyses. Leukemia 1994; 8:968-973.

67. Drach D, Zhao S, Drach J, et al. Low incidence of MDR1 expression in acute promyelocytic leukemia. Br J Haematol 1995; 90:369-374.

68. Claxton D, Reading C, Nagarian L, et al. Correlation of CD2 expression with PML gene breakpoints in patients with acute promyelocytic leukemia. Blood 1992 80:582-586.

69. Biondi A, Luciano A, Bassan R, et al. CD2 expression in acute promyelocytic leukemia is associated with microgranular morphology (FAB M3v) but not with any PML gene breakpoint. Leukemia 1995; 9:1461-1466.

70. Li S-W, Tang D, Ahrens K, et al. All-trans-retinoic acid includes CD52 expression in acute promyelocytic leukemia. Blood 2003; 101:1977-1983.

71. Murray C, Estey E, Paietta E, et al. CD56 expression in acute promyelocytic leukemia: A possible indicator of poor treatment outcome. J Clin Oncol 1999; 17:293-297.

72. Ferrara F, Morabito F, Martino B, et al. CD56 expression is an indicator of poor clinical outcome in patients with acute promyelocytic leukemia treated with simultaneous ATRA and chemotherapy. J Clin Oncol 2000; 18:1295-1300.

73. Scott A, Head D, Kopecky K, et al. HLA-DR-CD33+, CD56+, CD16- myeloid/natural killer cell acute leukemia: a previously unrecognized form of acute leukemia potentially misdiagnosed as French-American-British acute myeloid leukemia-M3. Blood 1994; 84:244-255.

74. Paietta E, Gallagher R, Wiernik P. Myeloid/natural killer cell acute leukemia: a previously unrecognized form of acute leukemia potentially misdiagnosed as FAB-M3 acute myeloid leukemia. Blood 1994; 84(8):2824-2825.

75. Tallman M, Hakimian D, Kwaan H, et al. New insights into the pathogenesis of coagulation dysfunction in acute promyelocytic leukemia. Leuk Lymphoma 1993; 11:27-36.

76. Barbui T, Falanga A. The management of bleeding and thrombosis in leukemia, in Henderson E, Greaves M (eds): Leukemia. Philadelphia, 1996, pp 291

77. Di Bona E, Avvisati G, Castaman G, et al. Early haemorrhagic morbidity and mortality during remission induction with or without all -trans retinoic acid in acute promyelocytic leukemia. Br J Haematol 2000; 108:689-695.

78. Falanga A, Iacoviello L, Evangelista V, et al. Loss of blast cell procoagulant activity and improvement of hemostatic variable in patients with acute promyelocytic leukemia administered all-trans-retinoic acid. Blood 1995; 86:1072-1081.

79. Dombret H, Scrobohaci M, Ghorra P, et al. Coagulation disorders associated with acute promyelocytic leukemia: corrective effect of all-trans retinoic acid treatment. Leukemia 1993; 7:2-9.

80. Barbui T, Finazzi G, Falanga A. The impact of all trans-retinoic acid on the coagulopathy of acute promyelocytic leukemia. Blood 1998; 91:3093-3102.

81. Tallman M, Nabhan C, Feusner J, et al. Acute promyelocytic leukemia: evolving therapeutic strategies. Blood 2002; 99:759-767.

82. Fenaux P, Chastang C, Chevret S, et al. A randomized comparison of all-trans retinoic acid (ATRA) followed by chemotherapy and ATRA plus chemotherapy and the role of maintenance therapy in newly diagnosed acute promyelocytic leukemia. Blood 1999; 94:1192-1200.

83. Tallman M, Andersen J, Schiffer C, et al. All-trans retinoic acid in acute promyelocytic leukemia. N Engl J Med 1997; 337:1021-1028.

84. Warrell R, De The H, Wang Z, et al. Acute promyelocytic leukemia. N Engl J Med 1993; 329:177-189.

85. Vahdat L, Maslak P, Miller Jr W, et al. Early mortality and the retinoic acid syndrome in acute promyelocytic leukemia: impact of leukocytosis, low-dose chemotherapy, PMN/RARa isoform, and CD 13 expression in patients treated with all-trans retinoic acid. 1994; Blood 84:3843-3849.

86. De Botton S, Dombret H, Sanz M, et al. Incidence, clinical features, and outcome of all-trans retinoic acid syndrome in 413 cases of newly diagnosed acute promyelocytic leukemia. Blood 1998; 92:2712-2718.

87. Tallman M, Anderson A, Schiffer C, et al. Clinical description of 44 patients with acute promyelocytic leukemia who developed the retinoic acid syndrome. Blood 2000; 95:90-94.

88. Sanz M, Martin G, Rayon C, et al. A modified AIDA protocol with anthracycline-based consolidation results in high antileukemic efficacy and reduced toxicity in newly diagnosed PML/RARa-positive acute promyelocytic leukemia. Blood 1999; 94:3015-3021.

89. Sanz M, LoCoco F, Martin G, et al. Definition of relapse risk and role of nonanthracycline drugs for consolidation in patients with acute promyelocytic leukemia: a joint study of the PETHEMA and GIMEMA cooperative groups. Blood 2000; 96:1247-1253.

90. Estey E, Thall P, Pierce S, et al. Treatment of newly diagnosed acute promyelocytic leukemia without cytarabine. J Clin Oncol 1997; 15:483-490.

91. Bocci G, Nicolaou K, Kerbel R, et al. Protracted low-dose effects on human endothelial cell proliferation and survival in vitro reveal a selective antiangiogenic window for various chemotherapeutic drugs. Cancer Res 2002; 62:6938-6943.

92. Kini A, Peterson L, Tallman M, et al. Angiogenesis in acute promyelocytic leukemia: induction by vascular endothelial growth factor and inhibition by all-trans retinoic acid. Blood 2001; 97:3919-3924.

93. Avvisati G, Petti M, Lo Coco F, et al: AIDA: the Italian way of treating acute promyelocytic leukemia: The final act (abstr). Blood 2003; 102:487.

94. Mandelli F, Diverio D, Avvisati G, et al. Molecular remission in PML/RAR alpha-positive acute promyelocytic leukemia by combined all-trans retinoic acid and idarubicin (AIDA) therapy. Gruppo Italiano-Malattie Ematologiche Maligne dell'Adulto and Associazione Italiana di Ematologia ed Oncologia Pediatrica Cooperative Groups. Blood 1997; 90:1014-1021.

95. Tallman M, Andersen J, Schiffer C, et al. All-trans retinoic acid in acute promyelocytic leukemia: long-term outcome and prognostic factor analysis from the North American Intergroup Protocol. Blood 2002; 100:4298-4302.

96. Lo Coco F, Diverio D, Falini B, et al. Genetic diagnosis and molecular monitoring in the management of acute promyelocytic leukemia. Blood 1999; 94:12-22.

97. Estey E, Giles F, Beran M, et al. Experience with gemtuzumab ozogamicin ("Mylotarg") and all-trans retinoic acid in untreated acute promyelocytic leukemia. Blood 2002; 99:4222-4224.

98. Shen Z-X, Chen G, Ni J, et al. Use of arsenic trioxide (As2O3) in the treatment of acute promyelocytic leukemia (APL): II. Clinical efficacy and pharmacokinetics in relapsed patients. Blood 1997; 89:3354-3360.

99. Soignet S, Maslak P, Wang Z, et al. Complete remission after treatment of acute promyelocytic leukemia with arsenic trioxide. N Engl J Med 1998; 339:1341-1348.

100. Soignet S, Frankel S, Douer D, et al. United States multicenter study of arsenic trioxide in relapsed acute promyelocytic leukemia. J Clin Oncol 2001; 19:3852-3860.

101. Niu C, Yan H, Yu T, et al. Studies on treatment of acute promyelocytic leukemia with arsenic trioxide: remission induction, follow-up and molecular monitoring in 11 newly diagnosed and 47 relapsed acute promyelocytic leukemia patients. Blood 1999; 94:3315-3324.

102. Meloni G, Diverio D, Vignetti G, et al. Autologous bone marrow transplantation for acute promyelocytic leukemia in second remission: prognostic relevance of pretransplant minimal residual disease assessment by reverse-transcription polymerase chain reaction of the PML/RAR alpha fusion gene. Blood 1997; 90:1321-1325.

103. Lo Coco F, Romano A, Mengarelli A, et al. Allogeneic stem cell transplantation for advanced acute promyelocytic leukemia results in patients with molecularly persistent disease. Leukemia 2003; 17:1930-1933.

104. Solary E, Casasnovas R-O, Campos L, et al. Surface markers in adult acute myeloblastic leukemia: Correlation of CD19+, CD34+ and CD14+ /DR - phenotypes with shorter survival. Leukemia 1992; 6:393-399.

105. Dinndorf P, Andrews R, Benjamin D, et al. Expression of normal myeloid-associated antigens by acute leukemia cells. Blood 1986; 67:1048-1053.

106. Griffin J, Linch D, Shabbath K, et al. A monoclonal antibody reactive with normal and leukemic human meyloid progenitor cells. Leuk Res 1984. 8:521-534.

107. van der Velden V, te Marvelde J, Hoogeveen P, et al. Targeting of the CD33-calicheamicin immunoconjugate Mylotarg (CMA-676) in acute myeloid leukemia: in vivo and in vitro saturation and internalization by leukemic and normal myeloid cells. Blood 2001; 97:3197-3204.

108. Sievers E, Appelbaum F, Spielberger R, et al. Selective ablation of acute myeloid leukemia using antibody-targeted chemotherapy: a phase I study of an anti-CD33 calicheamicin immunoconjugate. Blood 1999; 93:3678-3684.

109. Sievers E, Larson R, Stadtmauer E, et al. Efficacy and safety of gemtuzumab ozogamicin in patients with CD33-positive acute myeloid leukemia in first relapse. J Clin Oncol 2001; 19:3244-3254.

110. Giles F, Kantarjian H, Kornlau S, et al. Mylotarg (gemtuzumab ozogamicin) therapy is associated with hepatic venocclusive disease in patients who have not received stem cell transplantation. Cancer 2001; 92:406-413.

111.   Wadleigh M, Richardson P, Zahrieh D, et al. Prior gemtuzumab ozogamicin exposure significantly increases the risk of veno-occlusive disease in patients who undergo myeloablative allogeneic stem cell transplantation. Blood 2003; 102:1578-1582.

112.   Rajvanshi P, Shulman H, Sievers E, et al. Hepatic sinusoidal obstruction after gemtuzumab ozogamicin (Mylotarg) therapy. Blood 2002; 99:2310-2314.

113.   Kell W, Burnett A, Chopra R, et al. A feasibility study of simultaneous administration of gemtuzumab ozogamicin with intensive chemotherapy in induction and consolidation in younger patients with acute myeloid leukemia. Blood 2003; 102:4277-4283.

114.   De Angelo D, Stone R, Durant S, et al. Gemtuzumab ozogamicin (Mylotarg) in combination with induction chemotherapy for the treatment of patients with de novo acute myeloid leukemia: Two age-specific phase 2 trials (abstr). Blood 2003; 102:100a.

115.   Rombouts W, Blokland I, Lowenberg B, et al. Biological characteristics and prognosis of adult acute myeloid leukemia with internal tandem duplications in the Flt3 gene. Leukemia 2000; 14:675-683.

116.   Kottaridis P, Gale R, Frew M, et al. The presence of FLT3 internal tandem duplication in patients with acute myeloid leukemia (AML) adds important prognostic information to cytogenetic risk group and response to the first cycle of chemotherapy: analysis of 854 patients from the United Kingdom Medical Research Council AML 10 and 12 trials. Blood 2001; 98:1752-1759.

117.   Meshinchi S, Goods W, Stirewalt D, et al. Prevalence and prognostic significance of Flt3 internal tandem duplication in pediatric acute myeloid leukemia. Blood 2001; 97:89-94.

118.   Rombouts W, Lowenberg B, van Putten W, et al. Improved prognostic significance of cytokine-induced proliferation in vitro in patients with de novo acute myeloid leukemia of intermediate risk: impact of internal tandem duplications in the Flt3 gene. Leukemia 2001; 16:1046-1053.

119.   Schnittger S, Schoch C, Dugas M, et al. Analysis of FLT3 length mutations in 1003 patients with acute myeloid leukemia: correlation to cytogenetics, FAB subtype, and prognosis in the AMLCG study and usefulness as a marker for the detection of minimal residual disease. Blood 2002; 100:59-66.

120.   Thiede C, Steudel C, Mohr B, et al. Analysis of FLT3-activating mutations in 979 patients with acute myelogenous leukemia: association with FAB subtypes and identification of subgroups with poor prognosis. Blood 2002; 99:4326-4335.

121.   Shih L, Huang C, Wu J, et al. Internal tandem duplication of FLT3 in relapsed acute myeloid leukemia: a comparative analysis of bone marrow samples from 108 adult patients at diagnosis and relapse. Blood 2002; 100:2387-2392.

122.   Preudhomme C, Sagot C, Boissel N, et al. Favorable prognostic significance of CEBPA mutations in patients with de novo acute myeloid leukemia: a study from the Acute Leukemia French Association (ALFA). Blood 2002; 100:2717-2723.

123.   Schmid D, Heinze G, Linnerth B, et al. Prognostic significance of WT1 gene expression at diagnosis in adult de novo acute myeloid leukemia. Leukemia 1997; 11:639-643.

124.   King-Underwood L, Pritchard-Jones K. Wilms' Tumor (WT1) gene mutations occur mainly in acute myeloid leukemia and may confer drug resistance. Blood 1998; 91:2961-2968.

125.   Okutsu J, Tsunoda T, Kaneta Y, et al. Prediction of chemosensitivity for patients with acute myeloid leukemia, according to expression levels of 28 genes selected by

genome-wide complementary DNA microarray analysis. Mol Cancer Therapeutics 2002; 1:1035-1042.

Chapter 4

MOLECULAR CYTOGENETIC STUDIES FOR HEMATOLOGICAL MALIGNANCIES

Gordon W. Dewald, Stephanie R. Brockman, Sarah F. Paternoster
Cytogenetics Laboratory, Mayo Clinic, Rochester, MN

1.   INTRODUCTION

"FISH" is an acronym that is applied to genetic technology which uses fluorescent-labeled DNA probes. This acronym is derived from the ability to visualize fluorescent-labeled probes at the place of in situ hybridization with complementary DNA within a nucleus. Experts working with FISH often refer to their field as molecular cytogenetics because their work crosses the fields of molecular genetics (DNA probes) and cytogenetics (evaluation of chromosomes).[1]

FISH is widely used today in clinical practice to help diagnose and select appropriate treatments for patients with hematological malignancies.[2] This method permits analysis of proliferating (metaphase cells) and non-proliferating (interphase nuclei) cells, and is useful to establish the percentage of neoplastic cells before and after therapy (minimal residual disease).[3] Thus, FISH is helpful to assess the effectiveness of treatment and to monitor the durability of remission. In research, FISH studies are used to investigate the origin and progression of hematological malignancies, and to establish which hematopoetic compartments are involved in neoplastic processes.[4]

This chapter is intended for clinicians and hematopathologists who wish to use FISH in the workup and management of their patients with hematological malignancies. Information is provided about appropriate specimen collection and transportation, laboratory procedures and interpretation of results. A review of different FISH strategies to detect chromosome anomalies is presented to appreciate the strengths and limitations of this method. FISH studies are summarized for chronic myeloid leukemia (CML) and other myeloproliferative disorders (MPD), myelodysplastic syndromes (MDS), acute myeloid leukemia (AML), acute lymphoblastic leukemia (ALL), B-cell chronic lymphocytic leukemia (B-CLL), multiple myeloma, and lymphoma. Some algorithms for conventional cytogenetics and FISH are suggested to help accomplish appropriate application of FISH studies in clinical practice.

2.   CHROMOSOMAL BASIS OF MALIGNANCY[2]

2.1   Chromosome Anomalies[5]

The results of FISH can be used to detect neoplastic clones with either numeric or structural anomalies of chromosomes. The term polyploid refers to chromosome complements that are multiples of 23; the haploid number of chromosomes for humans. Diploid refers to 46 chromosomes, triploid to 69 chromosomes, and tetraploid to 92 chromosomes. In neoplastic disorders, most polyploid clones are associated with advanced stages of disease and are derived from fusion of neoplastic cells or endoreduplication. Aneuploid refers to chromosome complements that involve irregular multiples of the haploid chromosome number. Thus, any cell with trisomy 8 is characterized by 47 chromosomes and includes three number 8 chromosomes. A cell that is monosomy 7 contains 45 chromosomes and is lacking a chromosome 7. Aneuploid anomalies usually occur as a consequence of mitotic malfunction, such as chromosome nondisjunction.

The results of FISH can be used to discriminate among various anomalies of chromosome structure including translocations, deletions, inversions, duplications, or isochromosomes. Reciprocal translocations involve the interchange of parts of different chromosomes and are the most common type of translocation in hematological malignancies. Deletions involve loss of part of a chromosome and are either terminal or interstitial. Inversions produce a reversal in the direction of an interstitial part of a chromosome and are either pericentric or paracentric. Pericentric inversions involve both the short and long arms of any chromosome while paracentric inversions occur on only one of the arms of any chromosome. Duplications produce two or more copies of a particular DNA segment on the same chromosome. Amplification results in hundreds of copies of a gene or chromosomal segment, which can either occur within a chromosome as a homogenous staining region or as separate acentric double minutes within the nucleus. Isochromosomes produce a mirror-image band pattern with respect to the center of the chromosome and arise from a break and fusion of sister chromatids.

2.2   Variant Chromosome Anomalies

In clinical practice, it is important to detect common chromosome anomalies and their variant forms. This is best done by conventional cytogenetic studies, but FISH can also accomplish this goal because variant chromosomes possess the same underlying molecular abnormality as the more common anomaly. Most structural anomalies of chromosomes originate during replication or repair of DNA when chromosomes are uncoiled and different chromosomes are overlapped or in close association with one another. DNA breakage and re-fusion can involve multiple loci and occasionally several different chromosomes. The subsequent re-fusion or repair of broken DNA can result in the formation of variant translocations.

For example, results of conventional cytogenetic studies indicate several forms of translocations all resulting in BCR/ABL fusion. These forms include the classical t(9;22)(q34;q11.2), complex translocations involving chromosomes 9, 22 and other chromosomes, and masked translocations which result from submicroscopic insertion translocations. Molecular genetic studies provide evidence of further genetic variation of BCR/ABL fusion among patients with CML. In some patients, small deletions and duplications of DNA sequences have been detected within the BCR and ABL genes.[6,7] In addition, the DNA break and fusion point with the BCR can occur within the major or minor BCR region and sometimes elsewhere within the BCR region.[8]

FISH studies suggest even further genetic variation among BCR/ABL fusion loci.[3,9] An atypical FISH signal pattern at the ABL/BCR fusion site on the abnormal chromosome 9 occurs in at least 20% of patients with CML who have a t(9;22)(q34;q11.2). These patterns result from loss of portions of the BCR and/or ABL hybridization sites and some adjacent DNA sequences. This loss of DNA sequences most likely occurs during the formation of these translocations. FISH studies have demonstrated similar loss of DNA associated with t(8;21)(q22;q22), inv(16)(p13q22) and various translocations involving MLL (11q23) among patients with AML.[10-14] Similar loss of DNA has also been associated with t(11;18)(q21;q21) among patients with marginal zone lymphoma of mucosa associated lymphoid tissue.[15-17]

2.3   Demonstration of Clonality

Results of FISH studies demonstrate clonality of hematological malignancies. The concept of clonal expansion is based on the premise that the formation of each neoplastic clone begins with a chromosome anomaly in a single cell. This cell then proliferates to produce two cells, then four cells and so forth until millions of abnormal cells with the same chromosome anomaly occur. FISH probes that detect the primary chromosome anomaly associated with a neoplastic process will produce an abnormal signal pattern in all neoplastic cells.

As neoplastic cells proliferate, additional chromosome anomalies develop in sporadic malignant cells by "chromosome evolution". These cells then proliferate to produce subclones that contain the primary chromosome anomaly as well as one or more secondary chromosome anomalies. FISH assays that detect a secondary chromosome anomaly will produce an abnormal signal pattern in a subset of the neoplastic cells. For example, in CML a t(9;22)(q34;q11.2) is the primary chromosome anomaly. The observation of t(9;22)(q34;q11.2) and trisomy 8 in a subset of neoplastic cells is evidence of a subclone.

Chromosome evolution produces the complex karyotypes observed in many hematological malignancies. The mechanisms of chromosome evolution include nondisjunction, cell fusion, and a wide variety of structural anomalies. A general correlation does exist between the aggressiveness of hematological malignancies and the appearance of subclones. The number of chromosome anomalies in an abnormal clone may provide a crude measurement of tumor progression. CML and the 5q- syndrome are two well-studied disorders where chromosome evolution correlates with more aggressive stages of the disease.[18,19] Evidence is accumulating that suggests a similar correlation exists between karyotype complexity and disease progression in other hematological malignancies, especially among MPD and MDS.[20]

3.   FISH PROCEDURES

3.1   Specimen Collection

It is important that specimens referred for FISH studies include malignant cells. Bone marrow aspirates are best for patients with MPD, MDS and acute leukemia.[3,21] If the disease involves circulating cells, then a peripheral blood specimen can be collected. In some cases, FISH methods can be used to study blood in preference over bone marrow, especially for CML[22] and B-CLL[23]. Lymph node tissues can be studied using paraffin-embedded tissue, touch preparations or frozen cells.[24] In certain clinical situations, FISH may be used on various body fluids including pleural or ascitic effusions, spinal fluid, and rarely other specimens. FISH can be successful even on low volume specimens that appear to lack cells.

FISH studies are routinely performed on 0.25 to 0.50 mL of bone marrow collected in sodium heparin. FISH analysis of peripheral blood requires 7.0 to 10.0 mL collected in sodium heparin. The specimen should be transported to the cytogenetic laboratory at ambient temperature by the most expeditious means, along with a note indicating the FISH probes to be tested, comments regarding the patient's possible diagnosis and history of any treatment.

3.2   Laboratory Procedures

In the cytogenetic laboratory, various methods can be used to process specimens for FISH analysis. Bone marrow and blood specimens are usually processed using hypotonic solution (0.075 M KCl) for 15 minutes and fixed with 3:1 methanol-glacial acetic acid. These cells can be stored indefinitely at -70°C until FISH studies are needed. The laboratory method to perform FISH is summarized in Figure 4-1 and described in detail in various books[1] and publications[24,25]. Briefly, fixed cells are dropped on a microscope slide and allowed to air-dry. To denature specimen DNA, the slide preparation is processed with 70% formamide solution at 74°C for 1 to 2 minutes. The probe DNA is denatured separately in a micro-centrifuge tube for 5 minutes in a 74°C water bath. The slide preparation is then flooded with denatured probe DNA and incubated in a humidified chamber at 37°C for 8 to 20 hours to allow probe DNA and specimen DNA to hybridize. The slide preparation is first washed with 0.4xSSC at 74°C and then washed again with 2xSSC/0.1% NP40 solution at room temperature for 1 minute. The nucleus is counterstained with DAPI.

3.3   Microscope Analysis

FISH studies require the use of a high quality fluorescence microscope equipped with a 100-watt mercury lamp and appropriate filter sets. To observe FISH signals produced by a set of probes, one of which is red and the other which is green, it is best to use a combination of a single DAPI filter and a dual-pass SpectrumGreen[TM] and SpectrumOrange[TM] filter set. With this setup, the nucleus appears blue from the DAPI stain, and red and green FISH signals can be observed within the nucleus; the cytoplasm is not usually apparent. Normal and abnormal interphase or metaphase cells have different signal patterns depending upon the FISH strategy employed (Figure 4-2).

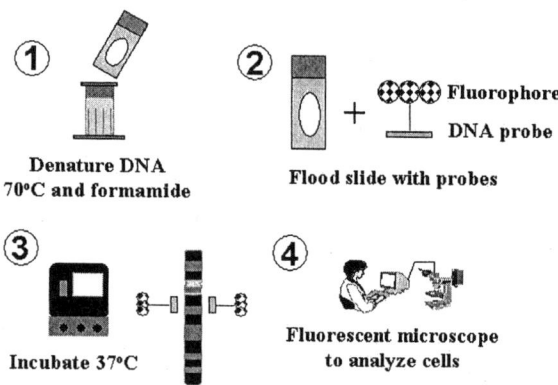

Figure 4-1. Summary of FISH method for bone marrow and blood specimens. The cells are fixed with methanol-glacial acetic acid and dropped on a microscope slide. 1) To denature specimen DNA, the slide preparation is incubated at 74°C with 70% formamide solution. 2) Fluorescent-labeled DNA is denatured and then added to the slide preparation. 3) Probe DNA and specimen DNA is allowed to hybridize together in an incubator at 37°C. Nuclei are then counter-stained with DAPI. 4) FISH signals are observed with a microscope using appropriate filters. See text for more information.

The typical interphase FISH study involves scoring 200 or more nuclei, but the sensitivity of some FISH assays to detect neoplastic cells is greatly increased by examining more cells. Most laboratories use two observers to independently score consecutive interphase cells from two or more separate areas of the hybridization site, and their results are averaged together to calculate the percentage of neoplastic cells. Some of the factors that interfere with effective analysis include overlapping nuclei, inconsistent hybridization, and variable morphology of the probe signal.

Accrediting agencies require that representative cells are documented by photographs or computer images for each case studied by FISH in clinical practice. Many laboratories use computer-assisted karyotype systems to capture FISH images and integrate data into their laboratory computer system.

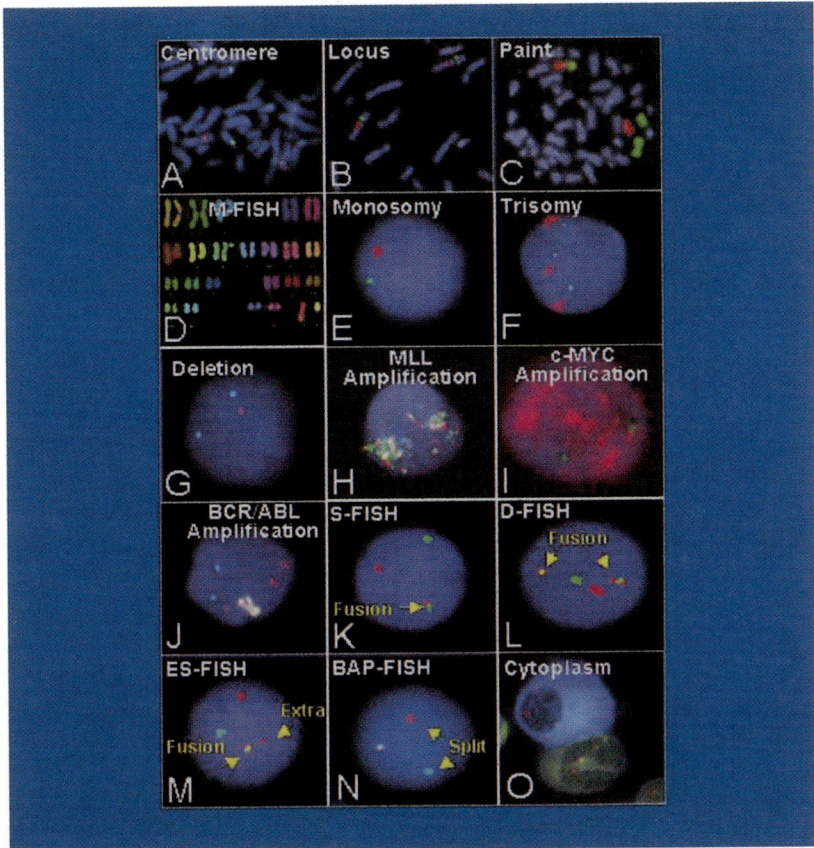

Figure 4-2. DNA probes for FISH are classified by where they hybridize. Some probes hybridize to specific centromeres (A) and others to specific gene loci (B). Some probes hybridize to unique DNA sequences producing a paint-like pattern for a specific chromosome (C). With M-FISH each of the chromosomes can be painted a different color (D). Using ND-FISH, cells with monosomy have one red and one green signal (E), cells with trisomy have three red and three green signals (F), and cells with deletion for part of a chromosome have one red and two green signals (G). Examples of amplification are shown for MLL in AML (H) c-MYC in leukemia (I), and BCR/ABL fusion in CML (J). S-FISH produces a single fusion signal (K). D-FISH produces double or two fusion signals (L). ES-FISH produces a single fusion signal and an extra small signal (M). BAP-FISH produces one red, one green and one yellow fusion signal in abnormal nuclei (N). Combined immunophenotyping and FISH using AMPCA bound to antibodies for cytoplasmic immunoglobulin and red and green FISH signals to detect t(11;14)(q13;q32) in multiple myeloma (O).

3.4   **Interpretation of Results**

Most FISH studies are informative about the chromosomal locus that they are designed to detect, but are not helpful to identify other chromosome anomalies. Thus, a normal FISH result does not rule out other chromosomal or genetic abnormalities that might be associated with a neoplastic clone.

The standard FISH definition of a clone requires the observation of more nuclei with neoplastic FISH signal patterns than is observed in normal individuals. This requires establishing strict scoring criteria, validation of probes, and defining a "normal cut-off" prior to using the technology in clinical practice (see validation of FISH probes). Because a normal cut-off is used with FISH, it is possible for a patient to have low level of disease that cannot be distinguished from technical artifact.

Although the agents used to treat malignancies may induce sporadic chromosome anomalies, treatment does not usually interfere with the detection of abnormal clones by FISH. It is important to perform a FISH study prior to treatment to establish a benchmark for the percentage of neoplastic nuclei and to accurately establish the signal pattern of the neoplastic clone.

Occasionally an abnormal FISH result will be different than is expected from the design of the test. For example, a patient may be studied with *BCR* and *ABL* probes to look for *BCR/ABL* fusion, but will show three *ABL* signals. It is tempting to conclude that the patient has a clone with trisomy 9. In these cases, it is important to avoid over interpreting the results. The FISH test only reveals three signals of the *ABL* locus and the results are not direct evidence for the presence of an entire chromosome 9. Certain translocations can also produce three *ABL* signals. The only confident conclusion an investigator can make about this result is that the patient has a neoplastic clone involving three *ABL* signals and does not have *BCR/ABL* fusion. Of course, the absence of *BCR/ABL* fusion is sufficient to rule out CML as a possible diagnosis.

Certain technical factors can introduce false signal patterns and interfere with accurate interpretation of FISH results. For example, the signals for some probes may split as a result of asynchronous DNA replication or incomplete saturation of the target DNA hybridization sequence. Some probes contain sequences that share homology with other DNA sequences in the genome. Unless washing stringency is perfect, these probes will produce false signal patterns due to cross-hybridization. Certain biological factors can also interfere with interpretation of the results. For example, sporadic cells in normal individuals may be aneuploid, but not part of any neoplastic process. Many of these problems can be addressed by performing appropriate probe validation studies (see validation of FISH probes).

Table 4-1. Some chromosome anomalies and FISH probes for ALL, AML, MPD, MDS, B-CLL, MM, and lymphoma

Disorder[1]	Chromosome anomaly[2]	FISH probes	Sensitivity	Strategy[3]
ALCL	t(2;var)(p23;var)	ALK	>3%	BAP
AML	t(8;21)(q22;q22) and variants	AML1/ETO	>1%	D
AML, pre-B-ALL, MDS	t(11;var)(q23;var)	MLL	>3%	BAP
AML	t(15;17)(q22;q21) and variants	PML/RARα	>1%	D
AML	inv(16)(p13q22) and variants	CBFβ	>3%	BAP
B-CLL, MM, MGUS	del(6)(q13q23)	D6Z1, MYB	>7%	ND
B-CLL, MM, MGUS	del(11)(q13q23)	D11Z1, ATM	>7%	ND
B-CLL, MM, MGUS	+12	D12Z3, MDM2	>2%	ND
B-CLL, MM, MGUS, MDS, MPD	del(13)(q12q14), -13	D13S319, 13q34	>7%	ND
B-CLL, MM	del(17)(p13)	D17Z1, P53	>7%	ND
BL, pre-B-ALL	t(8;14)(q24;q32) and variants	c-MYC/IGH	>1%	D
CML, pre-B-ALL, AML	t(9;22)(q34;q11.2) and variants	BCR/ABL	>1%	D
DLCL	t(3;var)(q27;var)	BCL6	>3%	BAP
FL	t(14;18)(q32;q21) and variants	BCL2/IGH	>1%	D
MALT	+3,+7,+12,+18	D3Z1, D7Z1, D12Z3, D18Z1	>4%	ND
MALT	t(11;18)(q21;q21) and variants	API2/MALT1	>1%	D
MALT	t(14;18)(q32;q21) and variants	MALT1/IGH	>1%	D
MALT	t(18;var)(q21;var)	MALT1	>3%	BAP
MCL, MM, MGUS	t(11;14)(q13;q32) and variants	CCND1/IGH	>1%	D
MDS, AML, MPD	del(5)(q13q33), -5	D5S23, D5S721, EGR1	>7%	ND
MDS, AML, MPD	del(7)(q22q34), -7	D7Z1, D7S486	>7%	ND
MDS, MPD, AML	+8	D8Z2, D10Z1	>4%	ND
MM, MGUS	t(4;14)(p16.3;q32) and variants	FGFR3/IGH	>1%	D
MM, MGUS	t(14;16)(q32;q23) and variants	c-MAF/IGH	>1%	D
MPD	+9	D9Z1, ABL	>4%	ND
MPD	del(12)(p12)	TEL/AML1	>10%	D
MPD, MDS	del(20)(q11q13), -20	D20S108	>10%	ND
Pre-B-ALL	t(12;21)(p13;q22) and variants	TEL/AML1	>3%	ES
Pre-B-ALL	+4, +10, +17	D4Z1, D10Z1, D17Z1	>4%	ND

[1]*Disorders:* AML, acute myeloid leukemia; ALCL, anaplastic large cell lymphoma; BL, Burkitt lymphoma; B-CLL, B-cell chronic lymphocytic leukemia; CML, chronic myeloid leukemia; DLCL, diffuse large B-cell lymphoma; FL, follicular lymphoma; MCL, mantle cell lymphoma; MDS, myelodysplastic syndrome; MM, multiple myeloma; MPD, myeloproliferative disorder; MGUS, monoclonal gammopathy of undetermined significance; MALT, marginal zone lymphoma of mucosa associated lymphoid tissue; pre-B-ALL, precursor B-cell acute lymphocytic leukemia. [2]*Anomalies: See text for information.*[3]*Strategies:* ND, numeric and/or deletions; D, double fusion for translocations; BAP, break-apart for translocations; ES, extra signal for translocations. *See text for more information.*

The United States Food and Drug Administration has not approved most FISH tests. Under these circumstances, the final report for any patient should indicate "this test was developed and its performance characteristics were determined by your Laboratory Name, and has not been approved by the United States Food and Drug Administration".[26]

4.　　FISH PROBES AND FISH NOMENCLATURE

The utility and accuracy of FISH probes to detect chromosome anomalies have been established for many hematological malignancies (Table 4-1). However, the United States Food and Drug Administration has approved only a few commercial FISH probes for this purpose. While many DNA probes can be purchased from commercial companies, "home-brew" probes can also be prepared. Commercial probes are usually preferred to avoid the rigorous quality control steps needed for making home-brew probes.

4.1　　Selection of DNA Probes

Most FISH probes contain two or more separate DNA sequences that collectively hybridizes over 200 to 600 kilobases of target DNA. The selection of fluorescent-labeled DNA probes to accurately detect any hematological neoplasm is critical for a successful FISH study. Oncogenes that are directly involved with the neoplastic process are excellent probe targets for FISH studies. Evidence indicates that one or more oncogenes are located near sites of chromosome breakage for several of the specific chromosome anomalies associated with hematological disorders.[27] These structural changes alter gene expression either by position effect or gene mutation leading to transcription of the oncogene. Tumor-suppressor genes are also important probe targets of FISH studies.[27] In normal cells, tumor-suppressor genes regulate cell proliferation. Loss of tumor suppressor genes can happen by chromosome loss or by structural rearrangements such as deletions and unbalanced translocations. For example, monosomy 7, del(5)(q13q33), del(6)(q14q32), and other losses of chromosomal material are candidates for FISH studies.

4.2　　Home-Brew Probes

Home-brew probes can be made from bacterial artificial chromosome (BAC) or yeast artificial chromosome (YAC) clone(s) containing the DNA covering the genome sequence of interest. The appropriate BACs and/or

YACs can be determined and purchased using Internet resources such as www.ncbi.nih.gov/ and www.sanger.ac.uk/. Polymerase chain reaction (PCR) primers are designed for the gene of interest and/or for markers in the genome target. Bacteria containing appropriate BACs are cultured and PCR is performed to ensure the presence of the desired DNA sequence. The plasmid DNA is then separated from the genomic DNA of the bacteria and purified. The concentration of DNA is determined and fluorescent-labeled nucleotide bases are incorporated into the clone using standard nick translation procedures. Each batch of probe is then validated using normal specimens to ensure the FISH signal appears at the right chromosome location and there is no cross-hybridization of the probe with any inappropriate loci. The probe is subsequently applied to known abnormal specimens to determine its efficacy to identify chromosome anomalies for which it was designed to detect.

4.3   Naming FISH Probes

FISH probes are given names in various ways according to information known about the DNA fragments.[28] All approved human gene symbols can be found in the Genew database.[29] Arbitrary DNA fragments and loci are assigned gene symbols by the Genome Database. The symbols are made up of four parts. For example, the probe D13S319 indicates D for DNA, 13 for chromosome 13, S for a unique DNA sequence and 319 for a sequential number to make the probe designation unique. FISH probes that hybridize to repetitive DNA, such as the alphoid DNA associated with different chromosomes, are given the symbol Z. For example, the probe D8Z2 is a DNA probe for chromosome 8, alphoid region and sequence number 2. Other probes are given the name of the gene they are intended to detect. For example, *BCR* is a FISH probe that hybridizes to the *BCR* locus on chromosome 22.

4.4   FISH Nomenclature

Standard nomenclature to communicate results of FISH among cytogeneticists were created in 1995 and published in the International System for Cytogenetic Nomenclature.[5] It is beyond the scope of this chapter to discuss FISH nomenclature in detail, but we provide a couple of examples here to help appreciate the language.

The nomenclature is different for interphase FISH than for metaphase FISH. The expression *nuc ish* indicates results for interphase FISH. For example, the following interphase FISH nomenclature indicates two copies of *ABL* and two copies of *BCR*, but one copy of *ABL* and one copy of *BCR* is connected i.e. fusion.

nuc ish 9q34(*ABL*x2),22q11.2(*BCR*x2)(*ABL* con *BCR*x1)

Nomenclature for metaphase FISH requires both karyotype and FISH results at the same time. The nomenclature for conventional cytogenetics and FISH is separated by a dot. The following nomenclature indicates a male karyotype with a t(9;22) that has been studied by FISH. The FISH nomenclature indicates that the *ABL* locus is missing from the derivative chromosome 9 and is present on the derivative chromosome 22 at a location that is distal to the *BCR* locus.

46,XY,t(9;22)(q34;q11.2).ish t(9;22)(*ABL*-;*BCR*+,*ABL*+)

Recent data from the College of American Pathologists and American College of Medical Genetics indicate that FISH is widely used by cytogenetic laboratories[30], but the consistent application of this nomenclature is problematic in routine practice[31]. Problems with writing FISH nomenclature arise when probes for the same clinical purpose are used with different names and different FISH strategies. To complicate things, several new FISH techniques have been developed for which the current nomenclature was not designed to communicate. These and other problems make it difficult for FISH laboratories to consistently apply the present nomenclature guidelines in clinical practice.[31]

5. FISH STRATEGIES

DNA probes are classified by where they hybridize.[1] Some FISH probes hybridize to specific centromeres (Figure 4-2A)[32,33] and others to gene loci (Figure 4-2B)[3,21,34,35]. Some probes hybridize to unique DNA sequences over the length of the entire chromosome to produce a paint-like pattern for a single chromosome (Figure 4-2C) or to paint all chromosome pairs a different color (Figure 4-2D).[36] DNA probes can be used individually or in combinations and can be labeled with different colored fluors.[23,24]

Because of a variety of attempts to reduce false-positive signal patterns in normal loci, multiple FISH strategies have become available. Over-lapping signals of the same color can be erroneously interpreted as loss of a chromosome locus. Over-lapping signals of different colors can be erroneously interpreted as a fusion of two different loci. Thus, the sensitivity to detect low levels of disease is not the same for all FISH assays.

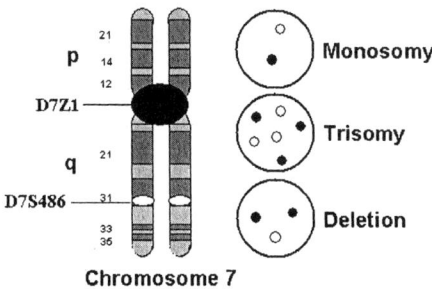

Chromosome 7

Figure 4-3. A FISH strategy to detect aneuploidy and deletions uses a probe of one color for the centromere and a probe of another color for an interstitial site on the chromosome. The most common colors of flours are red and green. This strategy produces two red and two green signals in normal interphase cells, cells with monosomy have one red and one green signal, cells with trisomy have three red and three green signals, and cells with deletion have one red and two green signals.

5.1 ND-FISH

The most common FISH strategy to detect aneuploidy and chromosome deletions uses a probe of one color for a control site and a probe of another color for an interstitial target site on the same chromosome.[2] For purposes of this chapter, this method is referred to as ND-FISH to indicate that this method detects numeric anomalies and/or deletions.

An illustration of ND-FISH is shown in Figure 4-3. The most common colors of fluors used with ND-FISH are red and green. This FISH strategy produces two red and two green signals in normal interphase cells. A cell with trisomy would have three control and three target signals. A cell with monosomy would have one control and one target signal. A cell with a deletion would have two control signals and one target signal.

The control and target chromosomal sites are selected for ND-FISH based on cytogenetic studies involving a large series of specimens with interstitial deletions such as del(5)(q13q33) or del(7)(q22q34). The control site is selected because it is seldom lost in association with a specific chromosome deletion. The target site is the most frequently lost DNA sequence associated with any given chromosome deletion.

False-positive signal patterns can occur when signals of the same color overlap in normal nuclei, any probe fails to hybridize, or there is cross-hybridization with inappropriate loci. In our experience, the sensitivity of ND-FISH to detect neoplastic clones in 200 nuclei is >5% for monosomy (Figure 4-2E), >3% for trisomy (Figure 4-2F), and >7% for deletions (Figure 4-2G).[23]

5.2   Amplification Detection by FISH

Certain hematological disorders are associated with gene amplification, which can be detected by observing many copies of a FISH probe signal for a gene. Figures 4-2H-J shows examples of amplification of *MLL* in AML, *c-MYC* in Burkitt leukemia, *BCR/ABL* fusion in CML and *TEL/AML1* fusion in ALL.

5.3   BAP-FISH

Some structural anomalies involve one locus that is involved in translocations with a variety of different chromosomal loci. One example is translocations involving *MLL* at 11q23. This locus has participated in translocations with more than 40 different chromosomal loci. Each of these translocations results in inappropriate activation of the *MLL* locus. The most common FISH method to detect these kind of translocations uses a probe strategy that we refer to in this chapter as BAP-FISH to indicate break-apart of the probe signal.

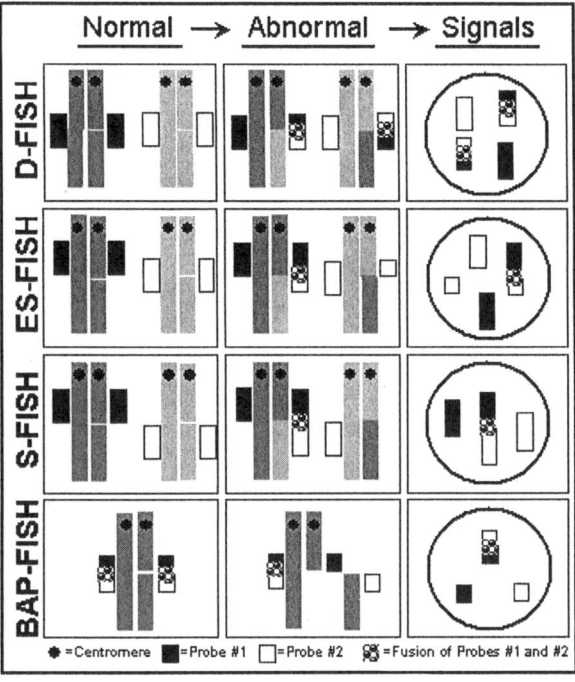

Figure 4-4. At least four different FISH strategies can be used to detect fusion of loci associated with chromosome translocations and inversions. D-FISH produces double or two fusion signals. ES-FISH produces a single fusion signal and an extra small signal. S-FISH produces a single fusion signal. BAP-FISH produces two fusion signals in a normal cell, but one of these signals separates or breaks apart in cells with a translocation or inversion. For more information see text, Table 4-1 and Figure 4-4.

An illustration of BAP-FISH is shown in Figure 4-4. With BAP-FISH, the probes hybridize to a specific region on only one chromosome. The probe is designed so that a red signal occurs on one side of the breakpoint cluster region and a green signal occurs on the other side. The breakpoint cluster region is small but is not represented in the probe set. When normal cells are observed, red and green signals merge to form a yellow fusion signal on each chromosome. A disruption in the breakpoint cluster region due to a translocation or inversion causes the fusion signal to break-apart and form separate red and green signals. In an abnormal interphase nucleus, one red, one green, and one yellow signal are observed (Figure 4-2N).[13]

False-positive cells occasionally occur in interphase when the red and green signals separate more than usual because of DNA decondensation in the breakpoint cluster region. In our experience, the sensitivity of BAP-FISH to detect neoplastic clones in 200 nuclei is >3%.

5.4   D-FISH

The most sensitive FISH method to detect reciprocal translocations produces double or two fusion signals as a result of fusion of two loci on two different chromosomes.[3] We refer to this method as D-FISH.

An illustration of D-FISH is shown in Figure 4-4. This strategy usually uses red and green probes that hybridize to loci on different chromosomes.[3,25] The hybridization sites span the breakpoint on each chromosome. When normal cells are observed, there are two red and two green signals. The reciprocal translocation produces adjacent red and green hybridization sites on each abnormal chromosome. Thus, in an abnormal interphase nucleus one red, one green, and two yellow fusion signals are observed (Figure 4-2L).

False-positive signals are very rare with D-FISH, but can occur when the probe signals are extensively disrupted for technical reasons and there is coincidental overlap of some of the signals. In one of our early experiments, we observed only one false-positive nucleus among 18,000 consecutive nuclei.[22] The sensitivity of D-FISH to detect neoplastic clones in 500 nuclei is >1%, but it can be increased to >0.079% by analyzing 6,000 nuclei.[22]

5.5   ES-FISH

Another sensitive FISH method to detect reciprocal translocations produces a single fusion signal and an extra small signal as a result of fusion of two loci on different chromosomes.[37] We refer to this strategy as ES-FISH.

An illustration of ES-FISH is shown in Figure 4-4. This strategy usually uses red and green probes that hybridize to different loci. The hybridization site spans the breakpoint on one of the chromosomes. The hybridization site of the other chromosome is relegated to one side of the breakpoint. With this method normal cells have two red and two green signals. The reciprocal translocation produces a yellow fusion signal on one abnormal chromosome, and a small residual red signal on the other abnormal chromosome. Abnormal interphase nuclei have two red, one green, and one yellow fusion signal (Figure 4-2M).

False-positive nuclei occasionally occur when a red or green signal separates in interphase cells for technical reasons. In our experience, the sensitivity of ES-FISH to detect neoplastic clones in 200 nuclei is >3%.[9]

5.6 S-FISH

The earliest FISH strategy to detect reciprocal translocations produces a single fusion signal that results from the fusion of two chromosomal loci from a translocation.[38] We refer to this strategy as S-FISH.

An illustration of S-FISH is shown in Figure 4-4. This strategy usually uses red and green probes that hybridize to different loci.[38] The green hybridization site occurs on the centromeric side of the breakpoint cluster region, and the red hybridization site occurs on the telomeric side of the breakpoint cluster region. With this method, normal cells have two red and two green signals. The reciprocal translocation produces a yellow fusion signal on one of the abnormal chromosomes. Abnormal interphase nuclei have one red, one green, and one yellow fusion signal (Figure 4-2K).

False-positive cells with an S-FISH pattern are common because of the overlap of red and green signals in normal cells. This problem is the primary cause of the high normal cut-off associated with S-FISH and has lead to the emergence of other more sensitive methods such as D-FISH and ES-FISH. In our experience, the sensitivity of S-FISH to detect neoplastic clones in 200 nuclei is >10%.[2]

5.7   Whole Chromosome Paints and Multi-Color FISH

For cells in metaphase, whole chromosome paints can be used to identify most major structural anomalies of a few chromosomes at a time (Figure 4-2C).[39] A variant of whole chromosome paints is called M-FISH (multi-color FISH) because it paints each of the 24 types of human chromosomes a different color (Figure 4-2D). This method is particularly useful to characterize chromosomal anomalies in complex karyotypes that are difficult to define by conventional cytogenetic studies.[36] However, these paint methods are expensive, do not detect small chromosome anomalies and require proliferating cells for study.

6.   VALIDATION OF FISH PROBES

Validation of any new FISH assay is necessary to ensure safe and effective testing for the specific intended clinical purpose. The validation of

FISH assays is a systematic multi-step process designed to assess probe performance in normal and abnormal specimens. This process also provides important experience with many cases to assure consistent scoring criteria and accurate interpretation of results.[40-42]

The procedures to validate FISH assays vary significantly depending upon the specific clinical application and FISH methodology (i.e., whole chromosome paints, centromere specific or locus specific probes).[42,43] The extent of validation among laboratories varies depending on probe approval by the United States Food and Drug Administration and the extent of published work regarding the assay. Standards for validating and applying FISH tests in clinical practice are still in the formative stages. Some recommendations for performing FISH testing have been suggested by the American College of Medical Genetics.[42] In addition, certain accrediting agencies such as the College of American Pathologists[26] and New York State Department of Health[44] have defined certain quality assurance criteria. Probe manufacturers do extensive quality control testing on their products, but validation, analysis and interpretation of FISH results rests with the laboratory that performs the assay.

We use a system to validate new probes that begins with a familiarization phase. The process involves experiments with a few known normal and abnormal specimens. These experiments provide initial experience with the assay and help create preliminary scoring criteria, assess equipment, and evaluate potential interfering factors. We do pilot investigations on a small series of normal and abnormal specimens using scoring criteria that were formulated in the familiarization experiments. These pilot studies include experiments to calculate the analytical sensitivity and analytical specificity of the assay.

Finally, we perform a clinical-pathological study on a blinded series of specimens from a large number of normal and abnormal specimens. From this information we calculate the normal cut-off for different signal patterns, clinical sensitivity and clinical specificity of the assay. These experiments provide important experience with actual patient material before using the FISH assay in clinical practice. It is useful to share data from the clinical-pathological trial and pilot studies with appropriate clinical and laboratory peers to identify any unexpected problems and to assess the utility of the test in clinical practice.

In clinical practice, it is important to develop control charts, monitor technologist competency and maintain equipment appropriately. Accrediting agencies have published criteria for FISH in routine practice and at least one accrediting agency provides an on-going proficiency testing program for FISH.[30,42]

7.　　　FISH IN CLINICAL PRACTICE

Most treatment protocols for hematological malignancies require quantitative procedures to assess tumor burden and response to therapy. This can be done by using various genetic tests including quantitative cytogenetic studies, FISH and molecular genetic techniques. No single genetic testing procedure fulfills all the needs of clinical care for patients with hematological malignancies. Thus, it is important to use combinations of testing methods that are both accurate and cost-effective for each clinical situation. It is particularly important to utilize the results of genetic testing together with other clinical and laboratory results to provide the best care and management of the patient. Since all genetic tests are relatively expensive and genetic laboratories are busy, it is not reasonable to routinely perform all available genetic tests.

Conventional cytogenetic studies are the standard method to study proliferating cells in hematological malignancies. This method can detect most chromosome anomalies and determine the percentage of proliferating neoplastic cells.[2] FISH can be readily performed on the same specimen, and uses the same specimen collection and transportation requirements. Thus, FISH assays can be used in any cascade algorithm before or after conventional cytogenetic studies.

FISH methods are useful to study non-proliferating cells. Moreover, using FISH it is easy to analyze large numbers of cells and to detect masked chromosome anomalies that are not apparent by conventional cytogenetic studies. Most FISH tests can be performed on an overnight basis and so are useful in urgent medical conditions. The expense associated with many FISH assays is approximately half the cost of conventional cytogenetic studies. Table 4-1 summarizes many of the commercially available FISH probes, their FISH strategies and sensitivity to detect neoplastic cells in specific hematological malignancies.

7.1　　Bone Marrow Transplantation

Various FISH strategies are available to monitor patients after bone marrow transplantation. FISH probes for the X and Y chromosome can be used for opposite-sex bone marrow transplantation to detect levels >0.3% XY cells in females and >0.6% XX cells in males.[33] This method defines the ratio of host versus donor cells, but does not directly establish the percentage of neoplastic cells. Alternatively, an appropriate FISH assay can be used to establish the percentage of neoplastic cells. The difficulty with this approach is that the sensitivity of most FISH assays for neoplastic disease is only 1 to 3% of all cells.

An elegant approach to increase the sensitivity of the FISH assay for patients with opposite sex bone marrow transplants is to combine aqua colored probes for the Y with red and green probes for the neoplastic process. For example, the use of a FISH assay for *BCR/ABL* fusion to score only Y bearing nuclei in the bone marrow of a male who has received a transplant from an XX donor can detect disease in >0.003% of all cells.

For same sex allogenic transplants or autologous transplants, the sensitivity of the FISH assay is only as good as the probe and FISH strategy employed. In some of these cases, molecular genetic methods can be used to detect residual recipient cells and/or disease. Conventional cytogenetic studies can help determine the presence of disease when relapse is related to the original clone or if any new malignancy emerges such as therapy-related neoplasms.

7.2   Chronic Myeloid Leukemia

Given the available successful treatments with imatinib mesylate, arsenic trioxide, interferon and/or bone marrow transplantation, CML is a particularly important disease to identify by genetic testing. About 95% of patients with CML have a t(9;22)(q34;q11.2) or a variant of this translocation. A similar translocation occurs in 6% of children with ALL, 17% of adults with ALL and 1% of patients with AML-M1.

The International System for Cytogenetic Nomenclature[5] designates the abnormal chromosome 22 in this translocation as the Philadelphia chromosome or Ph-chromosome. Nearly 2% of patients with CML have a complex variant Ph-chromosome that involves ≥3 chromosomes, but two are always chromosomes 9q34 and 22q11.2. The remaining 3% of patients with CML have a submicroscopic translocation that is not evident by conventional cytogenetic methods. Most cytogeneticists refer to these Ph-chromosomes as "masked". All forms of the Ph-chromosome are associated with fusion of the *BCR* and *ABL* loci.

Not all patients with CML respond to the same kind of therapy, and this outcome may be due to chromosome evolution. The appearance of additional chromosome anomalies together with a Ph-chromosome occurs in cells of bone marrow and peripheral blood in most patients with CML prior to the on-set of blast crisis. About 71% of patients with CML in blast crisis have at least one of the following anomalies: +8, i(17q), +19 or extra Ph-chromosomes. About 15% of patients with CML in blast crisis have -7, -17, +17, +21, -Y or t(3;21)(q26;q22). Although there are FISH assays to detect many of these chromosome anomalies, conventional cytogenetic studies may do this better and the focus of treatment today is to cure CML rather than predict blast crisis.

Many clinicians use a systematic method to classify remission based on the percentage of metaphases with Ph-chromosomes observed by conventional cytogenetic studies, e.g. no response, partial response and complete remission.[45,46] However, the goal for any treatment for CML should be to achieve a complete cytogenetic or FISH remission i.e. no Ph-positive metaphases and/or FISH results within normal limits. In our experience, the best testing method to detect all the various forms of the Ph-chromosome uses the D-FISH strategy for *BCR* and *ABL* fusion (Table 4-2).[3] Strict scoring criteria have been developed for D-FISH to reliably classify cells as either normal or abnormal.[3] With experience, D-FISH is highly sensitive, consistent and can be mastered by most laboratories.[47]

Table 4-2. Algorithm for conventional cytogenetic and FISH studies for CML

-At diagnosis perform quantitative cytogenetic analysis of 25 metaphases from bone marrow. In addition, perform FISH on 500 nuclei from bone marrow and 500 nuclei from blood.

-To monitor patients during therapy, use FISH to study blood or bone marrow to track changes in the percentage of cells with *BCR/ABL* fusion at 3 to 6-month intervals. It is important to compare results of blood with pre-treatment blood and results of bone marrow with pre-treatment bone marrow.

-D-FISH analysis of up to 6,000 nuclei can be performed to look for residual disease among patients in FISH remission.[22]

-At relapse perform a chromosome study to assess the karyotype of the neoplastic process to determine if a new disorder has developed or relapse of CML has occurred.

FISH analysis of interphase nuclei from bone marrow is useful to study patients before and after treatment to assess response to therapy.[3,22,48-50] With FISH the percentage of Ph-positive nuclei in bone marrow prior to treatment is usually 85% to 99%. When treatment is successful, the post-treatment percentage of neoplastic nuclei progressively decreases to less than 1%.

Several investigations have studied the efficacy of FISH to examine blood to monitor response to therapy in CML.[22,48,51] One such study involved 37 paired sets of bone marrow and blood specimens collected within 24 to 96 hours of each other, from 10 patients before and during treatment of CML with interferon.[22] Results of this investigation indicated that analysis of 500 nuclei with D-FISH from bone marrow and peripheral blood can detect less than 1% neoplastic cells and produced results that were more sensitive than conventional quantitative cytogenetic studies. Consequently, analysis of interphase nuclei from blood with D-FISH can substitute for quantitative cytogenetic studies on bone marrow even when the patient is in complete cytogenetic remission. Based on analysis of 6,000 nuclei with D-FISH, very low levels of abnormal cells can be identified in both bone marrow and blood from patients in complete cytogenetic remission.[22]

Some patients with CML on imatinib mesylate become "drug resistant" due to amplification of the *BCR/ABL* fusion gene. This outcome can be detected in individual neoplastic cells with FISH by observing multiple or clusters of *BCR/ABL* fusion signals (Figure 4-2J). Organized studies of patients with imatinib mesylate drug resistant need to be performed to understand how to accurately score and learn the clinical relevancy of *BCR/ABL* fusion amplification.

Patients with complex Ph-chromosomes have a unique signal pattern by D-FISH. For example, consider a patient with a t(5;9;22)(q31;q34;q11.2). In an abnormal metaphase from this patient, a *BCR/ABL* fusion signal occurs on the Ph-chromosome, a small *ABL* signal occurs on the abnormal chromosome 9, and a small *BCR* signal occurs on the abnormal chromosome 5. The *ABL/BCR* fusion that is normally observed on the abnormal chromosome 9 with D-FISH does not occur in complex translocations.

Unusual *BCR/ABL* signals are also observed among patients with masked Ph-chromosomes. FISH studies show that masked Ph-chromosomes originate from small insertions involving the *BCR* and *ABL* loci. These chromosome insertions are not visible by conventional cytogenetic studies, but are readily detectable by FISH.[3] In our experience, 50% of patients with a masked Ph-chromosome have a *BCR/ABL* fusion signal on the abnormal chromosome 22. The remaining 50% have *BCR/ABL* fusion on the abnormal chromosome 9. It is important to use a FISH technique to monitor response to therapy for patients with a masked Ph-chromosome.

Nearly 20% of patients with a t(9;22)(q34;q11.2) have any one of three different forms of atypical D-FISH patterns.[9] Among these patients, there is loss of a portion of *BCR* or *ABL* or both of these hybridization sites normally associated with the break and fusion point on the abnormal chromosome 9. Laboratory personnel need to be aware of these variant signal patterns in order to adjust their scoring criteria and to utilize different cut-off values for normal. In our experience, the normal cutoff is 1.2 to 1.8% for two of these atypical signal patterns and 0.6% for the other atypical signal pattern.[52] It is useful to examine a few metaphases at diagnosis to establish the exact *BCR/ABL* signal pattern for each patient.

With D-FISH, approximately 10% of patients with a t(9;22)(q34;q11.2) have an atypical signal pattern due to loss of both the translocated BCR and residual ABL DNA on the derivative chromosome 9. This event produces one red, one green and one yellow fusion signal. Because it is difficult to distinguish between neoplastic cells with a yellow *BCR/ABL* fusion signal and normal cells with a yellow signal due to the coincidental overlap of a red and green signal, the cutoff for this signal pattern in 500 nuclei is 23%. For these patients, we recommend a new TD-FISH strategy that uses an aqua signal for the ASS locus located near the *ABL* locus.[52] With this FISH assay, the neoplastic cells lose an ASS signal, but normal cells retain two copies of the ASS signal. This method makes it possible to distinguish between overlapping *BCR* and *ABL* signals and nuclei with *BCR/ABL* fusion. In our experience, this TD-FISH assay can detect disease at >0.6% among patients with CML.

Several groups suggest that loss of DNA associated with the break and fusion point on chromosome 9 in cells with a t(9;22)(q34;q11.2) is associated with a poor prognosis and reduced response to treatment.[53] Sinclair et al[54] studied survival among 11 patients with CML who had abnormal chromosome 9 deletions in patients with t(9;22)(q34;q11.2). They found that the deletions spanned up to several megabases of DNA and had variable molecular breakpoints. Statistical analyses using Kaplan-Meier methods showed a median survival of 36 months among these patients compared with >90 months for patients without a detectable deletion. The difference in survival was statistically significant and multivariate analysis demonstrated that the prognostic importance of the molecular deletion was independent of age, sex, percentage of blasts in peripheral blood, and platelet count. Sinclair et al[54] suggested that these deletions may result in loss of one or more genes that influence progression of the disease.

Subsequently, Huntly et al.[55] studied 241 patients including 39 with deletions and 202 without deletions. The median survival was 38 months for patients with deletions and 88 months for patients without deletions. Kolomietz et al.[56] compared median survival among 186 patients including 23 with deletions and 163 without deletions. The median survival was 36 months for patients with deletions and 84 months for patients without deletions. In these investigations[55,56] and two other smaller studies[57,58], the results indicated that shorter survival was associated with a shorter duration of the chronic phase and with earlier disease progression.

The reported investigations of survival and deletions in CML have been based primarily on patients receiving various forms of treatment, but mostly interferon. The survival status for patients with allogenic transplantation is not yet known for certain, but in one small series of 12 patients the rate of relapse was increased among patients with deletions after transplantation.[56] Data concerning the deletion status and survival among patients receiving imatinib mesylate are not yet known, but will be important considering the wide spread use of this treatment for CML.

FISH strategies that detect deletions on the abnormal chromosome 9 will be particularly important if correlations between survival and *ABL/BCR* deletion status hold-up in studies of large series of patients with CML that have been treated with imatinib mesylate. Since D-FISH is the only strategy that detects all atypical signal patterns associated with the abnormal chromosome 9 in CML, this will be the method of choice in clinical practice.[9,48,54,59] ES-FISH will detect some of the atypical patterns, but this strategy does not detect those 25% of patients with atypical patterns that have loss of the portion of *BCR* that should be translocated to the abnormal chromosome 9.

7.3   Myeloproliferative Disorders Other Than CML

At least 27 chromosome anomalies have been associated with MPD.[60,61,62,63,64] Although not diagnostic, a relatively strong association exists between del(13)(q12q14) with myelofibrosis[65,66], t(5;12)(q33;p13) with eosinophilia[67], and del(20)(q11q13), +8, +9 with polycythemia vera [68]. These and other chromosome anomalies are readily detected by conventional cytogenetic studies, but good FISH probes are available to detect most of them as well. An algorithm for cytogenetic and FISH testing in MPD is summarized in Table 4-3.

Evidence is emerging that suggests fusion of the Fip1-like1 (FIP1L1) gene and the platelet derived growth factor receptor alpha (PDGFRα) gene is associated with chronic hypereosinophilia with systemic mast cell disease.[69] Pardanani et al[69] used a FISH probe to successfully detect the deletion of CHIC2 locus between FIP1L1 and PDGFRα as a surrogate marker for this anomaly. This microdeletion is not apparent by conventional cytogenetic studies. The FIP1L1 and PDGFRα fusion is a target for imatinib mesylate treatment for patients with these conditions.

Table 4-3. Algorithm for conventional cytogenetic and FISH studies for MPD other than CML

-At diagnosis perform conventional cytogenetic studies on bone marrow.[60]
-To monitor patients during therapy, use an appropriate FISH assay to detect chromosome anomalies identified at diagnosis. In most patients, blood or bone marrow can be studied before and after treatment to track changes in the percentage of neoplastic over time.
-A FISH assay for *BCR/ABL* fusion is sometimes useful to rule out CML in the diagnosis of essential thrombocythemia or polycythemia vera.

To compare the efficacy of conventional cytogenetic studies and FISH, Tefferi et al.[70] used both of these methods to study blood and bone marrow from 42 patients who had myelofibrosis with myeloid metaplasia. The FISH method used probes to detect common anomalies of chromosomes 5, 7, 8, 11, 13, 20 and 21. The results of these two methods were similar, but some patients had chromosome anomalies that were only detected by conventional cytogenetic studies. Although FISH analysis is not generally a substitute for conventional cytogenetics studies for most MPD, it is useful for patients with inadequate bone marrow specimens and for patients that would benefit from periodic testing to monitor disease status.

7.4   Myelodysplastic Syndromes

The MDS are a clinically heterogeneous group of hematological disorders.[71] The most common chromosome anomalies in MDS involve chromosomes 5, 7, 8, 11, 13, 17, 20, 21 and X.[72,73] Cytogenetic studies are important for these disorders as the results can provide both diagnostic and prognostic information.[20] Briefly, patients with MDS who have –Y alone, 5q- alone, 20q- alone or normal metaphases have a favorable prognosis. Patients with a complex karyotype (defined as ≥3 anomalies) or anomalies of chromosome 7 have an unfavorable prognosis. Patients with other chromosome anomalies generally have an intermediate prognosis.

Using conventional cytogenetic studies, a chromosomally abnormal clone can be detected in 60% of patients with aggressive MDS such as refractory anemia with excess blasts or refractory anemia with excess blasts in transformation.[72,73] In contrast, a chromosomally abnormal clone can be detected in 35% of patients with less aggressive MDS such as refractory anemia or refractory anemia with ringed sideroblasts. Although no specific chromosome anomaly is associated with any MDS in the World Health Organization classification[71], there is a strong association between del(5)(q13q33) and 5q- syndrome[74], and idic(X)(q13) and refractory anemia with ringed sideroblasts[75].

Results of several investigations indicate that conventional cytogenetic studies and FISH have relatively similar sensitivities to detect an abnormal clone among patients with MDS. A reasonable panel FISH assay for MDS would utilize probes to detect numeric and/or structural anomalies of chromosome 5, 7, 8, 11, 13 and 20.[76,77] Occasional patients with normal chromosomes will show an occult neoplastic clone by FISH. Vice versa, occasional patients will show a neoplastic clone by conventional cytogenetic studies that are normal by FISH. An algorithm for cytogenetic and FISH testing in MDS is summarized in Table 4-4.

Table 4-4. Algorithm for conventional cytogenetic and FISH studies for MDS

-At diagnosis, the best genetic test is conventional cytogenetic studies.
-FISH is useful for some clinical situations such as bone marrow samples lacking analyzable metaphases, or to follow the percent of abnormal cells with known cytogenetic anomalies for patients undergoing treatment.[76]
-Useful FISH probes for patients with MDS include EGR1, D7S486, D8Z2, *MLL*, D13S319 and D20S108 (Table 4-1).[76,77]

Ketterling et al.[76] studied 32 patients with primary MDS and a normal karyotype to determine if interphase-FISH and/or multi-color FISH could detect chromosome anomalies that were not apparent by conventional cytogenetic studies. These investigators found that one patient had a chromosome 13q deletion, while the remaining 31 patients had normal results. These results indicate that many patients with MDS have a normal karyotype, and owe their disease to submicroscopic gene mutations or other biological causes. These results also suggest that mutations responsible for "MDS with normal cytogenetics" are undetectable by current cytogenetic methodologies and that more sophisticated molecular analysis will be required to determine the genetic aberrations responsible for this subtype of MDS.

7.5   Acute Myeloid Leukemia

Four cytogenetic risk categories of AML are widely applied in clinical practice: favorable, intermediate, unfavorable, and unknown.[78,79] Consequently, it is important to perform appropriate cytogenetic and FISH studies to establish the correct cytogenetic risk category to decide appropriate treatment. The favorable cytogenetic risk category anomalies include t(15;17)(q22;q21) and variants with or without other chromosome anomalies, inv(16)(p13q22)/t(16;16)(p13;q22)/del(16q)(q22) with or without other chromosome anomalies and t(8;21)(q22;q22) without either del(9q) or part of a complex karyotype. These patients are generally younger, have a good response to chemotherapy and a favorable duration of remission.

The intermediate risk category anomalies include +8, −Y, +6, del(12p) and normal karyotype. The most common chromosome anomalies of the unfavorable risk categories are -5/del(5q), -7/del(7q), inv(3)(q21q26), del(9q), t(6;9)(p23;q34), t(9;22)(q34;q11.2), or any abnormality of 11q, 17p, 20q, or 21q, or complex karyotype defined as ≥3 anomalies. Many of these chromosome anomalies are also associated with MDS or AML arising from chemotherapy, radiotherapy or exposure to environmental clastogens. All other clonal anomalies with less than three anomalies are classified as unknown prognosis.

Approximately 80% of patients with AML have a chromosomally abnormal clone that is detected by conventional cytogenetic studies. Many investigators believe that all patients with AML may actually have a neoplastic clone involving a chromosome anomaly. Sampling error, cryptic chromosome anomalies or technical error may miss the neoplastic clone in "normal karyotype" patients with AML. Although only a few investigations have been done, FISH may prove to be a more consistent and cost-effective method to detect "hidden" chromosome aberrations among patients with AML and to monitor treatment.

FISH can identify many of the chromosome anomalies associated with AML in both metaphase and interphase cells. FISH may be particularly valuable to detect *AML1/ETO* fusion among patients with variants of t(8;21)(q22;q22) or complex karyotypes in which detection of t(8;21)(q22;q22) is difficult by conventional chromosome studies.[80,81] Interphase-FISH is also an effective technique to detect anomalies of CBFβ associated with inv(16)(p13q22), especially when the patient has a variant inversion or translocations of chromosome 16.[82-84] FISH is also useful to detect *MLL* gene rearrangements including translocations, deletions and amplifications of the 11q23 locus.[85,86]

Among patients with acute promyelocytic leukemia, the t(15;17)(q22;q21) is sometimes missed in conventional cytogenetic studies because of technical problems.[21] In some instances, the *PML/RARα* fusion is masked and cannot be detected by conventional cytogenetic studies. Using a D-FISH method, Brockman et al.[25] accurately detected *PML/RARα* in all patients with either a t(15;17)(q22;q21) or variant forms of this translocation. In addition, this D-FISH method detected all alternate translocations involving *RARα* and not *PML*. These investigators suggest this D-FISH method can be used both for the accurate diagnosis of acute promyelocytic leukemia and to monitor low levels of disease in treated patients.

Fischer et al[86] used sets of DNA probes with interphase-FISH to detect common chromosome anomalies associated with AML and compared the results with conventional cytogenetic studies. Interphase-FISH proved to be more sensitive to detect AML-specific gene fusion anomalies and some partial trisomies.[86] Some reports indicate that interphase-FISH is particularly valuable to detect monosomy 7 (36%) and trisomy 8 (12%) in AML.[85,87] However, Richkind et al.[88] used DNA probes for selected anomalies associated with AML and found that neoplastic cells were detectable in only 2.4% of patients with AML who had normal cytogenetic results. The different outcomes of these studies may be due to differences among patients studied and variations in methods among cytogenetic laboratories.

Cytogenetic studies are valuable to assess the effectiveness of therapy. For patients with AML in remission, the predominant cells have normal chromosomes. When the disease of these patients relapses, the cells with the original chromosome anomalies re-emerge. Nevertheless, if a FISH assay is available to quantify disease, these are the genetic tests of choice to predict relapse. These FISH methods are less expensive and more sensitive than conventional cytogenetic studies. If therapy-related AML is suspected, it is also useful to perform a cytogenetic study because these hematological malignancies can be recognized by their characteristic chromosome anomalies.[89] An algorithm for cytogenetic and FISH studies for patients with AML is shown in Table 4-5.

Table 4-5. Algorithm for conventional cytogenetic and FISH studies for AML

-At diagnosis, conventional cytogenetic studies should be performed on bone marrow.[79]

-FISH can be performed on bone marrow at diagnosis to establish a benchmark for the percentage of neoplastic cells and again after treatment to help assess the effectiveness of therapy.

-To help identify patients with favorable or unfavorable cytogenetic risk chromosome anomalies, FISH is useful using probes for *AML1/ETO*, CBFβ, *MLL*, PML/RARα, *EGR1*, D7S486, D8Z2, and *BCR/ABL* (Table 4-1).

7.6 Acute Lymphoblastic Leukemia

Most published series of patients with ALL indicate that more than 85% have an abnormal clone by conventional cytogenetic studies. At least 36 chromosome anomalies are common in ALL. The most common karyotype among children with ALL is hyperdiploidy. This karyotype is associated with a good prognosis in the absence of any structural anomalies and when associated with trisomies of chromosomes 4, 10 and 17.[90] The most common chromosome translocations in pediatric ALL include t(9;22)(q34;q11.2), t(12;21)(p13;q22),   t(1;19)(q23;p13),   t(8;14)(q24;q32),   and t(11;var)(q23;var).[90] These anomalies are important to detect as they are critical prognostic markers, such that the decision for early transplantation may be made if t(9;22)(q34;q11.2) is detected. In contrast, if t(12;21)(p13;q22) is detected, the patient has a favorable prognosis and transplantation is rarely considered.

FISH can detect many of these abnormalities in interphase nuclei, but little has been published on this subject. We compared the efficacy of conventional cytogenetic methods and interphase-FISH to study bone marrow from 83 patients with ALL. Among this series of patients, 18 had T-cell, 64 had precursor B-cell and 1 had Burkitt leukemia. We used FISH with commercial probes for *BCR/ABL*, D4Z1 and D10Z1, *MLL*, *TEL/AML1*, and IGH to detect t(9;22)(q34;q11.2), +4 and +10 together, t(11;var)(q23;var), t(12;21)(p13;q22), and t(14;var)(q32;var), respectively. For patients with an abnormal signal pattern for IGH, further FISH studies were done with *c-MYC*, *BCL2*, and *CCND1* for t(8;14)(q23;q32), t(14;18)(q32;q21), and t(11;14)(q13;q32), respectively. We did not have FISH probes for t(1;19)(q23;p13).

Among 18 patients with T-cell ALL, the results of conventional cytogenetics studies were abnormal in 14 (78%). For these same specimens, FISH was normal in all 18 patients for the primary anomaly each probe was designed to detect, but 7 (39%) showed aneuploidy for one or more of the probes. None of the four chromosomally normal patients were aneuploid by FISH. Thus, conventional cytogenetic studies are more useful for patients with T-cell ALL, than the panel FISH test that we employed.

Among 65 patients with precursor B-cell ALL or Burkitt leukemia, results of conventional cytogenetic studies were abnormal in 53 (82%), FISH was abnormal in 57 (88%), and either FISH or cytogenetics was abnormal in 62 (95%). FISH was abnormal in 9 of 12 patients who were normal by cytogenetics. FISH was particularly valuable to detect *TEL/AML1* fusion. This gene fusion was detected in 6 patients: 1 had a normal karyotype, and 5 had a complex karyotype with no apparent t(12;21)(p13;q22). The t(12;21)(p13;q22) is associated with *TEL/AML1* fusion and can be very difficult to detect by conventional cytogenetic studies.

Algorithms for conventional cytogenetics and FISH are still experimental, but a possible strategy is summarized in Table 4-6. If a t(9;22)(q34;q11.2), 11q23 anomaly or 14q32 anomaly is detected by conventional cytogenetic studies, the specimen can be tested with appropriate FISH probes to verify the anomaly and establish a baseline percentage of abnormal cells. FISH can be used to monitor the effectiveness of therapy among these patients. If a complex karyotype without a t(9;22)(q34;q11.2), 11q23 anomaly or 14q32 anomaly is observed, the complete panel FISH test for precursor B-cell ALL can be performed. Conventional cytogenetic studies sometimes detect abnormalities of 11q23, but FISH is a useful adjunct to be certain that *MLL* is abnormal.

Table 4-6. Algorithm for conventional cytogenetic and FISH studies for ALL.

-Useful FISH probes for patients with ALL include *BCR/ABL*, D4Z1 and D10Z1, *MLL*, *TEL/AML1*, and IGH.
-For patients with IGH abnormalities, it is useful to follow-up with FISH studies for c-*MYC*/IGH, *BCL2*/IGH and *CCND1*/IGH.

7.7 B-cell Chronic Lymphocytic Leukemia

The prognosis and clinical course of patients with B-CLL are highly variable. Studies with conventional cytogenetics, FISH, molecular genetics, immunophenotyping, and mutation analysis of the immunoglobulin heavy chain variable regions have all been used to study B-CLL.[23,91-95,96] Each of these approaches helps to assess prognosis in this disease, but the oncogenic events that lead to the origin of B-CLL remain unknown.

Based on conventional cytogenetic studies, the most common anomalies in B-CLL involve chromosomes 6, 11, 12, 13, 14 and 17. These same chromosome anomalies are observed in small cell lymphocytic leukemia. In B-CLL, these anomalies have been associated with differing prognoses and lengths of survival.[91,92,97,98,99] Using various mitogens to stimulate neoplastic B-cells, conventional cytogenetic studies have detected abnormal clones in 50% of patients with progressive B-CLL.[91,92,100,101] Conventional cytogenetic studies using these same methods have been less successful for early and indolent B-CLL.

FISH has been used to detect common chromosome anomalies in interphase nuclei among patients with B-CLL. In one investigation of 325 patients the median survival for patients with 17p deletion, 11q deletion, trisomy 12, normal or 13q deletion was 32, 79, 114, 111 and 133 months, respectively, and the treatment-free interval was 9, 13, 33, 49 and 92 months, respectively.[96] Some investigators have compared known prognostic features of B-CLL with results of interphase FISH.[23] The results indicate that FISH-detected anomalies are frequent in B-CLL even in Rai stages 0-1, but are more frequent among patients with progressive disease (88%) than patients with stable disease (66%).[23]

In our experience, conventional cytogenetic studies are much less informative, more expensive and more difficult to use in clinical practice than panel FISH testing for common chromosome anomalies. A suggested algorithm for FISH testing in B-CLL is summarized in Table 4-7.

Table 4-7. Algorithm for FISH studies of B-CLL

-Interphase FISH on peripheral blood can be used in lieu of conventional cytogenetic studies as it is less expensive and identifies a clinically significant clone in most patients.
-FISH studies for common chromosome anomalies should be done at least once in the course of a patient's disease to obtain prognostic information, but may also be useful at any time when there is progression of the patients condition.
-A good panel FISH test for B-CLL includes probes for *MYB, ATM*, D13S319, *P53*, D12Z3 and IGH (Table 4-1).
-This FISH test can distinguish between patients with B-CLL and patients with the leukemic phase of certain lymphomas such as mantle cell lymphoma with t(11;14)(q13;q32), follicular lymphoma with t(14;18)(q32;q21), t(14;19)(q32;q13.1) with low grade lymphoma and others.

7.8   Myeloma

The karyotype of myeloma is typically hyperdiploid and involves numerous chromosome anomalies, but occasional patients have a hypodiploid chromosome number. Most likely all patients with myeloma have a chromosomally abnormal clone, but results of conventional cytogenetic studies at diagnosis are abnormal in only 20 to 30% of patients.[102,103] The observation of an abnormal clone by conventional cytogenetics is an indication of active disease and is associated with a poor prognosis, especially when there are deletions or loss of chromosome 13.[102,103]

Based on interphase FISH studies, chromosome anomalies can be detected in nearly all patients with multiple myeloma. Several investigators have demonstrated a different prognosis for anomalies of chromosome 13 and 17 as well as for t(11;14)(q13;q32), t(4;14)(p16.3;q32) and t(14;16)(q32;q23).[104-107,108,109] Consequently, if results of conventional cytogenetic studies are normal, interphase FISH studies may provide further prognostic information about patients with myeloma.

Detecting an abnormality by FISH for myeloma is difficult when the percentage of plasma cells is less than 20%. The sensitivity of FISH is significantly improved by plasma cell enrichment by sorting cells with CD138 magnetic beads or combined immunophenotyping for cytoplasmic immunoglobulin (Figure 4-2O).[109,110,111] It is important to use an IGH FISH probe that will break-apart when there is any translocation that involves this locus. This FISH assay does not detect translocations involving the immunoglobulin light chains. These translocations are expected to occur in at least some patients with myeloma. FISH probes to detect these translocations and other chromosome anomalies associated with myeloma are under development by various investigators. An algorithm for conventional cytogenetic and FISH studies for myeloma is summarized in Table 4-8.

Table 4-8. Algorithm for conventional cytogenetic and FISH studies for myeloma

-Conventional cytogenetic studies of bone marrow are useful at diagnosis. Interphase FISH studies can also be used to detect translocations involving the IGH locus, deletions of chromosome 13q and/or 17p.

-FISH studies on patients with less than 20% plasma cells are best done directly on plasma cells.[111]

-A good panel FISH test for myeloma might include probes to detect loss of D13S319 at 13q14 (13q-) and *P53* at 17p13.1 (17p-), and to detect common translocations involving the IGH locus such as *CCND1* for t(11;14)(q13;q32), *FGFR3* for t(4;14)(p16.3;q32) and *c-MAF* for t(14;16)(q32;q23).

7.9   Lymphoma

The World Health Organization recognizes that genetic anomalies are one of the most reliable criteria for classification of malignant lymphomas.[62]

Conventional cytogenetic studies can detect many of these anomalies but this method is difficult, expensive and requires fresh tissues for analysis. Thus, many investigators today use FISH to study cells from touch preparations or paraffin-embedded lymphoid tissue.[24,112,113,114]

All patients with Burkitt lymphoma have a t(8;14)(q24;q32) or a variant of this translocation involving *c-MYC* and one of the light chain immunoglobulin loci at 22q11 or 2p12.[62] With D-FISH it is easy to detect the *c-MYC*/IGH fusion associated with t(8;14)(q24;q32). When there is either a t(8;22)(q24;q11) or t(2;8)(p12;q24), the *c-MYC* signal breaks-apart, but there is no fusion of *c-MYC*/IGH.[24,114] To distinguish between trisomy 8 and a translocation involving the *c-MYC* locus, one FISH strategy uses a set of different colored probes, one for the chromosome 8 centromere and the other for the *c-MYC* locus. Cells with a t(8;22) or t(2;8) have two centromere signals, one normal sized *c-MYC* signal, and two small *c-MYC* signals. Cells with trisomy 8 have three signals for the centromere and 3 normal sized signals for *c-MYC*.

An estimated 70 to 95% of patients with follicular lymphoma have a t(14;18)(q32;21) associated with *BCL2*/IGH fusion.[115,116] Approximately 15% of patients with follicular lymphoma also have loss of the P53 locus at 17p13.[117] Many patients also have loss of the P16 locus at 9p21 and these patients are particularly prone to disease progression to diffuse large B-cell lymphoma.[118,119] Translocations involving 3q27 involving the *BCL6* locus have been described in 15% of follicular lymphomas.[120] FISH probes are available to detect fusion of *BCL2* and IGH, breakapart of the *BCL6* locus, and loss of P53 at 17p13 and/or loss of P16 at 9p21.[24,114]

Approximately 70% of patients with mantle cell lymphoma have a t(11;14)(q13;q32) by conventional cytogenetics.[121] This is surely an underestimate of the actual incidence of this chromosome anomaly because FISH can detect fusion of *CCND1* and IGH in nearly 100% of these patients.[35,114,122-124] A FISH assay to detect *CCND1*/IGH fusion is particularly valuable to detect the leukemia phase of mantle cell lymphoma by studying bone marrow or blood, even in the absence of lymphadenopathy. Some patients with mantle cell lymphoma will also have deletions in 11q, 17p, and/or 9p.[125,126] These same chromosome anomalies are also seen in other B-cell neoplasms such as B-cell chronic lymphocytic leukemia, follicular lymphoma and diffuse large B-cell lymphoma.[62]

Anaplastic large cell lymphoma is associated with several different translocations all involving the *ALK* locus at 2p23.[127] A BAP-FISH assay is useful to detect translocations involving the *ALK* locus. In our experience, the sensitivity of the FISH assay can be increased by scoring only the large mottled nuclei as these represent the neoplastic cells in this disease.

Recent cytogenetic reports dealing with marginal zone lymphoma of mucosa associated lymphoid tissue (MALT) suggest at least three different translocations are associated with this disease; t(1;14)(p22;q32), t(11;18)(q21;q21) and t(14;18)(q32;q21).[128-130] In addition, several aneuploidies have been associated with this disorder, especially +3, +7, +12 and +18.[129] These aneuploidies can be readily detected with FISH probes for the centromeres of these chromosomes. The t(11;18)(q21;q21) can be detected with FISH by looking for the fusion of *API2* and *MALT1*. FISH can detect the t(14;18)(q32;q21) by looking for fusion of *MALT1* and IGH (Table 4-1). By conventional cytogenetic studies, the t(14;18)(q32;q21) appears similar in MALT and follicular lymphoma, but the former is associated with the MALT locus whereas the latter is linked with the *BCL2* locus.[130] These translocations can be readily distinguished between one another by using separate FISH assays, one to look for fusion of *MALT1* and IGH, and the other to detect the fusion of *BCL2* and IGH.

The results of genetic studies for diffuse large B-cell lymphoma suggest this is a heterogeneous group of diseases. Up to 30% of these patients have translocations involving *BCL6* at 3q27; the most common translocation is t(3;14)(q27;q32).[131] BAP-FISH is used to detect translocations involving *BCL6* since multiple chromosome partners are involved. Another 20 to 30% of patients with diffuse large B-cell lymphoma have *BCL2*/IGH fusion.[132,133] These are patients who may have follicular lymphoma with disease progression to diffuse large B-cell lymphoma. The fusion of *c-MYC*/IGH, amplification of *c-MYC* and/or aneuploidy involving *c-MYC* is also observed in diffuse large cell lymphoma. Patients with these anomalies are generally associated with poor prognosis.[134]

FISH studies are relatively easy to perform on touch preparations. A fresh biopsy is touched to a dry slide to create a layer of cells that adhere to the slide. The slide is allowed to dry at room temperature for 30 minutes. The specimen is then fixed in a Coplin jar containing fresh fixative made-up of 3 parts methanol and 1 part glacial acetic acid. The standard FISH procedure can then be applied to these cells.

When fresh tissue samples are not available FISH can be performed on nuclei isolated from paraffin-embedded tissues by using a needle core biopsy method.[24,135] This method was used in one investigation to study 6 normal lymph nodes or tonsils and 32 malignant lymphomas. The lymphomas included 5 mantle cell, 5 follicular, 5 Burkitt, 5 MALT, 5 anaplastic large cell, and 7 diffuse large B-cell. Many of these specimens were known to have anomalies by previous genetic and/or FISH studies.[35,113,127] The results of FISH studies for chromosome anomalies involving *BCL6*, *BCL2*, *c-MYC*, *CCND1*, *ALK*, IGH, *MALT1* and *API2* were consistent with the type of lymphoma investigated. For these cases, the sensitivity of the method was

100%. Since each of the six normal tissues studied had a normal FISH pattern with each probe, this method has a high specificity as well. A variant FISH pattern associated with *c-MYC* break-apart was detected in one patient with Burkitt lymphoma due to a t(2;8)(p12;q24) and was confirmed by previous cytogenetic studies.

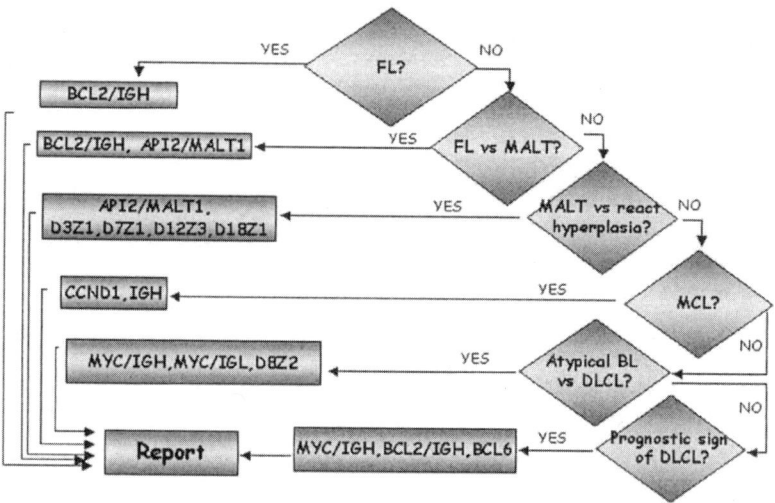

Figure 4-5. Algorithm for FISH testing in lymphoma. For more information see text and Table 4-1.

Clearly FISH can be used to detect certain important chromosome anomalies with high specificity and high sensitivity in many lymphomas. FISH is helpful to hematopathologists to diagnose and classify lymphomas (Table 4-9 and Figure 4-5).

Table 4-9. Algorithm for FISH studies for lymphoma.

-FISH can be done on touch preparations or paraffin-embedded tissue. [24,35]
-FISH assays have been successfully performed for *BCL6, BCL2, c-MYC, CCND1, ALK, IGH, MALT1* and *API2* (Figure 4-5).[24]
-In order to study the malignant cells, it is important to interact with a hematopathologist to identify neoplastic tissue.

REFERENCES

1. Fan Y-S: Molecular Cytogenetics. *In* Methods Mol Biol. 2002; Vol 204, pp 411.
2. Dewald G, Ketterling RP, Wyatt WA, Stupca P. Cytogenetic Studies in Neoplastic Hematologic Disorders. *In* Clinical Laboratory Medicine. Edited by K McClatchey, 2nd edition. Baltimore, Williams and Wilkens, 2002; pp 658-685.
3. Dewald GW, Wyatt WA, Juneau AL, Carlson RO, Zinsmeister AR, Jalal SM, Spurbeck JL, Silver RT. Highly sensitive fluorescence in situ hybridization method to detect double BCR/ABL fusion and monitor response to therapy in chronic myeloid leukemia. Blood 1998; 91:3357-3365.
4. Tefferi A, Schad CR, Pruthi RK, Ahmann GJ, Spurbeck JL, Dewald GW. Fluorescent in situ hybridization studies of lymphocytes and neutrophils in chronic granulocytic leukemia. Cancer Genet Cytogenet 1995; 83:61-64.
5. (1995) I. An international system for human cytogenetic nomenclature. Edited by F Mitelman. Basel, S. Karger, 1995
6. Shtalrid M, Talpaz M, Kurzrock R, Kantarjian H, Trujillo J, Gutterman J, Yoffe G, Blick M. Analysis of breakpoints within the bcr gene and their correlation with the clinical course of Philadelphia-positive chronic myelogenous leukemia. Blood 1988; 72:485-490.
7. Gonzalez F, Anguita E, Mora A, Asenjo S, de Miguel D, Villegas A: Deletion of the 3' bcr side in chronic myelogenous leukaemia. Educational Book for the Fourth Congress of the European Haematology Association held in Barcelona, Spain, on June 9-12, 1999. (Abstract). Haematologica 1999; 84:93.
8. Groffen J, Stephenson JR, Heisterkamp N, de Klein A, Bartram CR, Grosveld G. Philadelphia chromosomal breakpoints are clustered within a limited region, bcr, on chromosome 22. Cell 1984; 36:93-99.
9. Dewald GW, Wyatt WA, Silver RT. Atypical BCR and ABL D-FISH patterns in chronic myeloid leukemia and their possible role in therapy. Leuk Lymphoma 1999; 34:481-491.
10. Marlton P, Claxton DF, Liu P, Estey EH, Beran M, LeBeau M, Testa JR, Collins FS, Rowley JD, Siciliano MJ. Molecular characterization of 16p deletions associated with inversion 16 defines the critical fusion for leukemogenesis. Blood 1995; 85:772-779.
11. Kuss BJ, Deeley RG, Cole SP, Willman CL, Kopecky KJ, Wolman SR, Eyre HJ, Lane SA, Nancarrow JK, Whitmore SA, et al. Deletion of gene for multidrug resistance in acute myeloid leukaemia with inversion in chromosome 16: prognostic implications. Lancet 1994; 343:1531-1534.
12. Shimizu K, Miyoshi H, Kozu T, Nagata J, Enomoto K, Maseki N, Kaneko Y, Ohki M. Consistent disruption of the AML1 gene occurs within a single intron in the t(8;21) chromosomal translocation. Cancer Res 1992; 52:6945-6948.
13. Konig M, Reichel M, Marschalek R, Haas OA, Strehl S. A highly specific and sensitive fluorescence in situ hybridization assay for the detection of t(4;11)(q21;q23) and concurrent submicroscopic deletions in acute leukaemias. Br J Haematol 2002; 116:758-764.
14. Godon C, Proffitt J, Dastugue N, Lafage-Pochitaloff M, Mozziconacci MJ, Talmant P, Hackbarth M, Bataille R, Avet-Loiseau H. Large deletions 5' to the ETO breakpoint are recurrent events in patients with t(8;21) acute myeloid leukemia. Leukemia 2002; 16:1752-1754.
15. Morgan JA, Yin Y, Borowsky AD, Kuo F, Nourmand N, Koontz JI, Reynolds C, Soreng L, Griffin CA, Graeme-Cook F, Harris NL, Weisenburger D, Pinkus GS, Fletcher JA, Sklar J. Breakpoints of the t(11;18)(q21;q21) in mucosa-associated lymphoid tissue

(MALT) lymphoma lie within or near the previously undescribed gene MALT1 in chromosome 18. Cancer Res 1999; 59:6205-6213.

16. Akagi T, Motegi M, Tamura A, Suzuki R, Hosokawa Y, Suzuki H, Ota H, Nakamura S, Morishima Y, Taniwaki M, Seto M. A novel gene, MALT1 at 18q21, is involved in t(11;18) (q21;q21) found in low-grade B-cell lymphoma of mucosa-associated lymphoid tissue. Oncogene 1999; 18:5785-5794.

17. Baens M, Steyls A, Dierlamm J, De Wolf-Peeters C, Marynen P. Structure of the MLT gene and molecular characterization of the genomic breakpoint junctions in the t(11;18)(q21;q21) of marginal zone B-cell lymphomas of MALT type. Genes Chromosomes Cancer 2000; 29:281-291.

18. Mitelman F: The cytogenetic scenario of chronic myeloid leukemia. Leuk Lymphoma 1993; 11:11-15.

19. Dewald GW, Davis MP, Pierre RV, O'Fallon JR, Hoagland HC. Clinical characteristics and prognosis of 50 patients with a myeloproliferative syndrome and deletion of part of the long arm of chromosome 5. Blood 1985; 66:189-197.

20. Greenberg P, Cox C, LeBeau MM, Fenaux P, Morel P, Sanz G, Sanz M, Vallespi T, Hamblin T, Oscier D, Ohyashiki K, Toyama K, Aul C, Mufti G, Bennett J. International scoring system for evaluating prognosis in myelodysplastic syndromes. 1997; Blood 89:2079-2088.

21. Schad CR, Hanson CA, Paietta E, Casper J, Jalal SM, Dewald GW. Efficacy of fluorescence in situ hybridization for detecting PML/RARA gene fusion in treated and untreated acute promyelocytic leukemia. Mayo Clin Proc 1994; 69:1047-1053.

22. Buno I, Wyatt WA, Zinsmeister AR, Dietz-Band J, Silver RT, Dewald GW. A special fluorescent in situ hybridization technique to study peripheral blood and assess the effectiveness of interferon therapy in chronic myeloid leukemia. Blood 1998; 92:2315-2321.

23. Dewald G, Brockman S, Paternoster S, Bone N, O'Fallon J, Allmer C, James C, Jelinek D, Tschumper R, Hanson C, Pruthi R, Witzig T, Kay N. Chromosome anomalies detected by interphase FISH: correlation with significant biological features of B-cell chronic lymphocytic leukemia. Br J Haematol 2003; 121(2): 287-295.

24. Paternoster SF, Brockman SR, McClure RF, Remstein ED, Kurtin PJ, Dewald GW. A new method to extract nuclei from paraffin-embedded tissue to study lymphomas using interphase fluorescence in situ hybridization. Am J Pathol 2002; 160:1967-1972.

25. Brockman SR, Paternoster SF, Ketterling RP, Dewald GW. New highly sensitive fluorescence *in situ* hybridization method to detect PML/RARα fusion in acute promyelocytic leukemia. Cancer Genet Cytogenet 2003; 145:144-151.

26. CAP: College of American Pathologists Cytogenetics Inspection Checklists. Northfield, IL, College of American Pathologists, 2000.

27. Friend SH, Dryja TP, Weinberg RA. Oncogenes and tumor-suppressing genes. N Engl J Med 1988; 318:618-622.

28. Wain HM, Bruford EA, Lovering RC, Lush MJ, Wright MW, Povey S. Guidelines for human gene nomenclature. Genomics 2002; 79:464-470.

29. Wain HM, Lush M, Ducluzeau F, Povey S: Genew. The human gene nomenclature database. Nucleic Acids Res 2002; 30:169-171.

30. Dewald GW, Brothman AR, Butler MG, Cooley LD, Patil SR, Saikevych IA, Schneider NR. Pilot studies for proficiency testing using fluorescence in situ hybridization with chromosome-specific DNA probes: a College of American Pathologists/American College of Medical Genetics Program. Arch Pathol Lab Med 1997; 121:359-367.

31. Mascarello JT, Cooley LD, Davison K, Dewald GW, Brothman AR, Herrman M, Park JP, Persons DL, Rao KW, Schneider NR, Vance GH. As currently formulated, ISCN FISH nomenclature is not practical for use in clinical test reports or cytogenetic databases. Genet Med 2003; 5:370-377.

32. Jenkins RB, Le Beau MM, Kraker WJ, Borell TJ, Stalboerger PG, Davis EM, Penland L, Fernald A, Espinosa R, 3rd, Schaid DJ, et al. Fluorescence in situ hybridization: a sensitive method for trisomy 8 detection in bone marrow specimens. Blood 1992; 79:3307-3315.

33. Dewald GW, Schad CR, Christensen ER, Law ME, Zinsmeister AR, Stalboerger PG, Jalal SM, Ash RC, Jenkins RB. Fluorescence in situ hybridization with X and Y chromosome probes for cytogenetic studies on bone marrow cells after opposite sex transplantation. Bone Marrow Transplant 1993; 12:149-154.

34. Juneau AL, Kaehler M, Christensen ER, Schad CR, Zinsmeister AR, Lust J, Hanson C, Dewald GW. Detection of RB1 deletions by fluorescence in situ hybridization in malignant hematologic disorders. Cancer Genet Cytogenet 1998; 103:117-123.

35. Remstein ED, Kurtin PJ, Buno I, Bailey RJ, Proffitt J, Wyatt WA, Hanson CA, Dewald GW. Diagnostic utility of fluorescence in situ hybridization in mantle-cell lymphoma. Br J Haematol 2000; 110:856-862.

36. Jalal SM, Law ME, Stamberg J, Fonseca R, Seely JR, Myers WH, Hanson CA. Detection of diagnostically critical, often hidden, anomalies in complex karyotypes of haematological disorders using multicolour fluorescence in situ hybridization. Br J Haematol 2001; 112:975-980.

37. Sinclair PB, Green AR, Grace C, Nacheva EP. Improved sensitivity of BCR-ABL detection: a triple-probe three-color fluorescence in situ hybridization system. Blood 1997; 90:1395-1402.

38. Dewald GW, Schad CR, Christensen ER, Tiede AL, Zinsmeister AR, Spurbeck JL, Thibodeau SN, Jalal SM. The application of fluorescent in situ hybridization to detect Mbcr/abl fusion in variant Ph chromosomes in CML and ALL. Cancer Genet Cytogenet 1993; 71:7-14.

39. Jalal S, Law M, Dewald G: Atlas of Whole Chromosome Paint Probes. Normal Patterns and Utility for Abnormal Cases. Rochester, MN, Mayo Foundation for Medical Education and Research, 1996, pp 145.

40. Schad CR, Dewald GW. Building a new clinical test for fluorescence in situ hybridization. Appl Cytogenet 1995; 21:1-4.

41. Dewald G. Interphase FISH Studies of Chronic Myeloid Leukemia. *In* Molecular Cytogenetics: Protocols and Applications. Edited by YS Fan. Vol 204. Totowa, NJ, Humana Press, 2002, pp 311-342.

42. ACMG: American College of Medical Genetics Laboratory Practice Committee Standards and Guidelines for Clinical Genetics Laboratories. Edited by ACMG, 2nd edition. Bethesda, ACMG, 1999.

43. American College of Medical Genetics Laboratory Practice Committee. Metaphase fluorescence in situ hybridization (FISH). *In* Standards and Guidelines: Clinical Genetics Laboratories, 1996, pp 1

44. NYDH: New York Dept. of Health, Wadsworth Center for Laboratories and Research Genetics Laboratory Checklists. New York, New York State Department of Health, 2002

45. Talpaz M, Kantarjian H, Kurzrock R, Trujillo JM, Gutterman JU. Interferon-alpha produces sustained cytogenetic responses in chronic myelogenous leukemia. Philadelphia chromosome-positive patients. Ann Intern Med 1991; 114:532-538.

46. Leukemia. ICSGoCM. Interferon alfa-2a as compared with conventional chemotherapy for the treatment of chronic myeloid leukemia. N Engl J Med 1994; 330:820-825.

47. Dewald G, Stallard R, Alsaadi A, Arnold S, Blough R, Ceperich TM, Rafael Elejalde B, Fink J, Higgins JV, Higgins RR, Hoeltge GA, Hsu WT, Johnson EB, Kronberger D, McCorquodale DJ, Meisner LF, Micale MA, Oseth L, Payne JS, Schwartz S, Sheldon S, Sophian A, Storto P, Van Tuinen P, Zenger-Hain J, et al. A multicenter investigation with D-FISH BCR/ABL1 probes. Cancer Genet Cytogenet 2000; 116:97-104.

48. Le Gouill S, Talmant P, Milpied N, Daviet A, Ancelot M, Moreau P, Harousseau JL, Bataille R, Avet-Loiseau H. Fluorescence in situ hybridization on peripheral-blood specimens is a reliable method to evaluate cytogenetic response in chronic myeloid leukemia. J Clin Oncol 2000; 18:1533-1538.

49. Cuneo A, Bigoni R, Emmanuel B, Smit E, Rigolin GM, Roberti MG, Bardi A, Piva N, Scapoli G, Castoldi G, Van Den Berghe H, Hagemeijer A. Fluorescence in situ hybridization for the detection and monitoring of the Ph-positive clone in chronic myelogenous leukemia: comparison with metaphase banding analysis. Leukemia 1998; 12:1718-1723.

50. Nolte M, Werner M, Ewig M, von Wasielewski R, Wilkens L, Link H, Ganser A, Georgii A. Fluorescence in situ hybridization (FISH) is a reliable diagnostic tool for detection of the 9;22 translocation. Leuk Lymphoma 1996; 22:287-294.

51. Muhlmann J, Thaler J, Hilbe W, Bechter O, Erdel M, Utermann G, Duba HC. Fluorescence in situ hybridization (FISH) on peripheral blood smears for monitoring Philadelphia chromosome-positive chronic myeloid leukemia (CML) during interferon treatment: a new strategy for remission assessment. Genes Chromosomes Cancer 1998; 21:90-100.

52. Smoley SA, Brockman SR, Paternoster SF, Meyer RG, Dewald GW. A novel tricolor, dual-fusion fluorescence in situ hybridization method to detect BCR/ABL fusion in cells with t(9;22)(q34;q11.2) associated with deletion of DNA on the derivative chromosome 9 in chronic myelocytic leukemia. Cancer Genet Cytogenet 2004; 148:1-6.

53. Huntly B, Bench A, Green AR. Double jeopardy from a single translocation: deletions of the derivative chromosome 9 in chronic myeloid leukemia. Blood 2003; 102:1160-1168.

54. Sinclair PB, Nacheva EP, Leversha M, Telford N, Chang J, Reid A, Bench A, Champion K, Huntly B, Green AR. Large deletions at the t(9;22) breakpoint are common and may identify a poor-prognosis subgroup of patients with chronic myeloid leukemia. Blood 2000; 95:738-743.

55. Huntly BJ, Reid AG, Bench AJ, Campbell LJ, Telford N, Shepherd P, Szer J, Prince HM, Turner P, Grace C, Nacheva EP, Green AR. Deletions of the derivative chromosome 9 occur at the time of the Philadelphia translocation and provide a powerful and independent prognostic indicator in chronic myeloid leukemia. Blood 2001; 98:1732-1738.

56. Kolomietz E, Al-Maghrabi J, Brennan S, Karaskova J, Minkin S, Lipton J, Squire JA. Primary chromosomal rearrangements of leukemia are frequently accompanied by extensive submicroscopic deletions and may lead to altered prognosis. Blood 2001; 97:3581-3588.

57. Storlazzi CT, Specchia G, Anelli L, Albano F, Pastore D, Zagaria A, Rocchi M, Liso V. Breakpoint characterization of der(9) deletions in chronic myeloid leukemia patients. Genes Chromosomes Cancer 2002; 35:271-276.

58. Cohen N, Rozenfeld-Granot G, Hardan I, Brok-Simoni F, Amariglio N, Rechavi G, Trakhtenbrot L. Subgroup of patients with Philadelphia-positive chronic myelogenous leukemia characterized by a deletion of 9q proximal to ABL gene: expression profiling,

resistance to interferon therapy, and poor prognosis. Cancer Genet Cytogenet 2001; 128:114-119.

59. Popenoe DW, Schaefer-Rego K, Mears JG, Bank A, Leibowitz D. Frequent and extensive deletion during the 9,22 translocation in CML. Blood 1986; 68:1123-1128.

60. Dewald GW, Wright PI. Chromosome abnormalities in the myeloproliferative disorders. Semin Oncol 1995; 22:341-354.

61. Bench AJ, Cross NC, Huntly BJ, Nacheva EP, Green AR. Myeloproliferative disorders. [Review] [145 refs]. Bailliere's Best Practice in Clinical Haematology 2001; 14:531-551.

62. Jaffe ES, Harris NL, Stein H, Vardiman J. World Health Organization of Tumours. Pathology and Genetics of Tumours of Haematopoietic and Lymphoid Tissues. Lyon, France, International Agency for Research on Cancer, 2001.

63. Bain BJ. Chronic Myeloproliferative Disorders: Cytogenetic and Molecular Genetic Abnormalities. Unionville, CT, S. Karger Publishers, Inc, 2003, pp 132.

64. Adeyinka A, Dewald G. Cytogenetics of Chronic Myeloproliferative Disorders and Related Myelodysplastic Syndromes. Hematol Oncol Clin North Am, 2003; 17(5): 1129-1149.

65. Borgstrom GH, Knuutila S, Ruutu T, Pakkala A, Lahtinen R, de la Chapelle A. Abnormalities of chromosome 13 in myelofibrosis. Scand J Haematol 1984; 33:15-21.

66. Johnson DD, Dewald GW, Pierre RV, Letendre L, Silverstein MN. Deletions of chromosome 13 in malignant hematologic disorders. Cancer Genet Cytogenet 1985; 18:235-241.

67. Bain BJ. Eosinophilic leukaemias and the idiopathic hypereosinophilic syndrome. Br J Haematol 1996; 95:2-9.

68. Diez-Martin JL, Graham DL, Petitt RM, Dewald GW. Chromosome studies in 104 patients with polycythemia vera. Mayo Clin Proc 1991; 66:287-299.

69. Pardanani A, Ketterling RP, Brockman SR, Flynn HC, Paternoster SF, Shearer BR, Reeder TL, Li CY, Cross NC, Cools JD, Gilliland DG, Dewald GW, Tefferi A. *CHIC2* deletion, a surrogate for FIP1L1-PDGFRA fusion, occurs in systemic mastocytosis associated with eosinophilia and predicts response to imatinib mesylate therapy. Blood 2003; 102:3093-3096.

70. Tefferi A, Meyer R, Wyatt WA, Dewald G. Comparison of peripheral blood interphase cytogenetics with bone marrow karyotype analysis in myelofibrosis with myeloid metaplasia. Br J Haematol 2001; 115:316-319.

71. Harris NL, Jaffe ES, Diebold J, Flandrin G, Muller-Hermelink HK, Vardiman J, Lister TA, Bloomfield CD. The World Health Organization classification of hematological malignancies report of the Clinical Advisory Committee Meeting, Airlie House, Virginia, November 1997. Mod Pathol 2000; 13:193-207.

72. Knapp RH, Dewald GW, Pierre RV. Cytogenetic studies in 174 consecutive patients with preleukemic or myelodysplastic syndromes. Mayo Clin Proc 1985; 60:507-516.

73. Pierre RV, Catovsky D, Mufti GJ, Swansbury GJ, Mecucci C, Dewald GW, Ruutu T, Van Den Berghe H, Rowley JD, Mitelman F, et al. Clinical-cytogenetic correlations in myelodysplasia (preleukemia). Cancer Genet Cytogenet 1989; 40:149-161.

74. Mathew P, Tefferi A, Dewald GW, Goldberg SL, Su J, Hoagland HC, Noel P. The 5q-syndrome: a single-institution study of 43 consecutive patients. Blood 1993; 81:1040-1045.

75. Dewald GW, Brecher M, Travis LB, Stupca PJ. Twenty-six patients with hematologic disorders and X chromosome abnormalities. Frequent idic(X)(q13) chromosomes and Xq13 anomalies associated with pathologic ringed sideroblasts. Cancer Genet Cytogenet 1989; 42:173-185.

76. Ketterling RP, Wyatt WA, VanWier SA, Law M, Hodnefield JM, Hanson CA, Dewald GW. Primary myelodysplastic syndrome with normal cytogenetics: utility of 'FISH panel testing' and M-FISH. Leuk Res 2002; 26:235-240.

77. Cherry AM, Brockman SR, Paternoster SF, Hicks GA, Higgins RR, Bennett JM, Greenberg PL, Miller K, Rowe J, Tallman MS, Dewald GW. Comparison of interphase FISH and metaphase cytogenetics to study myelodysplasia: an Eastern Cooperative Oncology Group (ECOG) study. Leuk Res 2003; 27:1085-1090.

78. Grimwade D, Walker H, Oliver F, Wheatley K, Harrison C, Harrison G, Rees J, Hann I, Stevens R, Burnett A, Goldstone A. The importance of diagnostic cytogenetics on outcome in AML: analysis of 1,612 patients entered into the MRC AML 10 trial. The Medical Research Council Adult and Children's Leukaemia Working Parties. Blood 1998; 92:2322-2333.

79. Slovak ML, Kopecky KJ, Cassileth PA, Harrington DH, Theil KS, Mohamed A, Paietta E, Willman CL, Head DR, Rowe JM, Forman SJ, Appelbaum FR. Karyotypic analysis predicts outcome of preremission and postremission therapy in adult acute myeloid leukemia: a Southwest Oncology Group/Eastern Cooperative Oncology Group Study. Blood 2000; 96:4075-4083.

80. Harrison CJ, Radford-Weiss I, Ross F, Rack K, le Guyader G, Vekemans M, Macintyre E. Fluorescence in situ hybridization analysis of masked (8;21)(q22;q22) translocations. Cancer Genet Cytogenet 1999; 112:15-20.

81. Taviaux S, Brunel V, Dupont M, Fernandez F, Ferraz C, Carbuccia N, Sainty D, Demaille J, Birg F, Lafage-Pochitaloff M. Simple variant t(8;21) acute myeloid leukemias harbor insertions of the AML1 or ETO genes. Genes Chromosomes Cancer 1999; 24:165-171.

82. Dierlamm J, Stul M, Vranckx H, Michaux L, Weghuis DE, Speleman F, Selleslag D, Kramer MH, Noens LA, Cassiman JJ, Van den Berghe H, Hagemeijer A. FISH identifies inv(16)(p13q22) masked by translocations in three cases of acute myeloid leukemia. Genes Chromosomes Cancer 1998; 22:87-94.

83. Mancini M, Cedrone M, Diverio D, Emanuel B, Stul M, Vranckx H, Brama M, De Cuia MR, Nanni M, Fazi F, Mecucci C, Alimena G, Hagemeijer A. Use of dual-color interphase FISH for the detection of inv(16) in acute myeloid leukemia at diagnosis, relapse and during follow-up: a study of 23 patients. Leukemia 2000; 14:364-368.

84. Reddy KS, Wang S, Montgomery P, Grove W, Robertson LE. Fluorescence in situ hybridization identifies inversion 16 masked by t(10;16)(q24;q22), t(7;16)(q21;q22), and t(2;16)(q37;q22) in three cases of AML-M4Eo. Cancer Genet Cytogenet 2000; 116:148-152.

85. Avet-Loiseau H, Godon C, Li JY, Daviet A, Mellerin MP, Talmant P, Harousseau JL, Bataille R. Amplification of the 11q23 region in acute myeloid leukemia. Genes Chromosomes Cancer 1999; 26:166-170.

86. Fischer K, Scholl C, Salat J, Frohling S, Schlenk R, Bentz M, Stilgenbauer S, Lichter P, Dohner H. Design and validation of DNA probe sets for a comprehensive interphase cytogenetic analysis of acute myeloid leukemia. 1996; Blood 88:3962-3971.

87. Cuneo A, Bigoni R, Roberti MG, Bardi A, Rigolin GM, Piva N, Mancini M, Nanni M, Alimena G, Mecucci C, Matteucci C, La Starza R, Bernasconi P, Cavigliano P, Genini E, Zaccaria A, Testoni N, Carboni C, Castoldi G. Detection and monitoring of trisomy 8 by fluorescence in situ hybridization in acute myeloid leukemia: a multicentric study. Haematologica 1998; 83:21-26.

88. Richkind KE, Mowery-Rushton PA, Chen Z, Lytle CA. Clinical utility of FISH analysis when cytogenetic studies are normal - Prospective analysis of 800 patients at diagnosis and after treatment for leukemia. Blood 2000; 96:707a.

89. Rowley JD, Olney HJ. International workshop on the relationship of prior therapy to balanced chromosome aberrations in therapy-related myelodysplastic syndromes and acute leukemia: overview report. Genes Chromosomes Cancer 2002; 33:331-345.

90. Look AT. Oncogenic transcription factors in the human acute leukemias. Science 1997; 278:1059-1064.

91. Han T, Ozer H, Sadamori N, Emrich L, Gomez GA, Henderson ES, Bloom ML, Sandberg AA. Prognostic importance of cytogenetic abnormalities in patients with chronic lymphocytic leukemia. N Eng J Med 1984; 310:288-292.

92. Juliusson G, Oscier DG, Fitchett M, Ross FM, Stockdill G, Mackie MJ, Parker AC, Castoldi GL, Guneo A, Knuutila S, et al. Prognostic subgroups in B-cell chronic lymphocytic leukemia defined by specific chromosomal abnormalities. N Engl J Med 1990; 323:720-724.

93. Brito-Babapulle V, Garcia-Marco J, Maljaie SH, Hiorns L, Coignet L, Conchon M, Catovsky D. The impact of molecular cytogenetics on chronic lymphoid leukaemia. Acta Haematol 1997; 98:175-186.

94. Fais F, Ghiotto F, Hashimoto S, Sellars B, Valetto A, Allen SL, Schulman P, Vinciguerra VP, Rai K, Rassenti LZ, Kipps TJ, Dighiero G, Schroeder HW, Jr, Ferrarini M, Chiorazzi N. Chronic lymphocytic leukemia B cells express restricted sets of mutated and unmutated antigen receptors. J Clin Invest 1998; 102:1515-1525.

95. Damle RN, Wasil T, Fais F, Ghiotto F, Valetto A, Allen SL, Buchbinder A, Budman D, Dittmar K, Kolitz J, Lichtman SM, Schulman P, Vinciguerra VP, Rai KR, Ferrarini M, Chiorazzi N. Ig V gene mutation status and CD38 expression as novel prognostic indicators in chronic lymphocytic leukemia. Blood 1999; 94:1840-1847.

96. Dohner H, Stilgenbauer S, Benner A, Leupolt E, Krober A, Bullinger L, Dohner K, Bentz M, Lichter P. Genomic aberrations and survival in chronic lymphocytic leukemia. N Engl J Med 2000; 343:1910-1916.

97. Zhang Y, Weber-Matthiesen K, Siebert R, Matthiesen P, Schlegelberger B. Frequent deletions of 6q23-24 in B-cell non-Hodgkin's lymphomas detected by fluorescence in situ hybridization. Genes Chromosomes Cancer 1997; 18:310-313.

98. Neilson JR, Auer R, White D, Bienz N, Waters JJ, Whittaker JA, Milligan DW, Fegan CD. Deletions at 11q identify a subset of patients with typical CLL who show consistent disease progression and reduced survival. Leukemia 1997; 11:1929-1932.

99. El Rouby S, Thomas A, Costin D, Rosenberg CR, Potmesil M, Silber R, Newcomb EW. p53 gene mutation in B-cell chronic lymphocytic leukemia is associated with drug resistance and is independent of MDR1/MDR3 gene expression. Blood 1993; 82:3452-3459.

100. Finn WG, Kay NE, Kroft SH, Church S, Peterson LC. Secondary abnormalities of chromosome 6q in B-cell chronic lymphocytic leukemia: a sequential study of karyotypic instability in 51 patients. Am J Hematol 1998; 59:223-229.

101. Peterson LC, Lindquist LL, Church S, Kay NE. Frequent clonal abnormalities of chromosome band 13q14 in B-cell chronic lymphocytic leukemia: multiple clones, subclones, and nonclonal alterations in 82 midwestern patients. Genes Chromosomes Cancer 1992; 4:273-280.

102. Dewald GW, Kyle RA, Hicks GA, Greipp PR. The clinical significance of cytogenetic studies in 100 patients with multiple myeloma, plasma cell leukemia, or amyloidosis. Blood 1985; 66:380-390.

103. Sawyer JR, Waldron JA, Jagannath S, Barlogie B. Cytogenetic findings in 200 patients with multiple myeloma. Cancer Genet Cytogenet 1995; 82:41-49.

104. Fonseca R, Oken MM, Harrington D, Bailey RJ, Van Wier SA, Henderson KJ, Kay NE, Van Ness B, Greipp PR, Dewald GW. Deletions of chromosome 13 in multiple myeloma identified by interphase FISH usually denote large deletions of the q arm or monosomy. Leukemia 2001; 15:981-986.

105. Avet-Loiseau H, Facon T, Grosbois B, Magrangeas F, Rapp MJ, Harousseau JL, Minvielle S, Bataille R. Oncogenesis of multiple myeloma: 14q32 and 13q chromosomal abnormalities are not randomly distributed, but correlate with natural history, immunological features, and clinical presentation. Blood 2002; 99:2185-2191.

106. Fonseca R, Harrington D, Oken MM, Dewald GW, Bailey RJ, Van Wier SA, Henderson KJ, Blood EA, Rajkumar SV, Kay NE, Van Ness B, Greipp PR. Biological and prognostic significance of interphase fluorescence in situ hybridization detection of chromosome 13 abnormalities (delta13) in multiple myeloma: an eastern cooperative oncology group study. Cancer Res 2002; 62:715-720.

107. Fonseca R, Blood EA, Oken MM, Kyle RA, Dewald GW, Bailey RJ, Van Wier SA, Henderson KJ, Hoyer JD, Harrington D, Kay NE, Van Ness B, Greipp PR. Myeloma and the t(11;14)(q13;q32); evidence for a biologically defined unique subset of patients. Blood 2002; 99:3735-3741.

108. Moreau P, Facon T, Leleu X, Morineau N, Huyghe P, Harousseau JL, Bataille R, Avet-Loiseau H. Recurrent 14q32 translocations determine the prognosis of multiple myeloma, especially in patients receiving intensive chemotherapy. Blood 2002; 100:1579-1583.

109. Fonseca R, Blood E, Rue M, Harrington D, Oken M, Kyle R, Dewald G, Van Ness B, Van Wier S, Henderson K, Bailey R, Greipp P. Clinical and biologic implications of recurrent genomic aberrations in myeloma. Blood 2003; 101:4569-4575.

110. Ahmann GJ, Jalal SM, Juneau AL, Christensen ER, Hanson CA, Dewald GW, Greipp PR. A novel three-color, clone-specific fluorescence in situ hybridization procedure for monoclonal gammopathies. Cancer Genet Cytogenet 1998; 101:7-11.

111. Fonseca R, Coignet L, Dewald G. Cytogenetic abnormalities in multiple myeloma. *In* Hematol Oncol Clin North Am. Edited by R Kyle and M Gertz. Philadelphia, W. B. Saunders Co, 1999, pp 1169-1179.

112. Andreeff M, Pinkel D. Introduction to fluorescence in situ hybridization - principles and clinical applications, 1st edition. New York, John Wiley & Sons, Inc, 1999, pp 455.

113. Remstein E, Kurtin P, James C, Wang X, Meyer R, Dewald G. Detection of t(11;18)(q21;q21) in extranodal marginal zone B-cell lymphomas of MALT type by two-color fluorescence in situ hybridization. Presented at the Annual Meeting of the United States and Canadian Academy of Pathology. Mod Pathol 2001; 14:177A.

114. Haralambieva E, Kleiverda K, Mason DY, Schuuring E, Kluin PM. Detection of three common translocation breakpoints in non-Hodgkin's lymphomas by fluorescence in situ hybridization on routine paraffin-embedded tissue sections. J Pathol 2002; 198:163-170.

115. Horsman DE, Gascoyne RD, Coupland RW, Coldman AJ, Adomat SA. Comparison of cytogenetic analysis, southern analysis, and polymerase chain reaction for the detection of t(14;18) in follicular lymphoma. Am J Clin Pathol 1995; 103:472-478.

116. Rowley JD. Chromosome studies in the non-Hodgkin's lymphomas: the role of the 14;18 translocation. J Clin Oncol 1988; 6:919-925.

117. Sander CA, Yano T, Clark HM, Harris C, Longo DL, Jaffe ES, Raffeld M. p53 mutation is associated with progression in follicular lymphomas. Blood 1993; 82:1994-2004.

118. Pinyol M, Cobo F, Bea S, Jares P, Nayach I, Fernandez PL, Montserrat E, Cardesa A, Campo E. p16(INK4a) gene inactivation by deletions, mutations, and hypermethylation is

associated with transformed and aggressive variants of non-Hodgkin's lymphomas. Blood 1998; 91:2977-2984.

119.   Elenitoba-Johnson KS, Gascoyne RD, Lim MS, Chhanabai M, Jaffe ES, Raffeld M. Homozygous deletions at chromosome 9p21 involving p16 and p15 are associated with histologic progression in follicle center lymphoma. Blood 1998; 91:4677-4685.

120.   Peng HZ, Du MQ, Koulis A, Aiello A, Dogan A, Pan LX, Isaacson PG. Nonimmunoglobulin gene hypermutation in germinal center B cells. Blood 1999; 93:2167-2172.

121.   Vandenberghe E, De Wolf-Peeters C, van den Oord J, Wlodarska I, Delabie J, Stul M, Thomas J, Michaux JL, Mecucci C, Cassiman JJ, et al. Translocation (11;14): a cytogenetic anomaly associated with B-cell lymphomas of non-follicle centre cell lineage. J Pathol 1991; 163:13-8.

122.   Li JY, Gaillard F, Moreau A, Harousseau JL, Laboisse C, Milpied N, Bataille R, Avet-Loiseau H. Detection of translocation t(11;14)(q13;q32) in mantle cell lymphoma by fluorescence in situ hybridization. Am J Pathol 1999; 154:1449-452.

123.   Vaandrager JW, Schuuring E, Zwikstra E, de Boer CJ, Kleiverda KK, van Krieken JH, Kluin-Nelemans HC, van Ommen GJ, Raap AK, Kluin PM. Direct visualization of dispersed 11q13 chromosomal translocations in mantle cell lymphoma by multicolor DNA fiber fluorescence in situ hybridization. Blood 1996; 88:1177-1182.

124.   Paternoster S, Rodacker M, Powell C, Hanson C, Wyatt WA, Dewald G. Comparison of karyotype and results of FISH using probes for five common chromosome anomalies in acute lymphoblastic leukemia. Association of Genetic Technologists Meeting Minneapolis 2001.

125.   Williams ME, Whitefield M, Swerdlow SH. Analysis of the cyclin-dependent kinase inhibitors p18 and p19 in mantle-cell lymphoma and chronic lymphocytic leukemia. Ann Oncol 1997; 8:71-73.

126.   Williams M, Woytowitz D, Finkelstein S, Swerdlow S. MTS1/MTS2 (p15/p16) deletions and p53 mutations in mantle cell (centrocytic) lymphoma. Blood 1995; 86:747a.

127.   Cataldo KA, Jalal SM, Law ME, Ansell SM, Inwards DJ, Fine M, Arber DA, Pulford KA, Strickler JG. Detection of t(2;5) in anaplastic large cell lymphoma: comparison of immunohistochemical studies, FISH, and RT-PCR in paraffin-embedded tissue. Am J Surg Pathol 1999; 23:1386-1392.

128.   Sanchez-Izquierdo D, Buchonet G, Siebert R, Gascoyne RD, Climent J, Karran L, Marin M, Blesa D, Horsman D, Rosenwald A, Staudt LM, Albertson DG, Du MQ, Ye H, Marynen P, Garcia-Conde J, Pinkel D, Dyer MJ, Martinez-Climent JA. MALT1 is deregulated by both chromosomal translocation and amplification in B-cell non-Hodgkin lymphoma. 2003; Blood 30:30.

129.   Remstein ED, Kurtin PJ, James CD, Wang X, Meyer RG, Dewald GW. Mucosa-associated lymphoid tissue lymphomas with t(11;18)(q21;q21) and mucosa-associated lymphoid tissue lymphomas with aneuploidy develop along different pathogenetic pathways. Am J Pathol 2002; 161:63-71.

130.   Streubel B, Lamprecht A, Dierlamm J, Cerroni L, Stolte M, Ott G, Raderer M, Chott A. T(14;18)(q32;q21) involving IGH and MALT1 is a frequent chromosomal aberration in MALT lymphoma. Blood 2002; 24:24.

131.   Yunis JJ, Mayer MG, Arnesen MA, Aeppli DP, Oken MM, Frizzera G. bcl-2 and other genomic alterations in the prognosis of large-cell lymphoma. N Engl J Med 1989; 320:1047-1054.

132.   Weiss LM, Warnke RA, Sklar J, Cleary ML. Molecular analysis of the t(14;18) chromosomal translocation in malignant lymphomas. N Engl J Med 1987; 317:1185-1189.

133. Lipford E, Wright JJ, Urba W, Whang-Peng J, Kirsch IR, Raffeld M, Cossman J, Longo DL, Bakhshi A, Korsmeyer SJ. Refinement of lymphoma cytogenetics by the chromosome 18q21 major breakpoint region. Blood 1987; 70:1816-1823.
134. McClure RF, Macon W, Remstein ED, Dewald G, Kurtin PJ. Burkitt-like lymphoma and diffuse large B-cell lymphoma in adults form a continuum that is distinct from classical Burkitt lymphoma. J Clin Pathol 2002; 55(Suppl I):A21-A22.
135. Pickering D, Nelson M, Chan W, Huang J, Dave B, Sanger W. Paraffin tissue core sectioning: An improved technique for whole nuclear extraction and interphase FISH. J Assoc Genet Technol 2001; 27:38-39.

Chapter 5

THE PLASMA CELL DYSCRASIAS

Carla S. Wilson
Department of Pathology, University of New Mexico Health Sciences Center, Albuquerque, NM

1.   INTRODUCTION

The plasma cell dyscrasias are a group of disorders that are related by the finding of an expanded monoclonal plasma cell population. The type and quantity of the secreted monoclonal immunoglobulin (M-protein), best determined by serum and urine protein electrophoresis (SPEP, UPEP) and immunofixation (IFE) studies, in conjunction with the clinicopathologic findings helps to classify these disorders into: monoclonal gammopathy of undetermined significance (MGUS), plasmacytoma, multiple myeloma (MM), monoclonal immunoglobulin deposition diseases, and heavy chain diseases.   While other B-cell lymphoproliferative disorders may be associated with an M-protein, especially lymphoplasmacytic lymphoma (Waldenstrom's macroglobulinemia), only the pure plasma cell disorders are discussed. Multiple myeloma is emphasized as it is the second most common hematopoietic malignancy and has been most extensively studied.

With recent advances in the understanding of genetic mechanisms underlying plasma cell tumorgenesis and the importance of the bone marrow microenvironment, the role of the oncologist and hematopathologist is changing. This chapter details how the identification of specific genetic events, in conjunction with pathologic findings, and newer prognostic indicators are being utilized in patient management. With the rapidity of these new discoveries, the past five years has seen the plasma cell disorders at the forefront of Phase I, II or III clinical trials of new and emerging therapies that target the plasma cell as well as the bone marrow microenvironment.

1.1   Normal Plasma Cell Differentiation

In normal plasma cell differentiation, immature B-cells, that have undergone VDJ recombination, migrate from the bone marrow to lymphoid tissues (Figure 5-1). Within the lymph node, the immature B-cells either: 1) mature into short lived plasma cells that remain in the local tissue, secrete IgM, and have a half life of approximately three days; or, 2) enter follicular germinal centers and undergo programmed cell death unless rescued by antigen selection. Cells selected for survival undergo IgH switch recombination, after multiple rounds of somatic hypermutation of the IgH and IgL V(D)J sequences. Upon differentiation into post-germinal center plasmablasts/plasma cells or memory B-cells, they home to the bone marrow to reside as long lived terminally differentiated plasma cells that produce large amounts of immunoglobulin. These plasma cells normally account for less than 5% of total bone marrow cellularity.

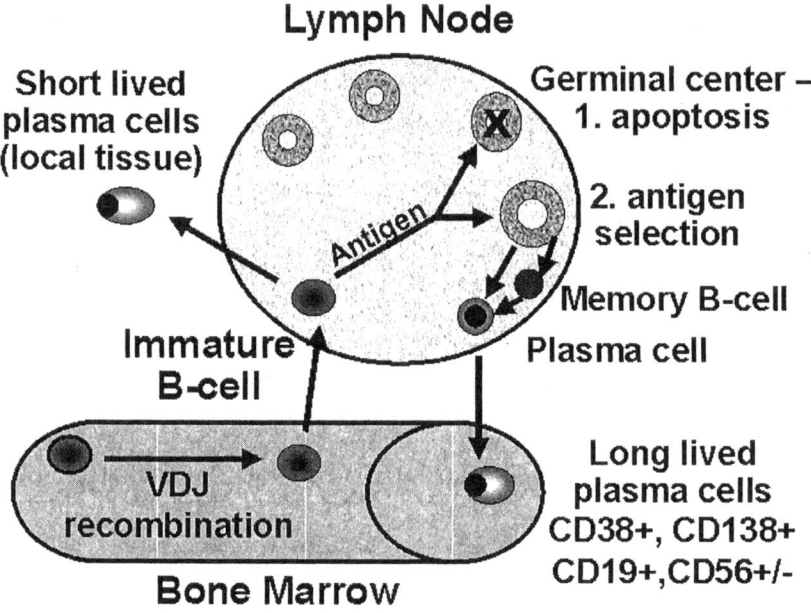

Figure 5-1. Normal plasma cell differentiation

1.2 Neoplastic Plasma Cell Differentiation

Germinal center B-cells that survive antigen selection during normal plasma cell differentiation have marked intrinsic genetic instability. This leads to errors in IgH switch recombination or less frequently somatic hypermutation. Many of the errors involve the immunoglobulin (Ig) locus and likely represent the initial immortalizing event in plasma cell tumorgenesis. For example, juxtaposition of the IgH gene next to an oncogene is common, resulting in oncogene dysregulation.[1] Genetically abnormal plasma cells return to the bone marrow and through a multistep transformation process, undergo additional genetic alterations that prevent normal cell differentiation and apoptosis, with ultimate immortalization of the plasma cell clone (Figure 5-2). The finding of multiple numeric chromosomal abnormalities in plasma cells from patients with MGUS provides the first evidence for karyotypic instability.[2,3] Additional genetic aberrations, with complex translocations and insertions, occur with disease progression.[4] Clearly, not all cases go through this orderly succession of events as only 15-25% of MGUS become MM and many MM patients have no evidence of an earlier MGUS.[5] Nonetheless, prior to a diagnosis of MM approximately one-third of patients have a recognized plasma cell proliferative process, including primarily MGUS but also smoldering myeloma, plasmacytoma or primary amyloidosis.[6]

As more is being learned about the genetic features of plasma cell dyscrasias other than MM, parallels are being found that support a similar pathway of neoplastic plasma cell development.[2,7] Underlying genetic variations likely explain the significant differences in biologic and clinical behavior between the different plasma cell disorders, as well as the great variation in clinical outcome among patients with MM.

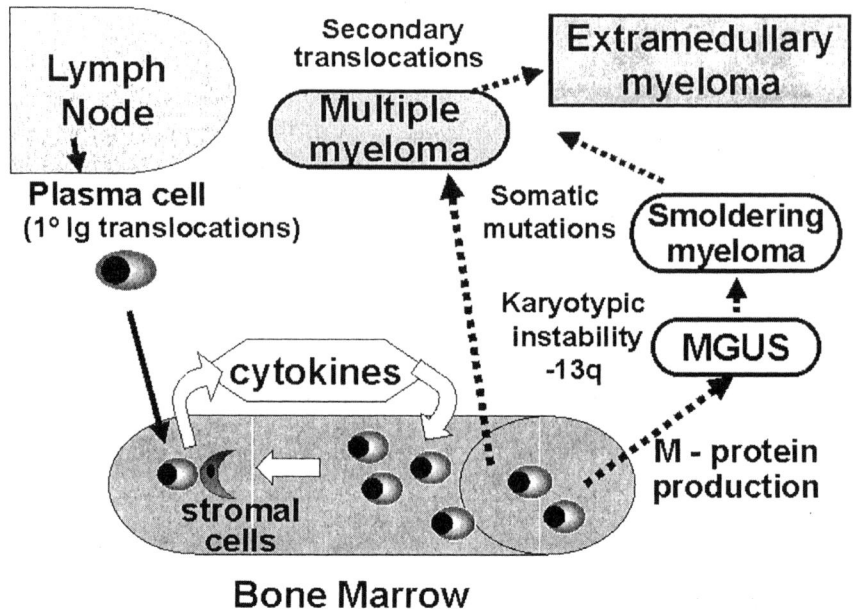

Figure 5-2. Neoplastic plasma cell differentiation

2.   MULTIPLE MYELOMA

2.1   Epidemiology

Multiple myeloma, also termed plasma cell myeloma, is a currently incurable neoplastic disorder. MM accounts for slightly more than 10% of hematopoietic malignancies and has a slight predilection for males (male:female, 3:2). The disease is rare in individuals less than 35 years of age; the peak incidence is in the eighth decade of life. Approximately 14,400 new patients present annually in the United States, with approximately 50,000 total patients affected.[8] The incidence of myeloma is increasing as the population is aging, although some reports suggest an increased incidence among younger individuals as well. The cause for this increase may relate in part to improved access to health care and improved diagnostic techniques.[6] A genetic propensity seems likely given the higher incidence among African Americans (9.5/100,000) as compared to Caucasian Americans (4.1/100,000), and the report of familial clustering.[9,10] Additionally, a family history of cancer in first-degree relatives is found in approximately 40% of cases, with approximately 10% of these representing hematologic malignancies.[6] A declining immune system and increased accumulation of certain chemicals and toxins, such as herbicides, insecticides, asbestosis, and rubber, plastic, wood, or petroleum products, may increase susceptibility among older individuals or people with increased occupational exposure.[11,12] Radiation exposure from the atomic bomb in Hiroshima and Nagasaki, or occupation related in nuclear plant workers or radiologists also increases the risk.[13]

The role for an underlying viral etiology is controversial. In 1997, DNA sequences belonging to human herpesvirus-8 (HHV8) were identified in bone marrow dendritic cells and bone marrow biopsy sections of MM patients, analyzed by polymerase chain reaction (PCR) assay and in situ hybridization.[14,15] Subsequent studies have yielded conflicting data; however, the preponderance of evidence from molecular and seroepidemiological studies suggests there is no definitive association between HHV8 infection and MM.[16,17]

2.2 Clinical Features

A unique triad of osteolytic bone lesions, atypical bone marrow plasmacytosis, and monoclonal gammopathy characterizes myeloma. Many of the clinical and laboratory findings at diagnosis reflect or are secondary to increased circulating immunoglobulin and bone destruction (Table 5-1).

The most common symptoms at presentation are bone pain (58% of cases), fatigue (32%), and weight loss (24%).[6] Osteolytic bone lesions are a major cause of morbidity and are therefore further discussed in section 2.8. Recurrent bacterial infections are a significant complication that result from the hypogammopathy and immunodeficiency that accompany displacement and suppression of normal cells by the myeloma clone. An increased suppressor T-cell response is also elicited to suppress the myeloma cells.[18]

2.3 Diagnosis

The bone marrow examination is essential for the diagnosis of MM, even when immunologic or radiographic studies are strongly supportive of this disease. Studies of bone marrow also provide prognostic information and a basis from which to measure therapeutic response. Adequate sampling, including obtaining both aspirate smears and a trephine biopsy, is critical as focal lesions may be widely spaced and irregularly distributed. In approximately 9% of myeloma, the bone marrow cannot be aspirated due to fibrosis, and touch imprints of the trephine biopsy are an important substitute for the aspirate smears. Plasma cell cytology is best appreciated on the aspirate smears and touch imprints; recognizable plasma cell features are usually found in even the most unusual appearing MMs. The biopsy sections provide an overview for the extent and distribution of myelomatous involvement. The most reliable morphologic criteria for making a diagnosis of MM are listed in Table 5-2 .[19,20]

Table 5-1. Laboratory and radiographic findings in myeloma patients at diagnosis (% cases).

Complete blood count and peripheral blood smear	Normochromic normocytic anemia (60%)
	Macrocytic anemia with vit B_{12} deficiency (8%)
	Rouleaux formation (55%)
	Plasma cells (>15%)
	Leukopenia or thrombocytopenia (<20%)
	Leukocytosis or thrombocytosis (rare)
Chemistry panel	Increased:
	B–2 microglobulin (75%)
	uric acid (>50%)
	creatinine (40%)
	calcium (<30%)
	Decreased:
	albumin (15%)
	alkaline phosphatase (occasional)
Serum and urine protein electrophoresis, immunofixation studies (97% abnormal)	Increased total gammaglobulin
	Monoclonal protein:
	IgG (50%), IgA (20-25%), light chain (20%),
	IgD (2%), biclonal (2%), nonsecretory (3%)
	IgE, IgM, (<1% each)
	Decreased uninvolved immunoglobulin (91%)
Radiographic skeletal survey	Lytic lesions or combination of osteoporosis, osteolysis, or pathologic fracture (75-80%)
MRI or CT scan	Small bone lesions
	Extramedullary plasma cell infiltrates

Table 5- 2. Morphologic features of multiple myeloma

Morphologic Criteria for MM	Features of Plasma Cell Atypia
1. Homogenous nodule or sheet of plasma cells measuring $\geq \frac{1}{2}$ of a 40x high power field	Cellular enlargement
	Nuclear enlargement
2. Monotypic plasma cell aggregates that fill at least one interfatty space	Nuclear pleomorphism
	Dispersed nuclear chromatin
	Prominent nucleoli
3. Bone marrow plasmacytosis with monotypic plasma cells and marked cytologic atypia (see text)	Cytoplasmic fraying or shedding
	Intranuclear inclusions
	Variety of cytoplasmic inclusions

Identification of only one of the three morphologic criteria listed in Table 5-2 is sufficient; however, the third criterion is subjective in the absence of a specific plasma cell percentage (BMPC%), and thus requires caution in interpretation. A specific BMPC% is not stipulated as it is often biased by bone marrow cellularity, distribution of plasma cell infiltrates, and bone marrow fibrosis. More than one-third of myeloma patients have <30% plasma cells and 4-14% have <10% plasma cells on initial bone marrow evaluation.[21] In general, the lower the BMPC%, the less likely a definitive diagnosis can be made solely by bone marrow evaluation. Nonetheless, monotypic plasma cells with marked cytologic atypia, displaying many of the cytologic features listed in Table 5-2, are strongly suggestive of MM even in lower numbers. Cells with enlarged nuclei, increased nuclear pleomorphism, and prominent nucleoli are particularly worrisome. Clonality must be confirmed either by immunohistochemistry (IHC) or *in situ* hybridization for kappa and lambda light chains on biopsy sections, or by flow cytometric (FCM) evaluation of plasma cell cytoplasmic immunoglobulin light chain in aspirate specimens. A light chain ratio of >16:1 is highly predictive of MM in biopsy sections[22]; flow cytometry is more sensitive but a value that best separates MM from MGUS has not been established.

If clonality is recognized but the BMPC% and cytologic atypia are borderline, a diagnosis of *plasma cell dyscrasia* is recommended with a comment that additional testing is required for definitive classification as outlined below. In the absence of clonality, a striking plasmacytosis (>10%) and plasma cell atypia may occur in certain chronic infections, especially HIV infection; autoimmune diseases; hypersensitivity disorders; aplastic anemia, cirrhosis and other inflammatory conditions.[23] Reactive plasma cells may be larger than normal, contain nucleoli and 1-5% may be binucleate or rarely trinucleate. Cytoplasmic immunoglobulin or glycoprotein inclusions can also be found, including Russell bodies, Mott cells, crystalline rods and pseudo-Gaucher cells.

Correlation of the bone marrow morphology with available radiographic and clinical laboratory findings (protein electrophoresis studies, quantitative Ig levels) is strongly recommended in all cases, and is required in those patients with non-diagnostic bone marrow evaluations. The diagnostic criteria for MM in the recently published WHO classification for tumors of haematopoietic and lymphoid tissues[24] are similar to previously published guidelines (Table 5-3).[25-28] The minor criteria are particularly useful for atypical presentations of MM, such as nonsecretory disease. When these criteria are not met, the main alternative diagnosis is MGUS (see Table 5-4)

Table 5-3. World Health Organization Classification: criteria for diagnosis of multiple myeloma (requires at least 1 major and 1 minor criterion, or 3 minor criteria [including 1 and 2])

Major Criteria	Minor Criteria
1. Bone marrow plasmacytosis (>30%)	1. Bone marrow plasmacytosis (>10%)
2. Plasmacytoma on biopsy	2. M-component present but less than values listed as a major criteria
3. M-component in serum (IgG>3.5 g/dl, IgA>2g/dl) or urine (light chain >1g/24hr)	3. Lytic bone lesions
	4. Reduced normal immunoglobulins (<50% normal): IgG<600 mg/dl, IgA <100 mg/dl, IgM <50mg/dl.

Table 5-4. World Health Organization Classification: criteria for diagnosis of monoclonal gammopathy of undetermined significance.

M-component present but less than myeloma levels
Marrow plasmacytosis <10%
No lytic bone lesions
No myeloma-related symptoms

Not all patients who fulfill the minimal criteria for MM require conventional chemotherapy for their disease, particularly patients with minimal (≤3) or no lytic bone lesions, anemia or hypercalcemia.[21] Criteria have been established to classify these patients as either smoldering myeloma or indolent myeloma, although the criteria are insufficient in many cases. Patients with smoldering myeloma exhibit no myeloma related organ or tissue impairment, as reflected by increased calcium, renal insufficiency, anemia or bone lesions. Smoldering MM is reported in only 5-9% of patients with MM at diagnosis and is associated with low tumor burden and lack of progression for months to years.[27] More sophisticated testing is now being used in large centers to better evaluate such patients and confirm the absence of more aggressive disease. Magnetic resonance imaging, positron emission tomography and computed tomography recognize lesions missed by conventional roentgenograms.[29,30] Radiographically directed aspiration or biopsy are being increasingly utilized to evaluate focal lesions to better assess disease status.[31] Patients may have stable disease for a prolonged period of time; however, the clinical course is often unpredictable, prompting many investigators to depend on additional prognostic indicators of disease in making treatment decisions (discussed in Section 2.6). New therapies are also being utilized earlier in the disease course.

2.4 Immunophenotype

Immunophenotyping of bone marrow or tissue sections has a number of roles in the evaluation of MM as outlined in Table 5-5.

Table 5-5. Role for immunophenotyping multiple myeloma by flow cytometric analysis or immunohistochemical techniques.

Role	Evaluate
Discriminate between neoplastic and reactive plasma cells	Immunoglobulin light chain restriction (or absence of light chain in rare cases)
Identify a neoplastic infiltrate as Myeloma	CD138, immunoglobulin light chain restriction, aberrant antigen expression
Evaluation for minimal residual disease after therapy	DNA ploidy versus cytoplasmic immunoglobulin, plasma cell immunophenotype profile (flow cytometry)
Prognostic indicator	Hypodiploid plasma cell population (flow cytometry) Proliferative activity Aberrant antigen expression (under investigation)
Utilize targeted therapy	CD20 (retuximab), CD52 (Campath 1H), CD117 (imatinib;STI571) (flow cytometry)

The transmembrane heparin sulphate proteoglycan, syndecan-1 (CD138), is the most specific marker for plasma cells and is recommended for evaluation by either IHC or FCM analysis. [32-35] Plasma cell immunoreactivity to the anti-CD138 antibodies B-B4 or MI15 in paraffin-embedded BM biopsy sections, is found in essentially all plasma cell dyscrasias and lymphoplasmacytic lymphomas.[35] CD138 staining may be seen in rare chronic lymphocytic leukemias (<10%), occasional classical Hodgkin lymphomas, and diffuse large B-cell lymphomas with plasmablastic or less commonly immunoblastic features (<10%).[34] Reports of lower sensitivity using FCM probably relate to technical and storage problems; CD138 is shed during plasma cell apoptosis and is lost when specimens are refrigerated prior to evaluation.[36,44]

CD138 does not distinguish between reactive and neoplastic plasma cells; Ig light chain must be concurrently evaluated for this purpose. Myeloma cells typically express monotypic cytoplasmic Ig, lack B-cell antigens (except CD79a) and are negative or only weakly positive for surface Ig. Cytoplasmic Ig is detectable by IHC or in situ hybridization on biopsy sections; permeablization of plasma cell membranes is required for the detection by FCM. Compared to normal plasma cells, neoplastic cells lose CD19 and CD45 (variable), and gain CD56 (65-80% of cases).[37-42] Strong immunoreactivity for CD38 membrane glycoprotein is characteristic but not specific, as bright CD38 expression may also be seen on activated T-cells, pre-B cells, immature T-cells, and monocytes. Malignant plasma cells often express dimmer CD38 than normal PCs, making them difficult to reliably gate or differentiate from these other cell populations. Because of these limitations, the most effective approach for plasma cell analysis by FCM is to gate based on the CD138/CD38/CD45 staining pattern. Once the plasma cell population is isolated, assessment of Ig light chain and phenotypic aberrations allows for identification of a neoplastic process.

Lineage infidelity is a feature of many MM as myelomonocytic antigens, mature B-cell antigens, and T-cell antigens are expressed in approximately 13%, 20%, and <5% of cases, respectively.[39,43,44] Expression of many additional antigens may be found, such as CD10, CD41, CD71 by FCM and CD30, CD43, CD45RO, EMA, vimentin, and rarely CEA and cytokeratin by IHC. While aberrant antigen expression helps to confirm MGUS or MM, it may also lead to an incorrect diagnosis when the immunophenotypic evaluation is limited, particularly if marked cytologic atypia is present such that a high-grade lymphoma, leukemia or metastatic carcinoma is a diagnostic consideration. For example, the presence of bright CD20 immunoreactivity in biopsy sections of 10-20% of MM is easily misinterpreted as lymphoma if insufficiently evaluated.

Approximately 80% of myelomas contain an abnormal amount of cellular DNA. Determination of DNA ploidy in the light chain restricted plasma cell population is a powerful method for evaluating minimal residual disease and relapse.[45] This test provides a unique MM cell descriptor for a given patient when an aneuploid plasma cell population is detected (60% of cases). The same aneuploid population is usually found early in relapse, with additional aneuploid populations arising during clonal evolution and disease progression. DNA ploidy is also a powerful prognostic indicator (see section 2.6). This test is technical difficulty and performed primarily in major centers specializing in the treatment of MM. Therefore, monitoring disease by multiparameter FCM with consideration of aberrant antigen expression is likely to play more of a role in the future as FCM techniques and reagents are becoming more specialized for plasma cell evaluation.[41,42,47] Plasma cell immunophenotype may also have prognostic implications. Initial reports suggest patients with CD45-negative myeloma cells have worse survivals after high dose therapy and autologous stem cell transplant (ASCT) than patients with weak to bright expression.[47] The absence of CD56 or presence of CD20 or CD10 have also been associated with a more aggressive disease course; the impact of these markers on patients receiving high dose therapy is under evaluation.[40,48]

A final role for immunophenotyping myeloma cells is that some patients may benefit from currently available immunotherapy, depending on whether the majority of their cells express specific targeted antigens such as CD20

(15-20% of cases), CD117 (15-35% of cases), or CD52 (14-52% of cases).[39,41,44]

2.5   Staging

For the past three decades, the Durie-Salmon staging system has been used for MM staging and prognosis.[49] A major drawback of this system is that important prognostic indicators are not included. Alternative staging systems have attempted to resolve this problem. The Southwest Oncology Group evaluates a combination of serum albumin and beta-2-microglobululin (β2M).[50] Investigators at the Mayo clinic examine β2M and plasma cell labeling index (PCLI),[51] while the University of Arkansas group uses a combination of β2M, karyotype, and c-reactive protein levels.[52] None of these systems is universally accepted; therefore, a group of leading myeloma researchers is currently developing an International Prognostic Index for staging MM that will include a combination of the most powerful, independent biologically relevant prognostic factors.[6]

2.6   Prognostic Factors

The most commonly used prognostic indicators estimate tumor burden (i.e. β2M) or intrinsic characteristic of the plasma cell clone (i.e. proliferative rate, genotype) (Table 5-6).

Prognostic factors utilized more commonly in the research setting, such as gene expression profiles (GEP), are making inroads into clinical practice and are beginning to influence treatment decisions.

2.6.1   Prognostic Relevance of Bone Marrow Morphology

Although increased tumor burden is associated with decreased patient survival; BMPC% is not predictive of survival for many of the same reasons that it is not a good diagnostic indicator. The volume percentage of plasma cells (bone marrow cellularity x BMPC%) appears to better estimate plasma cell burden and thus prognosis.[53,54]

The degree of plasma cell differentiation historically relates to survival of patients with MM; therefore, most MM classifications are based on plasma cell morphology.[55-59] The unifying finding in all classification schemes is that plasmablastic morphology is associated with more aggressive disease and shortened survival, regardless of therapy.[58,59] A problem for the hematologist/pathologist is that the definition of plasmablastic myeloma differs depending on the classification used.

Table 5-6. Laboratory tests used as prognostic indicators in patients with multiple myeloma.

Common Tests	Description	Favorable Value
Beta 2-microglobulin	Light chain of class I histocompatibility antigen on nucleated cell membranes	< 4 mg/L
C-reactive protein	Acute phase protein, surrogate for IL-6 levels or PCLI	<2 mg/dl
Albumin	Serum protein	
Plasma cell labeling index (PCLI)	Percentage of plasma cells in S-phase estimated by 5-bromo-2-deoxyuridine (BrdU) incorporation	<1%
Bone marrow morphology	Cell morphology, see section 2.6.1	Not plasmablastic morphology, decreased bone marrow plasma cell volume, absence of circulating plasma cells
Cytogenetic abnormalities	Evaluation of chromosomes after mitotic stimulation in vitro using G-banding techniques	Chromosome number either 46-80 or >91 No chromosome 13 abnormalities
RESEARCH		
DNA ploidy	DNA content of myeloma cells	Not hypodiploid (DNA index <1) or hypotetraploid
Fluorescent in situ hybridization (FISH)	Identify abnormalities in specific chromosome regions	No t(4;14), t(14;16), chromosome 13q or 17p13 deletions
Ki-67 or topoisomerase IIα immunoreactivity in biopsy sections	Alternative for PCLI, estimates proliferative activity	<5% Ki-67 positive cells, <10% topoisomerase IIα positivity
Vessel density	Number of CD34-positive vessels in biopsy sections	Low
Serum syndecan-1 levels	Transmembrane heparin sulphate proteoglycan shed from myeloma cells	Low
Gene expression profile	Myeloma cell gene expression by microarray technology	Similar to MGUS patients

Referral centers in the United States generally use the morphologic classification developed by either Greipp and coworkers at the Mayo clinic or by Bartl and colleagues in Germany.[54,59] The prior separates myeloma into mature, intermediate, immature, and plasmablastic cell types based solely on the appearance of plasma cells in bone marrow aspirate smears. Plasmablastic myeloma is defined by the presence of at least 10 unambiguous plasmablasts (2%) in a 500 plasma cell count. The areas counted on the smears are those that have been screened for cells with immature morphology. The definition of a plasmablast is outlined in Table 5-7.

Table 5-7. Morphologic features of plasmablasts in aspirate smears (per Greipp[59])
Large concentric nucleus (>10um) or large nucleolus (>2um)
Fine reticular chromatin, no or minimal chromatin clumping
Cytoplasm < ½ nuclear area
Absence or little perinuclear hof

The Bartl classification is easier to use in clinical practice and is based on both aspirate smear and trephine biopsy findings. The plasma cell type determines the grade (low, intermediate or high), although the degree and pattern of bone marrow infiltration and presence of fibrosis are also considered. Six plasma cell types are defined (see Figure 5-3). Blastic morphology (plasmablasts) is most easily recognized in biopsy sections as cells resemble immunoblastic lymphoma; they are always associated with an increase in mitoses. Areas with plasmablasts are often packed or fibrotic, and poorly represented in the aspirate smears. Patients with low grade MM (Bartl grade I) may have a better prognosis but this has not been fully substantiated in patients receiving high dose therapy.[60]

2.6.2   Proliferative Rate

The most commonly used indicator of proliferative activity in MM is the PCLI, performed on cultured bone marrow aspirate specimens. Patients with low pre-treatment PCLI (<1%) have longer survivals. High proliferative activity, found in rare cases at presentation or more commonly with disease progression, correlates with worse histologic grade and shortened patient survival.[51,61] FCM analysis can alternatively measure the S-phase in plasma cells but this does not correlate with outcome or with the PCLI. Surrogate markers of proliferation in paraffin embedded tissue sections better correlate with PCLI; these include monoclonal antibodies to nuclear proliferation antigens such as Ki-67, PCNA, and topoisomerase IIα.[62,63] These markers are easily performed in a majority of laboratories, particularly Ki-67. One caveat is that proliferation markers are best interpreted using dual staining with a light chain antibody to separate myeloma cells from proliferating erythroid progenitors in biopsy sections. The majority of MM have low proliferative activity (<5% Ki-67 positive cells).[62] Myelomas with intermediate and high proliferative rates (5-19% and >20% Ki-67 immunoreactivity, respectively) are associated with poorer patient survival.[63,64]

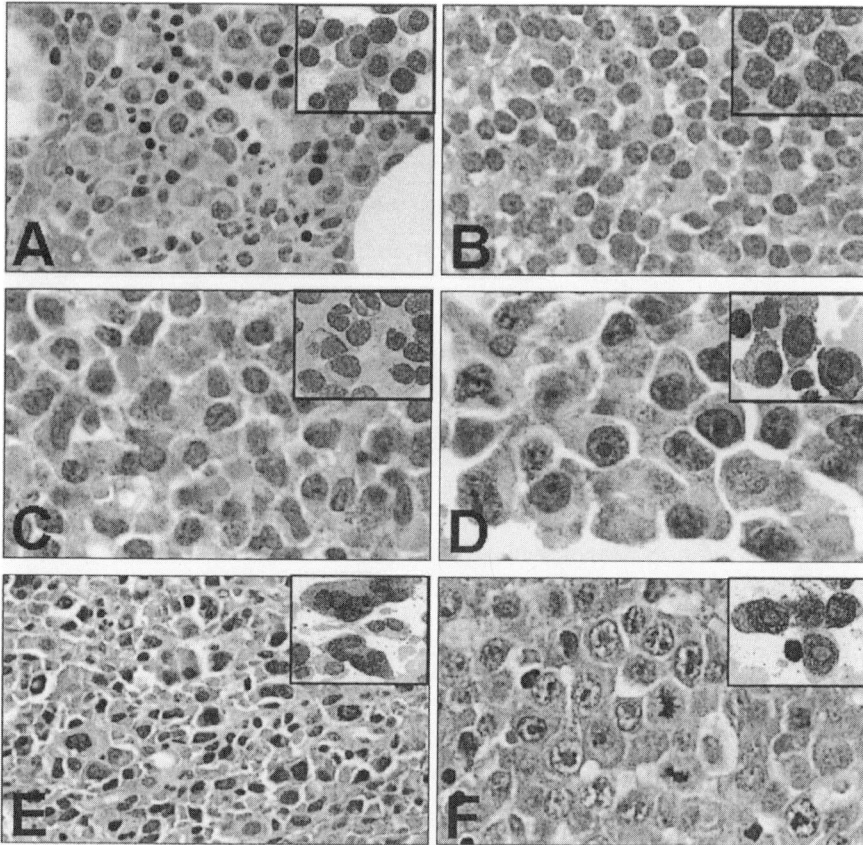

Figure 5-3. Bartl classification of multiple myeloma based on the type of plasma cells involving trephine biopsy sections and aspirate smears (inset). Low grade (Bartl grade I): **A,** Marschalko type – eccentric cartwheel nucleus, perinuclear hof, basophilic cytoplasm, few nucleoli; **B,** Small cell type – round lymphocyte- like nucleus, usually perinuclear hof, narrow rim of basophilic cytoplasm. Intermediate grade (Bartl grade II): **C,** Cleaved type – notched, cleaved or convoluted nuclei of variable size, high nuclear/cytoplasmic volume, small perinuclear hof; **D,** Asynchronous type – asynchronous nuclear/cytoplasmic maturation, >50% of cells have eccentric nuclei with prominent nucleoli; **E,** Polymorphous type – marked cellular pleomorphism, multinuclearity, 25% of cells with prominent nucleoli; High grade (Bartl grade III): **F,** Blastic type – plasmablasts with large nuclei, prominent centrally located (immunoblast-like) nucleoli, moderate rim of basophilic cytoplasm, increased mitoses.

2.6.3   Genetics

Cytogenetic evaluation of MM is hampered by the usually low proliferative rate of myeloma cells, as well as their poor growth in cell culture. Cytogenetic analysis is informative in only 30-50% of cases. Nonetheless, identification of a cytogenetic abnormality is a significant negative prognostic indicator in MM; the ability to detect an abnormality may indicate a more aggressive subtype of MM with genetic features that allow independent growth in culture conditions.[65,66] Cytogenetic findings are one of the most powerful predictors of outcome in both pre-treatment and relapse specimens. In particular, several studies have demonstrated the highly significant prognostic value of chromosome 13 abnormalities (primarily monosomy 13 but also deletion 13q and translocations involving 13q) and hypodiploidy (<46 chromosomes).[65,67,68] Patients with chromosome 13 abnormalities or hypodiploidy do poorly with current treatment regimens and should be considered for treatment protocols testing newer agents or therapeutic approaches.

Karyotypic abnormalities in MM are unusual in their complexity and resemble soft tissue tumors more than hematopoietic neoplasms, with a large number of numerical and structural aberrations. This genetic complexity supports the concept of a gradual accumulation of chromosomal abnormalities during neoplastic plasma cell differentiation (see section 1.2). Numerical chromosomal abnormalities occur early and are present in essentially all MM and most MGUS. Comparative genomic hybridization studies show that the most common chromosome gains are at 1q, 3q, 9q, 11q, and 15q with the most frequent loss at 13q. Primary immunoglobulin translocations also occur early and are likely initiating events in tumorgenesis.[1] Disease progression is associated with secondary translocations and genetic mutations, most frequently involving the ras oncogene.[69] Karyotypic abnormalities typically seen in a myelodysplastic syndrome may also be found in the MM karyotype (i.e. –5, 5q-, -7, 7q-, +8, del 20q, t(1;7)) in approximately 7% of cases; those with del 20 in particular have shortened survivals.[65]

Fluorescent in situ hybridization (FISH) is a technique that circumvents problems with proliferation and allows for targeting of specific recurrent chromosomal changes in a majority of MM. Using this technique, approximately 50% of MGUS and 60-75% of MM have IgH (14q32) rearrangements; the majority of these involve common partner chromosomes and their associated oncogenes listed in Table 5-8.[1,70-74]

The t(11;14)(q13q32) is the most common translocation identified, with at least one study showing a slightly higher prevalence in MGUS than in MM.[75] This translocation is associated with but not specific for increased plasma cell cyclin D1 immunoreactivity in biopsy sections.[61] Surprisingly, the t(11;14) is not a poor prognostic factor as initially suspected given the role of cyclin D1 in cell cycle regulation; instead, t(11;14) has either no effect or is associated with slightly improved survival depending on the study.[61,75,76]

Table 5- 8. Genetic loci involved in multiple myeloma.

	Gene locus	Oncogene product	Incidence (%)
Primary Ig translocations:	11q13	CCND1 (Cyclin D1)	15-20
Early event	4p16.3	FGFR3, MMSET	12-19
IgH locus on 14q32	16q23	c-MAF	5-10
Errors of IgH switch	12p13	Cyclin D2	5
recombination or somatic	6p21	Cyclin D3	5
hypermutation	20q11	MAFB	5
Secondary translocations:			
Late event	8q24	c-MYC	<10
Less often Ig associated	6p25	MUM/IRTA2	5
Usually complex	2p23	NMYC	<5

The next most common IgH translocation, t(4;14), detected by either FISH or reverse transcription-polymerase chain reaction (RT-PCR), has been associated with poor responses to primary chemotherapy and a very poor prognosis.[76,77] The t(4;14) is strongly associated with chromosome 13 abnormalities detected by FISH; they are seen together in up to 85% of MM.[78] The t(4;14) is also found in MGUS but at this point is of unclear significance in this disorder.[79] The t(14;16) is the third most common IgH translocation and has also been associated with shorter survivals.[74]

The secondary translocations are more complex and less often involve Ig rearrangements.[1] C-myc rearrangements are found in 15% of patients with MM; only 25% of these have an Ig partner, either t(8;14) or t(8;22).[80] Adverse patient outcome is associated with the finding of a 17p13.1 deletion, the genomic locus of the *p53* suppressor gene, seen in approximately 10% of MM.[74]

The respective value of detecting chromosome 13 abnormalities by interphase FISH versus cytogenetics is currently being debated. FISH detects chromosome 13 abnormalities in approximately 50% of cases versus 15% by conventional cytogenetic analysis.[81] While the majority of studies suggest identification of chromosome 13 abnormalities by FISH is an adverse prognostic factor, the results are dependent on the sets of probes used and the cutoff for calling a case positive.[82] Identification of abnormalities in 10% of cells is usually the definition of a chromosome 13 deletion; however, one study found only cases with greater than 20% of myeloma cells involved had shorter overall survivals.[83] In addition, the finding of chromosome 13 abnormalities by FISH in 15-50% of patients with MGUS does not predict which cases will evolve to MM.[79] Therefore, conventional cytogenetics appears to be the more powerful tool for assessing prognosis based on chromosome 13 abnormalities; it identifies an even worse subgroup of patients than FISH.[65,84]

2.6.4   Gene Expression Profiling

Gene expression profiling (GEP) by microarray analysis can be used to differentiate normal plasma cells from MM but cannot distinguish MGUS from MM.[85] GEP patterns confirm MM is composed of many distinct molecular entities, with variability in expression of early and late differentiation genes. On hierarchical clustering analysis, four distinct subgroups of MM have been identified. The subgroups show an association with survival; those with a GEP signature similar to MGUS have a better prognosis while those more similar to myeloma cell lines are more aggressive.[65,86]   Specific genes are also likely to have prognostic implications. For example, increased FGFR3, CCND1, or CCND3 gene expression correlate 100% with t(11;14), t(4;14), or t(6;14) detected by FISH analysis.[65,85]

The goal for GEP in MM is not simply for prognostication but rather to ultimately develop a classification for MM based on gene profiles that represent distinct stages of late B-cell development. A GEP-based classification is anticipated to help determine treatment by predicting which agents are likely to have the greatest probability of activity against a given tumor.   In this scenario, a bone marrow specimen obtained in the clinic would be sent to a microarray core facility to characterize the case and provide treatment recommendations based on the gene profile.

Preliminary GEP studies suggest that in addition to the clonal plasma cells, the gene profiles of the non-neoplastic cells in the bone marrow microenvironment have a major role in disease progression, particularly in the conversion of MGUS to overt MM[86] Upregulation of key adhesion molecules (i.e. UMAG3, a matrix metalloproteinase) influences myeloma cell growth and drug resistance.

2.7   Importance of the Bone Marrow Microenvironment

The bone marrow microenvironment plays a critical role in plasma cell survival, growth and differentiation. Adherence of plasma cells to the bone marrow extracellular matrix induces the production of numerous cytokines by stromal cells that have both autocrine and paracrine functions. Interleukin-6 (IL-6) is a key growth and survival factor for myeloma that additionally mediates many of the secondary effects of the malignancy, including osteolysis, anemia and immunodeficiency. Surprisingly, serum IL-6 levels have not been shown to have significant prognostic value.

A high level of syndecan-1 (CD138) in serum from MM patients is predictive of poor survival.[87,88] Syndecan-1 is a transmembrane heparin sulfate-bearing proteoglycan present on myeloma cells. Soluble syndecan-1 ectodomains, if present, are shed and trapped in the bone marrow matrix. The trapped syndecan 1 probably functions to bind heparin binding growth factors, such as fibroblast growth factor 2 (FGF 2) and hepatocyte growth factor.[33,89,90] This reservoir of syndecan-1 bound growth factors not only stimulates MM proliferation and growth, but also likely promotes disease relapse by nurturing residual tumor cells that survive chemotherapy.[33] Within this milieu are growth factors such as FGF 2 that stimulate angiogenesis. Increased vessel density in bone marrow biopsies of MM is a strong predictor of worse outcome, regardless of therapy.[64,91]

Research in recently developed mouse models confirms the requirement of the human bone microenvironment for growth of myeloma tumors.[92] An interesting observation in the mouse model is that MM cells depend on osteoclast activity for growth and survival. Growth factors normally present in latent form in the bone matrix are released in active form during bone resorption; these promote tumor cell growth. Current and emerging therapies (see section 2.10) rely on manipulation of this interaction to inhibit myeloma survival.

2.8   Bone Disease

Myeloma bone disease plays a profound role in patient morbidity. Bone marrow biopsy evaluation should document the presence of bony destruction and degree of osteoclastic activity. Bone lesions are found mainly in areas with adjacent myeloma cells and are caused by increased osteoclast activity and impaired osteoblast function. The myeloma cells either induce osteoblast apoptosis or block osteoblast differentiation. Myeloma cell binding to marrow stromal cells induces osteoclastogenic factors. Although a number of these factors have been described in myeloma cell lines and murine models of myeloma, their roles *in vivo* remain to be determined. Serum or secretory levels of these factors often show no correlation with severity of bone disease. Nonetheless, macrophage colony-stimulating factor (MIP-1α) and receptor activator of nuclear factor (kappa) B ligand (RANKL) are clearly two factors that are important. MIP-1α is a chemokine produced by MM cells that acts as an osteoclast chemoattractant and induces osteoclast formation. RANKL, secreted by activated T-cells, is a key mediator of osteoclastogenesis and plays a crucial role in bone destruction. A variety of cell types have osteoprotegerin (OPG) receptors that function as decoy receptors for RANKL and neutralize its biologic effects. An imbalance between RANKL expression and OPG levels in serum and bone marrow of MM patients favors osteoclast production and activation; the degree of the imbalance is associated with patient survival.[93] These primary osteoclastogenic factors are being investigated as therapeutic targets to block bone destruction, with the additional potential to secondarily decrease myeloma cell growth.

2.9   Current Therapies

Patients treated with conventional chemotherapy have a median survival of approximately 3 years.[6] Therapeutic failure in MM is multifactorial with the most significant problem being drug resistance. Current chemotherapy regimens attempt to use combinations of multiple drugs affecting different, non-overlapping, and non-cross resistant pathways.[94] Approximately 10 years ago, Barlogie and colleagues in Arkansas began tandem autologous stem cell transplantation (ASCT); randomized trials have confirmed the benefit of two transplants with prolongation of median survivals to at least 5 years.[95,96] Even for the older individuals who are most often afflicted with MM, ASCT appears to be a suitable option.[97] Nonetheless, the utility of performing double ASCT in patients who present with poor-risk factors, such as chromosome 13 abnormalities, is being questioned. Additional therapeutic options, with new drugs or mini-allotransplants should be considered in this group.

The role of the hematopathologist is to identify recurrent or residual disease as early as possible after ASCT, which may necessitate the use of flow cytometry, cytogenetic or FISH studies depending on characteristics of the original disease. Evaluation for myelodysplasia must also be considered as therapy related MDS/AML is a major complication of myeloma treatment.[98] Abnormal protein bands occur on serum and urine immunofixation studies in approximately 10% of patients after ASCT.[99] These may appear as monoclonal proteins and be misinterpreted as such but the immunoglobulin is usually of a different type or size than that seen in the original disease.

In 1998, we found that 30% of patients with relapsed and refractory disease responded to thalidomide.[100] The rationale for initially treating with the presumed antiangiogenic agent, thalidomide, was the finding of increased microvessel density in bone marrow biopsy sections from myeloma patients.[91] Several trials have now documented that thalidomide has significant activity in the treatment of relapse or refractory MM, with approximately one-third of patients having durable responses lasting approximately one year.[101,102] Interestingly, the primary action of thalidomide is probably not as a primary antiangiogenic agent.[103] Major side effects include somnolence, neuropathy, constipation, deep venous thrombosis and pulmonary emboli.[104,105] The realization that targeting factors in the bone marrow microenvironment acts to inhibit myeloma cell growth and survival, including chemoresistant myeloma, has changed the focus for emerging therapies.

2.10   Emerging Therapies

Table 5-9. Emerging Therapies for Multiple Myeloma

Thalidomide	Induces either apoptosis of MM cells or G1 growth arrest, blocks secretion of cytokines triggered by binding of MM cells to stromal cells (i.e. IL-6, VEGF), modulates tumor necrosis factor-alpha signaling potentiates natural killer cell activity against myeloma cells, possibly anti-angiogenic.
Immunomodulating derivative or ImiDs (Revimid, CC-5013)	Derivatives of thalidomide with similar actions but without significant side effects of somnolence, constipation or neuropathy. Additionally increases IL-2, IL-10, T-cell proliferation.
Proteasome inhibitors (Bortezomib, VELCADE ™, PS-341)	Targets proteasomes. Inhibits adhesion of myeloma cells to stromal cells. Blocks NF-κβ dependent genes involved in secretion of IL-6, VEGF, VCAM-1, counteracts IL-6 mediated effects on MM growth and survival, induces apoptosis of drug resistant myeloma cells.
Bcl-2 antisense oligonucleotide (oblimersen sodium, Genasense™)	Binds to bcl-2 mRNA and counteracts the anti-apoptotic effects of bcl-2 in myeloma cells treated with dexamethasone and doxorubicin.
Arsenic trioxide (As_2O_3)	Induces apoptosis via caspase 9 activation, decreased myeloma cell adhesion to stromal cells, blocks proliferation
Neovastat	Inhibits matrix metalloproteinases involved in cell growth, proliferation and apoptosis. Blocks VEGF receptors.
Bisphosphonates (zoledronate, pamidronate, etc.)	Inhibit osteoclast formation and activity to reduce bone disease. Possibly causes cell cycle arrest and apoptosis in MM cells. Currently used but investigating newer more potent agents.
Osteoprotegerin (AMGN-0007)	Antagonist of RANKL, inhibits osteoclastogenesis.
Alemtuzumab (Campath 1H)	Binds to and destroys cells with CD52 protein.
Monoclonal antibody to IL-6	Scheduled for clinical trial, questionable utility as IL-6 induces growth of MM in only approx 30% of patients
Immune therapy	Vaccination with idiotype, DNA, or tumor associated antigen, immunotherapy with idiotype pulsed dendritic cells.
Skeletal targeted radiotherapy (166 Holmium-DOTMP)	Radioactive high energy emitting beta particles attached to bone seeking drugs.

The majority of phase I, II, and III trials are targeting the myeloma cell interaction with its microenvironment. A number of the newer agents prevent adhesion of myeloma cells to the bone marrow stromal cells, acting to reduce cytokine secretion. Signaling pathways are also being targeted. A partial list of some of the newer therapeutic agents is provided in Table 5-9.

2.11   Multiple Myeloma Research Foundation (MMRF).

The MMRF was founded in 1998 by a drug company executive who was diagnosed with MM. This foundation is now the largest private source of money for myeloma specific research in the United States. Their website (www.multiplemyeloma.org) provides patient education and clinical updates for medical professionals, including information on current phase I, II, and III clinical trials.

3.   OTHER PLASMA CELL DYSCRASIAS

3.1   Monoclonal Immunoglobulin Deposition Diseases

Primary amyloidosis (AL) and light chain deposition disease (LCDD) are disorders caused by monoclonal plasma cell populations that over-synthesize free immunoglobulin light chains, which are deposited in tissues. Patients with these disorders most frequently present with symptoms of organ dysfunction due to the immunoglobulin deposition, along with weakness, fatigue, and weight loss. Kidney and liver involvement is common, while cardiac involvement has a particularly bad prognosis.[106]

A monoclonal immunoglobulin is detectable in approximately 80% of patients with AL or LCDD by immunofixation studies of the serum and urine. A definitive diagnosis depends on demonstration of immunoglobulin deposits in tissue from an involved organ. The subcutaneous fat pad is positive in 80% of patients with AL, while the bone marrow is positive in 55%.[107] AL amyloid is most commonly composed of lambda light chains with reduced folding stability, allowing for self-association into oligomers and fibrils, and the formation of distinct β-pleated sheets.[108] This is detectable by light microscopy; the amyloid fibrils take up Congo red stain and exhibit apple-green birefringence under polarized light. Although rarely warranted, the identification of fibrillary protein on electron microscopy is also diagnostic.[106] In contrast, LCDD more commonly involves kappa light chain, does not stain with Congo red, and has a granular appearance on electron microscopy.[109] Infrequently deposits in LCDD may be detected using immunofluorescent techniques; however, evaluation is limited by the inability to detect monoclonal kappa light chains that are associated with crystalline structures. In tissue sections, antibodies to light chains often give excess background staining, making them uninterpretable. Therefore, ultrastructural immunogold labeling or a similar technique may be required for a definitive diagnosis in LCDD.[110]

Approximately 10-15% of patients with MM have co-existing AL, while occasional patients with AL progress to overt MM.[111] Factors associated with worse survivals in patients with AL include increased serum β 2-microglobulin, increased BMPC%, cardiac amyloid involvement, and circulating peripheral blood plasma cells.[112] The molecular pathobiology of AL is similar to MM and MGUS. Translocations of the IgH locus, found in 46-72% of patients with systemic disease by interphase FISH, are early genetic events.[113,114] The chromosome partners are similar to those seen in MM, including 11q13 and 4p16. Multiple chromosomal numerical abnormalities are present; deletion 13q was found in 33% of systemic AL in one study.[7,113] Therapy requires treatment of the underlying plasma cell dyscrasia. In patients with AL, the agent I-DOX has been shown to promote amyloid resorption.[109]

3.2   Plasma Cell Leukemia

This rare aggressive variant of MM may occur de novo (primary PCL) or as a terminal event in refractory/relapsed MM (secondary PCL).[115] Patients with primary PCL, in contrast to MM, have a higher incidence of clinical stage III disease, extramedullary involvement, and immunoglobulin light chain (Bence Jones) disease. Criteria for the diagnosis of PCL are either a peripheral blood absolute plasma cell count >2 x 10^9/L or plasma cells >20% of white blood cells.[116] Circulating plasma cells in PCL often have a lymphoid appearance (i.e. small cell type, see Figure 5-3) and must be distinguished from a lymphoid neoplasm with plasmacytic features. This is best accomplished by identifying a CD138 positive population with cytoplasmic light chain restriction by FCM. A B-cell lymphoproliferative disorder can be excluded by the almost universal absence of CD19, minimal or absent surface light chain expression, and weak or negative CD45 expression.[117] The cells in a significant number of cases express CD20 (approximately 50%) and lack CD56 (>50%). CD117 expression has been linked to an especially unfavorable outcome.

PCL has many of the genetic abnormalities associated with poor prognosis in MM. For example, monosomy 13 or 13q deletions are found in 68-75% of cases by FISH analysis.[118,119] Complex chromosomal abnormalities are common with a majority of PCL having hypodiploid or diploid DNA.[117,119] Although the genetic abnormalities found in PCL are similar to MM, they are found at greater frequency. IgH gene rearrangements, t(11:14), and t(14:16) are found in approximately 80%, 33% and 13% of cases, respectively.[118] The t(11:14) may be associated with longer patient survivals. The optimal treatment for primary PCL has not been firmly established. Autologous SCT along with some of the newer treatment modalities, including the use of thalidomide, is the currently recommended treatment approach for eligible patients.[114,120]

3.3 Plasmacytoma

A plasmacytoma is a rare localized proliferation of clonal plasma cells involving a single bone (50% of cases) or extramedullary tissue site (often head and neck area).[121,122] Systemic MM must be excluded before this diagnosis is considered. Therefore, strict staging criteria including magnetic resonance imaging studies and negative bone marrow evaluations is required.[123] Extranodal marginal zone B-cell lymphoma with a predominant plasma cell component must also be excluded, particularly in the gastrointestinal tract. Plasmacytomas are most often found in males who are younger on average than patients with MM. The treatment of choice is localized radiotherapy.[124] Patients with solitary extramedullary plasmacytomas appear to have a better prognosis than those with bone disease. In particular, patients with persistent M-protein after definitive radiotherapy have a high likelihood of developing multiple myeloma.[121,122] The immunophenotypic and genetic features of the neoplastic plasma cells have not been extensively studied but appear to be similar to MM.

4. CONCLUSION

Recent advances in understanding the pathobiobiology of the plasma cell dyscrasias is allowing for better comprehension of this diverse group of disorders. In the process of understanding some of the basic genetic events that lead to plasma cell oncogenesis, a surprising finding is the similar molecular mechanisms of pathogenesis that unify these disorders. The clinical and biologic implications of these recurrent genomic aberrations are beginning to emerge. This knowledge is being translated into the clinical arena to help determine prognosis and predict responses to therapeutic interventions. While a heterogeneous clinical course is characteristic, particularly of MM, a number of prognostic indicators have been identified that help to determine the appropriate treatment approach. An important conceptual point in the treatment of these patients is that the microenvironment must be targeted in addition to the neoplastic plasma cells. With the increased use of transplantation, thalidomide, anti-osteogenic agents, and some of the newer therapies, survivals are improving along with optimism among clinicians and patients. Successful treatment approaches for the treatment of MM are beginning to translate to the other plasma cell dyscrasias. In addition, the work resulting from the increased allocation of research funding in this dynamic area will have implications in how all hematopoietic disorders are considered in the future.

REFERENCES

1. Kuehl WM, Bergsagel PL. Multiple myeloma: evolving genetic events and host inter-actions. Nat Rev Cancer 2002;2:175-187.
2. Fonseca R, Bailey RJ, Ahmann GJ, Rajkumar SV, Hoyer JD, Lust JA, Kyle RA, Gertz MA, Greipp PR, Dewald GW. Genomic abnormalities in monoclonal gammopathy of undetermined significance. Blood 2002;1000:1417-1424.
3. Zandecki M, Lai JL, Genevieve F, Bernardi F, Volle-Remy H, Blanchet O, Francois M Cosson A, Bauters F, Facon T. Several cytogenetics subclones may be identified within plasma cells of patients with monoclonal gammopathy of undetermined sig- nificance, both at diagnosis and during the indolent course of this condition. Blood 997;90:3682-3690.
4. Avet-Loiseau H, Facon T, Grosbois B, Magrangeas F, Rapp MJ, Harousseau JL, Min-vielle S, Bataille R; Intergroupe Francophone du Myelome. Oncogenesis of multiple myeloma: 14q32 and 13q chromosomal abnormalities are not randomly distributed, but correlate with natural history, immunological features, and clinical presentation. Blood 2002;99:2185-2191.
5. Kyle RA. "Benign" monoclonal gammopathy: after 20 to 35 years of follow-up. Mayo Clinic Proc. 1993;68:26-36.
6. Kyle RA, Gertz MA, Witzig TE, Lust JA, Lacy MQ, Dispenzieri A, Fonseca R, Raj-kumar SV, Offord JR, Larson DR, Plevak ME, Therneau TM, Greipp PR. Review of 1027 patients with newly diagnosed multiple myeloma. Mayo Clin Proc 2003;78:21- 33.
7. Fonseca R, Ahmann GJ, Jalal SM, Dewald GW, Larson DR, Therneau TM, Gertz MA, Kyle RA, Greipp PR. Chromosomal abnormalities in systemic amyloidosis. Br J Haematol 1998;103:704-710.
8. Greenlee RT, Hill-Harmon MB, Murray T, Thun M. Cancer statistics. CA Cancer J Clin. 2001;51:15-36.
9. Baris D, Brown LM, Silverman DT, Hayes R, Hoover RN, Swanson GM, Dosemeci M Schwartz AG, Liff JM, Schoenberg JB, Pottern LM, Lubin J, Greenberg RS, Fraumeni JF Jr. Socioeconomic status and multiple myeloma among US blacks and whites. Am J Public Health 2000;90:1277-1281.
10. Lynch HT, Sanger WG, Pirruccello S, Quinn-Laquer B, Weisenburger DD. Familial multiple myeloma: a family study and review of the literature. J Nat Cancer Inst 2001; 93:1497-1483.
11. Speer SA, Semenza JC, Kurosaki T, Anton-Culver H. Risk factors for acute myeloid leukemia and multiple myeloma: combination of GIS and case-control studies. J Environ Health 2002;64:9-16.

12. Khuder SA, Mutgi AB. Meta-analyses of multiple myeloma and farming. Am J Ind Med 1997;32:510-516.
13. Durie BG. The epidemiology of multiple myeloma. Semin Hematol 2001:38 (2 Suppl 3):1-5.
14. Rettig MB, Ma HJ, Vescio RA, Pold M, Schiller G, Belson D, Savage A, Nishikubo C, Wu C, Fraser J, Said JW, Berenson JR. Kaposi's sarcoma-associated herpesvirus infection of bone marrow dendritic cells from multiple myeloma patients. Science 1997;276:1851-1854.
15. Said JW, Rettig MR, Heppner K, Vescio RA, Schiller G, Ma HJ, Belson D, Savage A, Shintaku IP, Koeffler HP, Asou H, Pinkus G, Pinkus J, Schrage M, Green E, Ber- enson JR. Localization of Kaposi's sarcoma-associated herpesvirus in bone marrow biopsy samples from patients with multiple myeloma. Blood 1997;90:4278- 4282.
16. Tedeschi R, Kvarnung M, Knekt P, Schulz TF, Szekely L, De Paoli PD, Aromaa A, Teppo L, Dillner J. A prospective seroepidemiological study of human herpesvirus-8 infection and the risk of multiple myeloma. Br J Cancer 2001;84:122-125.
17. Drabick JJ, Davis BJ, Lichy JH, Flynn J, Byrd JC. Human herpesvirus 8 genome is not found in whole bone marrow core biopsy specimens of patients with plasma cell dy- scrasias. Ann Hematol 2002;81:304-307.
18. Raitakari M, Brown RD, Gibson J, Joshua DE. T cells in myeloma. Hematol Oncol. 2003;21(1):33-42.
19. Sukpanichnant S, Cousar JB, Oeelasiri A, Graber SE, Greer JP, Collins RD. Diagnostic criteria and histologic grading in multiple myeloma. Histologic and im- munohistologic analysis of 176 cases with clinical correlation. Hum Pathol 1994; 25:308-318.
20. Larson RS, Sukpanichnant S, Greer JP, Cousar JB, Collins RD. The spectrum of mul- tiple myeloma: diagnostic and biological implications. Hum Pathol 1997;28:1336- 1347.
21. Kyle RA. Diagnosis of multiple myeloma. Sem Oncol 2002;29(suppl 17):2-4.
22. Peterson LC, Brown BA, Crosson JT, Mladenovic J. Application of the immunoperoxidase technic to bone marrow trephine biopsies in the classification of patients with mono-clonal gammopathies. Am J Clin Pathol 1986;85:688-693.
23. Williams RL, Bailly RC, Howe RB. Studies of "benign" serum M-components. Am J Med Sci 1969;257:275-293.
24. Grogan TM, Van Camp B, Kyle RA, Muller-Hermelink HK, Harris NL. Plasma cell neoplasms, In Tumours of Haematopoietic and Lymphoid Tissues, World Health Organization Classification of Tumors, eds. Jaffe ES, Harris NL, Stein H, Vardiman JW. IARC Press, Lyon France 2001:142-156.
25. Salmon SE, Cassidy JR. Plasma cell neoplasms. In: Cancer, Principles and Practice of Oncology, DeVita VT, Hellman S, Rosenbers S, eds. J.B. Lippincott: Philadelphi 1988; 1854.
26. Alexian R. Localized and indolent myeloma. Blood 1980;56:521-525.
27. Kyle RA, Greipp PR. Smoldering multiple myeloma. N Engl J Med 1980;302:1347- 1349.
28. Durie BGM, Salmon SE. Multiple myeloma, macroglobulinemia and monoclonal gammopathies. In: Hoffbrand AV, Brian MC, Hirsch J eds. Recent advances in hema- tology. Edinburgh: Churchill Livingston, 1977:243.
29. Jadvar H, Conti PS. Diagnostic utility of FDG PET in multiple myeloma. Skeletal Radio 2002;31:690-694.

30. Mahnken AH, Wildberger JE, Gehbauer G, Schmitz-Rode T, Blaum M, Fabry U, Gunther RW. Multidetector CT of the spine in multiple myeloma: comparison with MR imaging and radiography. Am J Roentgenol 2002;178:1429-1436.

31. Avva R, Vanhemert RL, Barlogie B, Munshi N, Angtuaco EJ. CT-guided biopsy of focal lesions in patients with multiple myeloma may reveal new and more aggressive cyto-genetic abnormalities. AJNR Am J Neuroradiol 2001;22:781-785.

32. Witzig, TE, Kimlinger T, Stenson M, Therneau T. Syndecan-1 expression on malignant cells from blood and marrow of patients with plasma cell proliferative disorders and B-cell chronic lymphocytic leukemia. Leuk Lymphoma 1998;31:167-175.

33. Bayer-Garner IB, Sanderson RD, Dhodapkar MV, Owens RB, Wilson CS. Syndecan- 1 (CD138) immunoreactivity in bone marrow biopsies of multiple myeloma: Shed synde-can-1 accumulates in fibrotic regions. Mod Pathol 2001;14:1052-1058.

34. Costes V, Magen V, Legouffe E, Durand L, Baldet P, Rossi JF, Klein B. The Mi15 monoclonal antibody (anti-syndecan-1) is a reliable marker for quantifying plasma cells in paraffin-embedded bone marrow biopsy specimens. Human Pathology 1999;30:1405-1411.

35. Chilosi M, Adami F, Lestani M, Montagna L, Cimarosto L, Semenzato G, Pizzolo G Menestrina F. CD138/syndecan-1: a useful immunohistochemical marker of normal and neoplastic plasma cells on routine trephine bone marrow biopsies. Mod Pathol 1999:12:1101-1106.

36. Jourdan M, Ferlin M, Legouffe E, Horvathova M, Liautard J, Rossi JF, Wijdenes J, Brochier J, Klein B. The myeloma cell antigen syndecan-1 is lost by apoptotic myeloma cells. Br J Haematol 1998;100:637-646.

37. Harada H, Kawano MM, Huang N, Harada Y, Iwato K, Tanabe O, Tanaka H, Sakai A, Asaoku H, Kuramoto A. Phenotypic difference of normal plasma cells from mature myeloma cells. Blood 1993;81:2658-2663.

38. Lima M, Teixeira Mdos A, Fonseca S, Goncalves C, Guerra M, Queiros Santos AH, Coutinho A, Pinho L, Marques L, Cunha M, Ribeiro P, Xavier L, Vieira H, Pinto P, Justica B. Immunophenotypic aberrations, DNA content, and cell cycle analysis of plasma cells in patients with myeloma and monoclonal gammopathies. Blood Cells Mol Dis 2000;26:634-645.

39. Ruiz-Arguelles GJ, San Miguel JF. Cell surface markers in multiple myeloma. Mayo Clin Proc 1994;69:684-690.

40. Sahara N, Takeshita A, Shigeno K, Fujisawa S, Takeshita K, Naito K, Ihara M, Ono T, Tamashima S, Nara K. Clinicopathological and prognostic characteristics of CD56-negative multiple myeloma. Br J Haematol 2002;117:882-885.

41. San Miguel JF, Almeida J, Mateo G, Blade J, Lopez-Berges C, Caballero D, Hernandez J, Moro MJ, Fernandez-Calvo J, Diaz-Mediavilla J, Palomera L, Orfao A. Immunophenotypic evaluation of the plasma cell compartment in multiple myeloma: a tool for comparing the efficacy of different treatment strategies and predicting outcome. Blood 2002;99:1853-1856.

42. Rawston AC, Davies FE, DasGupta R, Ashcroft AJ, Patmore R, Drayson MT, Owen RG, Jack AS, Child JA, Morgan GJ. Flow cytometric disease monitoring in multiple myeloma: the relationship between normal and neoplastic plasma cells predicts outcome after transplantation. Blood 2002:100:3095-3100.

43. Petruch UR, Horny H-P, Kaiserling E. Frequent expression of haematopoietic and non-haematopoietic antigens by neoplastic plasma cells: an immunohistochemical study using formalin-fixed paraffin-embedded tissue. Histopathology 1992;20:35-40.

44. Lin P, Owens R, Tricot G, Wilson CS. Flow cytometry immunophenotypic analysis of

306 cases of multiple myeloma. Am J Clin Pathol 2004:(in press).

45. Kumar S, Kimlinger TK, Lust JA, Donovan K, Witzig TE. Expression of CD52 on plasma cells in plasma cell proliferative disorders. Blood 2003;102:1075-77.
46. Barlogie B, Alexanian R, Pershouse M, Smallwood L, Smith L. Cytoplasmic immunoglobulin content in multiple myeloma. J Clin Invest 1985;76:765-769.
47. Almeida J, Orfao A, Ocquetreau M, Mateo G, Corral M, Caballero MD, Blade J, Moro MJ, Hernandez J, San Miguel JF. High-sensitive immunophenotyping and DNA ploidy studies for the investigation of minimal residual disease in multiple myeloma. Br J Haematol 1999;107:121-131.
48. Pellat-Deceunynck C, Barille S, Jego G, Puthier D, Robillard N, Pineau D, Rapp MJ, Harousseau JL, Amiot M, Bataille R. The absence of CD56 (NCAM) on malignant plasma cells is a hallmark of plasma cell leukemia and of a special subset of multiple myeloma. Leukemia 1998;12:1977-1982
49. Durie BGM, Salmon SE. A clinical staging system for multiple myeloma. Correlation of measured myeloma cell mass with presenting clinical features, response to treatment and survival. Cancer 1975:36:842-854.
50. Jacobson JL, Hussein MA, Barlogie B, Durie BGM, Crowley JJ. Beta 2 microglobulin (B2M) and albumin define a new staging system for multiple myeloma: the Southwest Oncology Group (SWOG) experience (abstract). Blood 2001;98:155-156.
51. Greipp PR, Lust JA, O'Fallon WM, Katzmann JA, Witzig TE, Kyle RA. Plasma cell labeling index and beta 2-microglobulin predict survival independent of thymidine kinase and C-reactive protein in multiple myeloma. Blood 1993;81:3382-3387.
52. Desikan R. Barlogie B. Sawyer J, Ayers D, Tricot G, Badros A, Zangari M, Munshi NC, Anaissie E, Spoon D, Siegel D. Results of high dose therapy for 1000 patients with multiple myeloma: durable complete remissions and superior survival in the absence of chromosome 13 abnormalities. Blood 2000;95:4008-4010.
53. Bartl R, Frisch B, Burkhardt R, Rateh-Moghadam A, Mahl G, Gierster P, Sund M, Kettner G. Bone marrow histology in myeloma: its importance in diagnosis, prog- nosis, classification, and staging. Br J Haematol 1982;51:361-375.
54. Bartl R, Frisch B, Fateh-Moghadam A, Kettner G, Jaeger K, Sommerfeld W. Histologic classification and staging of multiple myeloma. A retrospective and pro- spective study of 674 cases. Am J Clin Pathol 1987;87:342-355.
55. Carter A, Hocherman I, Linn S, Cohen Y, Tatarsky I. Prognostic significance of plas- ma cell morphology in multiple myeloma. Cancer 1987;60:1060-1065.
56. Fritz E, Ludwig H, Kundi M. Prognostic relevance of cellular morphology in multiple myeloma. Blood 1984;63:1072-1079.
57. Sailer M, Vykoupil K-F, Peest D, Coldewey R, Deicher H, Georgii A. Prognostic relevance of a histologic classification system applied in bone marrow biopsies from patients with multiple myeloma: a histopathological evaluation of biopsies from 153 untreated patients. Eur J Haematol 1995;54:137-146.
58. Bartl R and Frisch B. Bone marrow histology in multiple myeloma: prognostic relevance of histologic characteristics. Hematology Reviews 1989:3:87-108.
59. Greipp PR, Leong T, Bennett JM, Gaillard JP, Klein B, Stewart JA, Oken MM, Kay NE, Van Ness B, Kyle RA. Plasmablastic morphology – an independent prognostic factor with clinical and laboratory correlates: Eastern Cooperative Oncology Group (ECOG) myeloma trial E9486 report by the ECOG Myeloma Laboratory Group. Blood 1998;91:2501-2507.

60.   Waldron J, Jazieh R, Jagannath S, Desikan KR, Siegel D, Fassas A,   Singhal S, Mehta J, Tricot G, Vesole D, Wilson C, Hough A, Nanucke S, Spoon D, Barlogie B.   Bone marrow morphology (BMM) adds critical prognostic information to other standard parameters (SP) including cytogenetics among newly diagnosed multiple myeloma (MM) patients   (PTS) receiving total therapy (TT). Blood 1997;90(suppl 1):90a.

61. Wilson CS, Butch AW, Lai R, Medeiros LJ, Sawyer JR, Barlogie B, McCourty A, Kelly K, Brynes RK. Cyclin D1 and E2F-1 immunoreactivity in bone marrow biopsy specimens of multiple myeloma; relationship to proliferative activity, cytogenetic abnormalities and ploidy. Br J Haematol 2001;112:776-782.

62. Wilson CS, Medeiros LJ, Lai R, Butch AW, McCourty A, Kelly K,   Brynes RK. DNA Topoisomerase IIα in multiple myeloma: A marker of proliferation and not drug resistance. Mod Pathol 2001;14:886-891.

63.   Rimsza LM, Campbell K, Dalton WS, Salmon S, Willcox G, Grogan TM. The major vault protein (MVP), a new multidrug resistance associated protein, is frequently expressed in multiple myeloma. Leuk Lymphoma 1999;34:315-324.

64. Xu JL, Lai R, Kinoshita T, Nakashima N, Nagasaka T. Proliferation, apoptosis, and intratumoral vascularity in multiple myeloma: correlation with the clinical stage and cytological grade. J Clin Pathol 2002;55:530- 534.

65. Shaughnessy J, Barlogie B, Sawyer J, McCoy J, Fassas A, Zhan F, Bumm K, Epstein J, Anaissie E, Jagannath S, Vesole D, Siegel D, Desikan R, Munshi N, Badros A,   Tian E, Zangari M, Jacobson J,   Crowley J, Tricot G. Continuous absence of metaphase-defined cytogenetic abnormalities especially of chromosome 13 and hypodiploidy assures long term survival in multiple myeloma treated with total therapy I: interpretation in the context of global gene expression. Blood 2003;101: 3849-3856.

66. Debes-Marun CS, Dewald GW, Bryant S, Picken E, Santana-Davila R, Gonzalez-Paz N, Winkler JM, Kyle RA, Gertz MA, Witzig TE, Dispenzieri A, Lacy MQ, Rajkumar SBV, Lust JA, Greipp PR, Fonseca R. Chromosome abnormalities clustering and its implications for pathogenesis and prognosis in myeloma. Leukemia 2003:17:427-436.

67. Shaughnessy J Jr, Tian E, Sawyer J, McCoy J, Tricot G, Jacobson J, Anaissie E, Zangari M, Fassas A, Muwalla F, Morris C, Barlogie B. Prognostic impact of cytogenetic and interphase fluorescence in situ hybridization-defined chromosome 13 deletion in multiple myeloma: early results of total therapy II. Br J Haematol. 2003;120:44-52.

68. Smadja NM, Bastard C, Brigaudeau C, Leroux D, Fruchart C. Hypodiploidy is a major prognostic factor in multiple myeloma. Blood 2001;98:2229-2238.

69. Bezieau S, Devilder MC, Avet-Loiseau H, Mellerin MP, Puthier D, Pennarun E, Rapp MJ, Harousseau JL, Moisan JP, Bataille R. High incidence of N and K-Ras activating mutations in multiple myeloma and primary plasma cell leukemia at diagnosis. Hum Mutat 2001;18:212-224.

70. Avet-Loiseau H, Li JY, Facon T, Brigaudeau C, Morineau N, Maloisel F,   Rapp   MJ, Talmant P, Trimoreau F, Jaccard A, Harousseau JL, Bataille R.   High incidence of translocations t(11;14)(q13;q32) and t(4;14)(p16;q32) in patients with plasma cell malignancies. Cancer Res. 1998;58:5640-5645.

71. Chesi M, Nardini E, Lim RS, Smith KD, Kuehl WM, Bergsagel PL. The t(4;14) translocation in myeloma dysregulates both FGFR3 and a novel gene, MMSET, resulting in IgH/MMSET hybrid transcripts. Blood 1998;92:3025-3034.

72. Avet-Loiseau H, Brigaudeau C, Morineau N, Talmant P, Lai JL, Daviet A, Li JY, Praloran V, Rapp MJ, Harousseau JL, Facon T, Bataille R. High incidence of cryptic translocations involving the Ig heavy chain gene in multiple myeloma as shown by fluorescence in situ hybridization. Genes Chromosomes Cancer. 1999;24:9-15.

73. Sawyer JR, Lukacs JL, Thomas EL, Swanson CM, Goosen LS, Sammartino G, Gilliland JC, Munshi NC, Tricot G, Shaughnessy JD, Jr, Barlogie B. Multicolour spectral karyotyping identifies new translocations and a recurring pathway for chromosome loss in multiple myeloma. Br J Haematol 2000;112:1-9.

74. Fonseca R, Blood E, Rue M, Harrington D, Oken MM, Kyle RA, Dewald GW, Van Ness B, Van Wier SA, Henderson KJ, Bailey RJ, Greipp PR. Clinical and biologic implications of recurrent genomic aberrations in myeloma. Blood 2003;101:4569- 4575.

75. Fonseca R, Blood EA, Oken MM, Kyle RA, Dewald GW, Bailey RJ, Van Wier SA, Henderson KJ, Hoyer JD, Harrington D, Kay NE, Van Ness B, Greipp PR. Myeloma and the t(11;14)(q13;q32); evidence for a biologically defined unique subset of patients. Blood 2002;99:3735-3741.

76. Moreau P, Facon T, Leleu X, Morineau N, Huyghe P, Harousseau JL, Bataille R, Av Avet- Loiseau H; Intergroupe Francophone du Myelome. Recurrent 14q32 translocations determine the prognosis of multiple myeloma, especially in patients receiving intensive chemotherapy. Blood 2002;100:1579-1583.

77. Keats JJ, Reiman T, Maxwell CA, Taylor BJ, Laratt LM, Mant MJ, Belch AR, Pilarski LM. In multiple myeloma, t(4;14)(p16;q32) is an adverse prognostic factor irrespective of FGFR3 expression. Blood 2003;101;1520-1529.

78. Fonseca R, Oken M, Greipp P. The t(4;14)(p16.3;q32) is strongly associated with chromosome 13 abnormalities (Δ13) in both multiple myeloma (MM) and MGUS. Blood 2001;98:1271-1272.

79. Fonseca R, Bailey RJ, Ahmann GJ, Rajkumar SV, Hoyer JD, Lust JA, Kyle RA Gertz MA Greipp PR, Dewald GW. Genomic abnormalities in monoclonal gammopathy of undetermined significance. Blood 2002;100:1417-1424.

80. Shou Y, Martelli ML, Tagrea A. Gabrea A, QI Y, Brents LA, Roschke A, Dewald G, Kirsch IR, Bergsagel PL, Kuel WM. Diverse karyotypic abnormalities of the c-myc locus associated with c-myc dysregulation and tumor progression in multiple myeloma. Proc Natl Acad Sci USA 2000;97:228-233

81. Zojer N, Konigsberg R, Ackermann J, Fritz E, Dallinger S, Kromer E, Kaufmann H, Riedl L, Gisslinger H, Schreiber S, Heinz R, Ludwig H, Huber H, Drach J. Deletion of 13q14 remains an independent adverse prognostic variable in multiple myeloma despite its frequent detection by interphase fluorescence in situ hybridization. Blood 2000;95:1925-1930.

82. Facon T, Avet-Loiseau H, Guillerm G, Moreau P, Genevieve F, Zandecki M, Lai JL, Leleu X, Jouet JP, Bauters F, Harousseau JL, Bataille R, Mary JY. Chromosome 13 abnormalities identified by FISH analysis and serum beta 2-microglobulin produce a powerful myeloma staging system for patients receiving high-dose therapy. Blood 2001;97:1566-1571.

83. Shaughnessy J, Tian E, Sawyer J, Bumm K, Landes R, Badros A, Morris C, Tricot G, Epstein J, Barlogie B. High incidence of chromosome 13 deletion in multiple myeloma detected by multiprobe interphase FISH. Blood;2000:96:1505-1511.

84. Tricot G, Barlogie B, Jagannath S, Bracy D, Mattox S, Vesole DH, Naucke S, Sawyer JR. Poor prognosis in multiple myeloma is associated only with partial or complete deletions of chromosome 13 or abnormalities involving 11q and not with other karyotype abnormalities. Blood 1995:86:4250-4256.

85. Zhan F, Hardin J, Kordsmeier B, Bumm K, Zheng M, Tian E, Sanderson   R,   Yang Y, Wilson C, Zangari M, Anaissie E, Morris C, Muwalla F, van   Rhee   F,   Fassas   A, Crowley J, Tricot G, Barlogie B, Schaughnessy J Jr. Global gene expression profiling of multiple myeloma, monoclonal gammopathy of undetermined significance, and normal bone marrow plasma cells. Blood 2002;99:1745-1757.

86. Zhan F, Tian E, Bumm K, Smith R, Barlogie B, Shaughnessy J Jr. Gene expression profiling of human plasma cell differentiation and   classification of multiple myeloma based on similarities to distinct stages of late-stage B-cell development. Blood 2003;101:1128-1140.

87. Seidel C, Sundan A, Hjorth M, Turesson I, Dahl IM, Abildgaard N,   Waage   A,   Borset M. Serum syndecan-1: a new independent prognostic   marker   in   multiple   myeloma. Blood 2000;95:388-392.

88. Yang Y, Yaccoby S, Liu W, Langford JK, Pumphrey Cy, Theus A, Epstein J, Sanderson RD. Soluble syndecan-1 promotes growth of myeloma tumors in vivo. Blood 2002:100:610-617.

89. Derksen PW, Keehnen RM, Evers LM, van Oers MH, Spaargaren M, Pals ST. Cell surface proteoglycan syndecan-1 mediates hepatocyte   growth   factor   binding   and promotes Met signaling in multiple myeloma. Blood 2002;99:1405-1410.

90. Kato M, Wang H, Kainulainen V, Fitzgerald ML, Ledbetter S, Ornitz DM, Bernfield   M. Physiological degradation converts the soluble syndecan-1 ectodomain from an inhibitor to a potent activator of FGF-2. Nat Med. 1998;4:691-697.

91. Munshi NC, Wilson C. Increased microvessel density in newly diagnosed multiple myeloma carries a poor prognosis. Semin Oncol   2001;28:265-269.

92. Yaccoby S, Epstein J. The proliferative potential of myeloma plasma cells manifest in the SCID-hu host. Blood 1999;94:3576-3582.

93. Terpos E, Szydlo R, Apperley JF, Hatjiharissi E, Poplitou M, Meletis J, Viniour N, Yataganas X, Goldman JM, Rahemtulla A. Soluble receptor activator of nuclear factor kappa B ligand-osteoprotegerin ratio predicts survival in multiple myeloma: proposal for a novel prognostic index. Blood 2003;102:1064-69.

94. Myeloma Trialists' Collaborative Group. Combination chemotherapy versus mel- phalan plus prednisone as treatment for multiple myeloma: an overview of 6,633   patients from 27 randomized trials. J Clin Oncol. 1998;16:3832-3842.

95. Attal M, Harousseau JL, Stoppa AM,   Sotto JJ,   Fuzibet JG, Rossi JF, Casassus P, Maisonneuve H, Facon T, Ifrah N, Payen C, Bataille R. A prospective randomized   trial of autologous bone marrow   transplantation and chemotherapy in multiple myeloma. Intergroupe Francais du Myelome. N Engl J Med. 1996;335:91-97.

96. Barlogie B, Shaughnessy J, Zangari M, Tricot G. High-dose therapy and immunomodulatory drugs in multiple myeloma. Semin Oncol 2002;29:26-33.

97. Badros A, Barlogie B, Siegel E, Morris C, Desikan R, Zangari M, Fassas A, Anaissie E, Munshi N, Tricot G. Autologous stem cell transplantation in elderly multiple   myeloma patients over the age of 70 years. Br J Haematol 2001;114:600-607.

98. Govindarajan R, Jagannath S, Flick JT, Vesole DY, Sawyer J, Barlogie B,   Tricot   G. Preceeding standard therapy is the likely cause of MDS after autotransplants for mul- tiple myeloma. Br J Haematol 1996;95:349-353.

99. Zent CS, Wilson CS, Tricot G, Jagannath S, Siegel D, Desikan KR, Munshi N, Bracy D, Barlogie B, Butch AW. Oligoclonal protein bands and immunoglobulin isotype switching in multiple myeloma patients treated with high dose therapy and hematopoietic cell transplantation.   Blood 1998;91:3518-2523.

100. Singhal S, Mehta J, Desikan R, Ayers D, Roberson P, Eddelmon P, Munshi N, Anaissie E, Wilson C, Dhodapkar M, Zeldis J, Barlogie B. Antitumor activity of thalidomide in refractory multiple myeloma. NEJM 1999;342:1565-1571.

101. Kumar S, Gertz MA, Dispenzieri A, Lacy MQ, Geyer SM, Iturria NL, Fonseca R, Hayman SR, Lust JA, Kyle RA, Greipp PR, Witzig TE, Rajkumar SV. Response rate, durability of response, and survival after thalidomide therapy for relapsed multiple myeloma. Mayo Clin Proc. 2003;78:34-39.

102. Tosi P, Zamagni E, Cellini C, Ronconi S, Patriarca F, Ballerini F, Musto P, De Raimondo F, Ledda A, Lauria F, Masini L, Gobbi M, Vacca A, Ria R, Cangini D, Tura S, Baccarini M, Cavo M. Salvage therapy with thalidomide in patients with advanced relapsed/refractory multiple myeloma. Haematologica 2002;87:408-414.

103. Matthews SJ, McCoy C. Thalidomide: a review of approved and investigational uses. Clin Ther 2003;25:342-395.

104. Zangari M, Anaissie E, Barlogie B, Badros A, Desikan R, Gopal AV, Morris C, Toor A, Siegel E, Fink L, Tricot G. Increased risk of deep vein thrombosis in patients with multiple myeloma receiving thalidomide and chemotherapy. Blood 2001;98:1614-1615.

105. Zangari M, Saghafifar F, Anaissie E, Badros A, Desikan R, Fassas A, Mehta P, Morris C, Toor A, Whitfield D, Siegel E, Barlogie B, Fink L, Tricot G. Activated protein C resistance in the absence of factor V Leiden mutation is a common finding in multiple myeloma and is associated with an increased risk of thrombotic complications. Blood Coagul Fibrinolysis 2002;13:187-192.

106. Pozzi C, Locatelli F. Kidney and liver involvement in monoclonal light chain disorder. Semin Nephrol. 2002;22:319-330.

107. Kyle RA. Clinical aspects of multiple myeloma and related disorders including amyloidosis. Pathol Biol 1999;47:148-157.

108. Bellotti V, Mangione P, Merlini G. Review: immunoglobulin light chain amyloidosis—the archetype structural and pathogenic variability. J Struct Biol 2000;130:280-289.

109. Dhodapkar MV, Merlini G, Solomon A. Biology and therapy of immunoglobulin deposition diseases. Hematol Oncol Clin North Am. 1997;11:89-110.

110. Gu X, Barrios R, Cartwright J, Font RL, Truong L, Herrera GA. Light chain crystal deposition as a manifestation of plasma cell dyscrasias: the role of immunoelectron microscopy. Hum Pathol. 2003;34:270-277.

111. Rajkumar SV, Gertz MA, Kyle RA. Primary systemic amyloidosis with delayed progression to multiple myeloma. Cancer 1998;82:1501-1505.

112. Pardanani A, Witzig TE, Schroeder G, McElroy EA, Fonseca R, Dispenzieri A, Lacy MQ, Lust JA, Kyle RA, Greipp PR, Gertz MA, Rajkumar SV. Circulating peripheral blood plasma cells as a prognostic indicator in patients with primary systemic amyloidosis. Blood 2003;101:827-830.

113. Harrison CJ, Mazzullo H, Ross FM, Cheung KL, Gerrard G, Harewood L, Mehta A, Lachmann HJ, Hawkins PN, Orchard KH. Translocations of 14q32 and deletions of 13q14 are common chromosomal abnormalities in systemic amyloidosis. Br J Haematol. 2002;117:427-435.

114. Hayman SR, Bailey RJ, Jalal SM, Ahmann GJ, Dispenzieri A, Gertz MA, Greipp PR, Kyle RA, Lacy MQ, Rajkumar SV, Witzig TE, Lust JA, Fonseca R. Translocations involving the immunoglobulin heavy-chain locus are possible early genetic events in patients with primary systemic amyloidosis. Blood 2001;98:2266-2268.

115. Hayman SR, Fonseca R. Plasma cell leukemia. Current Treatment Options Oncol. 2001;2:205-216.

116. Galton DA, Gralnick HR, Sultan C. Proposals for the classification of chronic (mature) B and T lymphoid leukaemias. French-American British (FAB) Cooperative Group. J Clin Pathol 1989;42:567-584.

117. Garcia-Sanz R, Orfao A, Gonzalez M, Tabernero MD, Blade J, Moro MJ, Fernandez-Calvo J, Sanz MA, Perez-Simon JA, Rasillo A, Miquel JF. Primary plasma cell leukemia: clinical, immunophenotypic, DNA ploidy, and cytogenetic characteristics. Blood 1999;93:1032-1037.

118. Avet-Loiseau H, Daviet A, Brigaudeau C, Callet-Bauchu E, Terre C, Lafage-Pochitaloff M, Desangles F, Ramond S, Talmant P, Bataille R. Cytogenetic, interphase, and multicolor fluorescence in situ hybridization analyses in primary plasma cell leukemia: a study of 40 patients at diagnosis, on behalf of the Intergroupe Francophone du Myélome and the Groupe Français de Cytogénétique Hématologique. Blood 2001;97:822-825.

119. Rasillo A, Tabernero MD, Sanchez ML, Perez de Andres M, MartinAyuso M, Hernandez J, Moro MJ, Fernandez-Calvo J, Sayagues JM,Bortoluci A, San Miguel JF, Orfao A. Fluorescence in situ hybridization analysis of aneuploidization patterns in monoclonal gammopathy of undetermined significance versus multiple myeloma and plasma cell leukemia. Cancer 2003;97:601-609.

120. Johnston RE, Abdalla SH. Thalidomide in low doses is effective for the treatment of resistant or relapsed multiple myeloma and for plasma cell leukaemia. Leukemia Lymphoma 2002;43:351-354.

121. Dimopoulos MA, Kiamouris C, Moulopoulos LA. Solitary plasmacytoma of bone and extramedullary plasmacytoma. Hematol Oncol Clin North Am 1999;13:1249-1257.

122. Dimopoulos MA, Hamilos G. Solitary bone plasmacytoma and extramedullary plasmacytoma. Curr Treat Options Oncol 2002;3:255-259.

123. Liebross RH, Ha CS, Cox JD, Weber D, Delasalle K, Alexanian R. Clinical course of solitary extramedullary plasmacytoma. Radiother Oncol 1999;52:245-249.

124. Liebross RH, Ha CS, Cox JD, Weber D, Delasalle K, Alexanian R. Solitary bone plasmacytoma: outcome and prognostic factors following radiotherapy. Int J Radiat Oncol Biol Phys 1998;41:1063-1067.

Chapter 6

ADVANCES IN THE DIAGNOSIS AND CLASSIFICATION OF CHRONIC LYMPHOPROLIFERATIVE DISORDERS

Eric D. Hsi and John L. Frater
Department of Clinical Pathology, Cleveland Clinic Foundation , Cleveland, OH (EDH), and Department of Pathology, Northwestern University Feinberg School of Medicine, Chicago, IL (JLF)

1.   INTRODUCTION

The diagnosis and classification of the chronic lymphoproliferative disorders (mature B, T, and NK-cell leukemias/lymphomas, CLPDs) is constantly undergoing revision and refinement as more is learned about the pathology and clinical behavior of these diseases. Research in immunology and molecular genetics has also driven laboratory medicine and transformed our practice of hematopathology as technological advances make their way into the clinical laboratory. Although many of the disease entities that are recognized in the World Health Organization (WHO) classification have long been known, our ability to recognize important subgroups based on immunophenotypic and/or molecular genetic features has grown.

Many of the CLPDs present or commonly involve the blood and appear as mature lymphoid leukemias. It is from this viewpoint that we approach this review. Rather than providing a compendium of all the known lymphoid leukemias, we focus on those disorders in which there have been recent advances in our understanding of either their pathogenesis or diagnosis. Specifically we address new developments in chronic lymphocytic leukemia (CLL), prolymphocytic leukemia (PLL) and its relationship to mantle cell lymphoma (MCL), splenic marginal zone lymphoma (SMZL)/splenic lymphoma with villous lymphocytes, T-prolymphocytic leukemia (T-PLL), Sezary syndrome (SS), and T-cell large granular lymphocytic leukemias (T-LGL).

2. CHRONIC LYMPHOCYTIC LEUKEMIA (CLL)

From a pathologist's standpoint, the diagnosis of CLL can be relatively straightforward from examination of the blood smear and immunophenotyping. Most cases demonstrate the typical morphology of mature lymphocytes with condensed, clumped nuclear chromatin, round nuclear contours, and scanty cytoplasm. Routine use of multiparameter flow cytometry confirms the morphologic impression when the typical phenotype of CD5+, CD19+, CD20+ (usually low level expression), CD23+, CD79b dim/negative, FMC7 dim/negative, and surface immunoglobulin light chain restricted (often low level expression). While most cases fit this description well, there is heterogeneity in the pathologic features of CLL. Some cases show increased numbers of prolymphocytes or morphologic deviation with clefted lymphocytes or lymphocytes with more abundant cytoplasm. Such cases have been termed "atypical CLL" by some investigators.[1] Although definitions have differed, atypical CLL has been shown to also deviate from the typical immunophenotype (brighter FMC7, surface immunoglobulin, and CD23 expression)[2,3] and is associated with trisomy 12.[1,2,4] Atypical features also appear to correlate with worse outcome for these patients.[1-5] This heterogeneity from the pathologist's perspective confirms what clinicians have long since known - that CLL is a heterogeneous disorder. Although clinical staging systems have proven useful in stratifying patients, there are still patients in intermediate stages that rapidly progress while others have stable disease for years.[6-8]

In the post-genomic era we have the ability to add molecular-genetic information to refine our diagnosis. It may no longer be sufficient to only correctly diagnose CLL. Important genetic prognostic information or assessment for the presence of certain molecules that are the targets of specific therapies may be required. Although not yet standard of care, we need to be aware of developments that might advance our understanding of CLL as a disease entity and lead to diagnostic tests that will add clinical value to the diagnosis of CLL. We will focus on three areas could impact pathologists – chromosomal abnormalities and the prognosis of CLL, immunoglobulin heavy chain gene (*IGH*) mutational analysis and CD38 expression, and cDNA microarray data.

Standard karyotyping and application of fluorescence in situ hybridization (FISH) has given us the ability to begin to dissect the heterogeneity of CLL. Because of the inability to routinely define clonal abnormalities cytogenetically due to failure of CLL cells to grow in short term culture, the application of interphase FISH probes has been helpful in demonstrating common abnormalities. More than half of CLL cases have chromosomal abnormalities including deletions at 13q14, deletions of the genomic region 11q22.3-q23.1, trisomy 12, deletions of 6q21-q23, or deletions/mutations of the TP53 tumor suppressor gene at 17p13.[9] Clinicopathologic studies now show that certain genetic abnormalities correlate with pathologic features. As noted above trisomy 12, the second most common karyotypic abnormality, has been shown to correlate with atypical morphology.[2,10] Döhner and colleagues have now clearly shown the frequency and prognostic significance of detecting these abnormalities (Table 6-1).[9,11] Deletion at chromosome 13q14 is the most common abnormality, followed by trisomy 12 and del 11q. Deletion of 17p portends a very poor prognosis for CLL patients and might identify a patient for whom alternate therapies may be beneficial. Given these data, it can be argued that routine FISH testing should now be performed in CLL.

Table 6-1. Frequency of chromosomal abnormalities*[11]

Aberration	Percentage of cases
13q deletion	55
11q deletion	18
Trisomy 12	16
17p deletion	7
6q deletion	6
Trisomy 8q	5
t(14q32)	4
Trisomy 3q	3
Normal	18

*defined by FISH, some cases may have more than one abnormality

Perhaps the most intriguing recent finding is that of Hamblin and Damle who, in tandem publications, showed that *IGH* mutational status defined two distinct types of CLL patients.[12,13] This finding contradicted the previous theory that CLL cells were all derived from naïve B-cells with unmutated *IGH* genes.[14] The authors found that patients whose CLL cells had >2% deviation from germline sequence had a better prognosis than those patients with germline IGH sequences in their CLL cells. Since somatic mutation of the IGH gene is considered a feature of post-germinal center cells, this suggested that CLL might actually be two diseases,[15] although expression profiling suggests a more unified concept since there appears to be a common gene signature.[16] Damle and colleagues also suggested that CD38 expression correlated with IGH mutational status, predicted for poor patient outcome, and therefore might be a surrogate for IGH mutational status.[12] Subsequently several other studies were published that demonstrated the predictive value of CD38 expression in CLL. Although cutoff values may vary (7%-30%), CD38 expression by flow cytometry identifies a group of CLL patients with a worse survival compared to those patients that lack CD38 expression.[17-20] It also appears that CD38 is not well-correlated with IGH mutational status.[21]

Two studies recently published at the time of this writing synthesize many of these new prognostic factors and begin to shed some light on what may become important factors to routinely consider in the CLL patient.[20,22] Lin and colleagues showed that IGH mutational status (<5% mutated), CD38 expression >20%, and TP53 dysfunction were associated with poor survival. The authors suggested that the poor prognosis of the unmutated cases was perhaps due to over-representation of cases with p53 dysfunction and CD38 expression. The CD38 negative and TP53 intact cases did well regardless of IGH mutation.[22] Korber et al, however, found that in multivariate analysis, only mutational status, del(17p), del(11q), age, WBC, and LDH were independent prognostic factors.[20] Given the ease of quantifying CD38 expression by flow cytometry, it is likely that measurement of this antigen will be widely used. Efforts at standardizing its expression levels are appearing in the literature with promising results that suggest antigen quantitation improves the prognostic value of CD38 expression.[23,24]

The discovery of mutated and unmutated IGH genes as a predictor of prognosis has resulted in microarray experiments that have attempted to determine a genetic profile that might be useful in predicting mutational status and providing insight into the biology of CLL. The results serve as a model for translating high-density expression array data to a useful, single parameter test applicable in a clinical laboratory. Rosenwald and colleagues studied a series of CLL samples with the Lymphochip cDNA microarray, consisting of over 17,000 human cDNAs.[16] A model for differentiating mutated from unmutated CLL was found that consisted of approximately 175 genes that were significantly differentially expressed. Remarkably, the most differentially expressed gene, zeta-associated protein-70 (ZAP-70), could discriminate the cases with 100% accuracy and recent studies confirm the prognostic significance of ZAP-70 protein expression by flow cytometry.[16,25,26] ZAP-70 is a molecule normally expressed in T-cells and is involved in T-cell receptor signaling. Further studies examining the function of this molecule in CLL cells may help elucidate the biologic explanation for the poor prognosis of these patients.

3. PROLYMPHOCYTIC LEUKEMIA (PLL) AND ITS RELATIONSHIP TO MANTLE CELL LYMPHOMA (MCL)

MCL is a B-cell lymphoma with a characteristic translocation t(11;14)(q13;q32) resulting in the juxtaposition of the *BCL1/CCND1* gene on chromosome 11q13 with the *IGH* gene on chromosome 14q32. This produces a constitutively upregulated *BCL1/CCND1*-encoded cyclin D1 protein, an important cell cycle regulator. Like CLL, the malignant cells characteristically aberrantly express the T-cell associated antigen CD5, but unlike most cases of CLL, the malignant population is CD23 negative. The cells of MCL are predominantly small and mature-appearing, lack nucleoli, and have prominent nuclear clefts and folds. A variant form (blastoid variant) has been described with an immature chromatin pattern and prominent nucleoli.[27] It is important to distinguish MCL from other B-cell lymphomas of small lymphocytes because of the more aggressive nature of this entity.[28]

Chronic leukemias with the morphologic and immunophenotypic characteristics of prolymphocytes are encountered in clinical practice, and these are oftentimes malignancies that have evolved from antecedent cases of chronic lymphocytic leukemia.[29] A survey of 20 cases of mature B cell leukemias with > 55% prolymphocytes showed that several entities can have a similar peripheral blood appearance of prolymphocytic leukemia.[30] Among these is d*e novo* PLL, a rare B-cell malignancy characterized clinically by marked splenomegaly without lymphadenopathy and a marked peripheral lymphocytosis.[31] The cells of both *de novo* and secondary PLL are larger than mature lymphocytes, with slightly open chromatin and prominent nucleoli.[32] The cells express a mature B-cell immunophenotype, and approximately one-third of cases are CD5 positive. Most cases are CD23 negative.[33] Like MCL, this is a clinically aggressive neoplasm.

With the application of molecular cytogenetics, our concept of PLL is evolving. Wong and colleagues reported a small series of patients with morphologic and clinical features of PLL but, upon further investigation were best considered as the pleomorphic blastoid variants of MCL mimicking PLL.[34] Likewise, Schlette and colleagues showed a subset of their cases harbored the t(11;14)(q13;q32), characteristic of MCL.[30] Thus, B-PLL of the past is a heterogenous group of disorders that includes transformation of pre-existing CLL, a leukemic variant of MCL (standard terminology has not been agreed upon but includes nucleolated variant of MCL and prolymphocytoid variant of MCL[35]), and B-PLL. The latter currently would be a diagnosis of exclusion after ruling out the former two possibilities.

4.   RECENT ADVANCES IN MOLECULAR GENETICS OF SPLENIC LYMPHOMA WITH VILLOUS LYMPHOCYTES (SLVL)

SLVL (splenic marginal zone lymphoma, SMZL) is a rare entity characterized by a proliferation of post-germinal center B cells present initially in the spleen and bone marrow, generally with a lack of lymph node involvement at presentation. The clinical course is generally indolent. The cytogenetic and molecular biologic findings of SLVL/SMZL have been recently reviewed.[36]   The most commonly encountered genetic lesions in this lymphoma include loss of chromosome 7q31-q32 (up to 40% of cases) and trisomy 3 (17% of cases).[36-38]   Although the translocation t(11;14)(q13;q32) was encountered in occasional cases of SLVL/SMZL in the past, such cases are probably best interpreted as mantle cell lymphoma.[39]

Investigators are attempting to identify genes important in the pathogenesis of SMZL and are focusing on 7q31-q32. Originally described using conventional cytogenetic analysis, deletions of 7q31-32 have also been identified by fluorescence in situ hybridization (FISH), loss of heterozygosity studies, and comparative genomic hybridization (CGH).[37,40,41] Abnormalities of chromosome 7q are particularly common in this entity and are quite rare in other non-Hodgkin lymphomas.[42]   Because they are so frequently encountered in SLVL/SMZL, abnormalities of chromosome 7q may be an early and possibly transforming genetic event.

Detailed mapping by FISH and microsatellite analysis has revealed several hotspots in this region and a number of cases have been shown to have biallelic deletions, suggesting the presence of genes of pathogenetic importance in this region.[43]   In addition to deletions, genes of potential importance in lymphomagenesis have been suggested at 7q21 due to the presence of translocations involving this locus. Corcoran et al studied a small group of cases with translocations involving chromosome 7q.[44]   In cases with t(2;7)(p11;q21-q22), the chromosome 7 breakpoint was upstream from *CDK6*. In a case with t(7;21)(q22;q22), the breakpoint also involved the *CDK6* locus. In the cases tested with the translocation, the *CDK6* protein product was overexpressed which may result in dysregulation of the normal cell cycle.[44] This may play a role in the pathogenesis of at least some cases of SMZL.

Examination of the *IGH* gene mutational status in SMZL has modified our concept of the cell of origin of this lymphoma. Given the presumed post-germinal cell origin of SLVL/SMZL cells, it would follow that most if not all cases would have mutated IgV$_H$, like their putative normal counterpart cell type, the memory B cell of the marginal zone. Algara et al examined IgV$_H$ mutational status in 35 cases of SLVL/SMZL and found that the cases fell into two separate categories.[45] The first group had mutated IgV$_H$, consistent with post-germinal center origin. Almost half of the examined cases had unmutated IgV$_H$, an unexpected finding in a tumor of supposed origin from the marginal zone of the lymphoid follicle. Bahler and colleagues reported similar findings with the unmutated cases expressing IgD, consistent with a naïve B-cell origin.[46] Of interest, the cases with unmutated V$_H$ sequences were highly associated with chromosome 7q deletion and a more aggressive disease course.[45] There also appears to be a non-random use of VH genes from the VH1 and VH4 familes (VH1-2, VH1-69, and VH4-34).[45,46] Thus, there appears to be two types of SMZL, arising from memory-type and naïve B-cells.

Further examination of the *IGH* gene sequence has shown that those cases with mutated *IGH* genes show ongoing mutations,[47] as has been seen on other lymphomas such as follicular lymphoma and MALT-type lymphoma.[48] Taken together, these *IGH* gene studies suggest that B-cell antigen receptor stimulation and antigen selection are important in the development of this lymphoma in at least a subset of cases.

5.   MYCOSIS FUNGOIDES AND SEZARY SYNDROME

SS is generally regarded as the leukemic form of epidermotropic cutaneous T-cell lymphoma (MF). Clinically, SS is characterized by erythroderma, palmoplantar keratoderma, partial alopecia, lymphadenopathy, and pruritis. Atypical lymphocytes are seen in the blood and take the form of lymphocytes with grooved, "cerebriform" nuclei of large (typical Sezary cells,) or small (so-called Lutzner cells) size. Although originally described in 1961 by Tasell and Winkelmann,[49] the exact definition of SS is still not uniformly agreed upon. Disagreement revolves around both clinical issues and laboratory issues. Clinically, distinction is made by some authors between classical SS, in which patients develop signs and symptoms over a rapid period of time usually without a prior history of

MF, and erythrodermic MF. The latter is regarded by some investigators as a secondary erythroderma. Others would view these two situations as erythrodermic cutaneous T-cell lymphomas with differing tumor burdens.[50] Regardless, it is clear that Sezary cells are found in many patients with MF, supporting a close biologic relationship (if not identity) between SS and MF.[51] Thus, SS is best considered as the leukemic and erythrodermic variant of mycosis fungoides.[50]

Superimposed on these differing clinical views are the advances in molecular genetic techniques and immunophenotyping that are now available in clinical laboratories, allowing a more objective determination of leukemic involvement by malignant T-cells. Circulating Sezary cells appear to correlate with high clinical stage and the presence of extracutaneous disease.[52] Their presence (>5% of lymphocytes) portends a worse prognosis in patients with erythrodermic MF and SS.[53,54]

Traditionally, Sezary cells have been enumerated by morphologic review of the peripheral smear with the number of Sezary cells/100 lymphocytes and/or leukocytes reported. Some have classified the Sezary cells by size. Small Sezary cells have a diameter of <12 μm (smaller than a resting lymphocyte). Large Sezary cells have a diameter of greater than or equal to 12 μm, and very large obviously malignant Sezary cells are >14 μm.[50] However, there is no clear consensus on the percentage of Sezary cells needed for the diagnosis of SS.

In the original TNM classification for MF, the criterion of >5% Sezary cells (as a percentage of lymphocytes) was used, although its clinical significance was not known.[55,56] Vonderheid and colleagues demonstrated the poor prognostic significance of the presence of Sezary cells, particularly large Sezary cells (>14 μm diameter), in the blood of patients with MF on multivariate testing.[57] More recently, Kim and colleagues also demonstrated that patients with greater than 5% Sezary cells in the blood had a worse outcome compared to those that did not in multivariate analysis.[54,58] Other clinical studies subsequently showed that >20% Sezary cells in patients with MF also identified a patient group with a poor outcome.[59] In a multivariate analysis, this effect was not found for all patients; however, when considering intermediate tumor grades (T2/T3), presence of blood involvement predicted a poor survival.[59]

Unfortunately, the morphologic identification of Sezary cells is somewhat subjective, with Sezary-like cells being seen frequently in some patients with benign dermatoses and also in patients with clinical features of SS who lack detectable T-cell clones in the blood.[60,61] Thus other criteria were proposed. An *absolute* Sezary cell count threshold of 1000/μl was used to identify pre-SS patients (less or equal to 1000/μl) and was felt to be more clinically reliable than percentage.[62,63] Scarisbrick and colleagues recently demonstrated the clinical significance of tumor burden in the blood of patients with erythrodermic cutaneous T-cell lymphoma.[54] The investigators found that hematologic stage (based on gene rearrangement studies and absolute Sezary counts) was associated with poor survival in univariate analysis. The addition of hematologic criteria for Sezary syndrome appears to have been accepted and has been adopted by both the European Organization for Research and Treatment of Cancer (EORTC) and the International Society for Cutaneous Lymphomas.[50,64] Patients who do not meet the criteria for SS are considered "pre-SS" or "erythrodermic MF" patients.

In order to supplement morphologic assessment, flow cytometric and molecular genetic studies of blood have been performed to determine whether these techniques could be helpful in diagnosis and prognosis of MF/SS. Basic immunophenotyping has already been incorporated into the criteria for SS.[50,64] In addition to >1000 Sezary cells/μl, a CD4:CD8 ratio of >10 is required for a diagnosis of SS. This is based on data from the EORTC showing a dismal 11% 5-year survival for patients meeting this criterion. Deletion of CD7 is also commonly used but is limited by the fact that many cases of MF/SS express CD7, small populations of cells in benign conditions can lack CD7, and that CD7 expression is variable.[65-67]

Diagnostically there have been two developments in flow cytometric immunophenotyping. CD26, dipeptidyl aminopeptidase IV, is a multifunctional molecule that is present on some types of non-Hodgkin lymphomas. Flow cytometric studies have shown that the great majority of cases of SS lack CD26 expression and that this is a diagnostic feature useful in identifying Sezary cells in blood samples.[68,69] Jones and colleagues found decreased CD26 expression in T-cells in 66/69 samples of blood from patients with morphological involvement by Sezary cells or enlarged nucleolated cells. An abnormal population was not seen in any of the 14 blood samples from patients with chronic dermatoses and in only 1/10 samples from patients with an atypical cutaneous lymphoid infiltrate where the abnormal population comprised only 1% of the cells.[69] In this study, loss of CD7 expression, while useful, was more variable.[69] Bernengo et al studied blood from a large series of patients with SS and mycosis fungoides with blood involvement and also demonstrated that CD4+CD26- cells had morphology of Sezary cells. The percentage of Sezary cells correlated well with the percentage of CD4+CD26- cells by flow cytometry. The percentage of CD4+CD26- cells was significantly higher in samples of MF with blood involvement compared to patients without circulating Sezary cells. All but one patient with MF and blood involvement had >30%

CD4+/CD26- cells and all cases of SS had >40% of theses cells.[68] Thus, flow cytometry for CD4+CD26- cells can be used objectively to detect blood involvement in SS and MF. However, it is still unclear whether the expression characteristics of CD26 in this setting are a stable feature.

Use of T-cell receptor Vβ family specific antibodies is now being explored as a way to document T-cell clones. We have found a panel of directly conjugated Vβ antibodies can be used to demonstrate the particular Vβ family usage of the neoplastic cells in the blood of patients of SS.[70] This approach has also been used to follow patients with SS on treatment with phototherapy.[71,72] These flow cytometric methods have the added value of being quantitative, as opposed to molecular methods. They are of potential benefit in the identification of leukemic cells in patients with MF/SS and phenotypes appear stable over time.[73]

Although there is not complete consensus in the literature, the documentation of monoclonal T-cells in the blood of patients with MF, particularly if the clone is identical to that detected in the skin, appears to be a prognostic marker in MF/SS. Combining clonality data with more traditional staging, Fraser-Andrews et al found the TCR clonality, Sezary counts, and lymph node status were of prognostic importance in SS. In their series of 74 patients, a set of 8 patients with non-clonal Sezary cells was found. None of these patients suffered death from disease whereas 40/66 patients with clonal SS died of disease.[60] However, in multivariate analysis, only absolute Sezary count and lymph node status were independent prognostic factors for survival. Beylot-Barry further demonstrated that detection of identical clones in the skin and blood of patients with cutaneous T-cell lymphoma (MF and SS) was an independent prognostic factor for survival.[74] Of course, detection of a monoclonal T-cell population by molecular methods may occur in some benign conditions and careful interpretation of results is needed.[75,76] Despite this caveat, it is becoming evident that TCR gene rearrangement studies in blood are helpful in the diagnosis and prognosis of MF and SS. TCR gene rearrangement has also been added to the list of criteria necessary for the diagnosis of SS by the both the EORTC and the International Society for Cutaneous Lymphomas.[50,64]

This wealth of morphologic, phenotypic, and genotypic data all point to the usefulness of examining the blood for Sezary cells, phenotypic abnormalities, and T-cell monoclonality. However, as noted at the beginning of this section, there is still no uniformly accepted definition of SS. Two multicenter groups have developed criteria that are summarized in Table 6-2. Because of the subjectivity of morphologic identification and quantification of Sezary cells, these groups require a *combination* of clinical features, morphologic findings, clonality information, and phenotypic data to define SS. Use of these criteria will help to uniformly define SS and therefore better predict prognosis in these patients. It should serve as the framework for definitions in clinical trials. Additional studies with newer phenotypic tools described above will be needed to determine whether they add additional clinical information in the setting of diagnosis and disease monitoring in MF and SS.

Table6- 2. Criteria for Sezary Syndrome

International Society for Cutaneous Lymphomas	EORTC
Generalized erythroderma and one or more of the following:	Generalized erythroderma
Sezary cells 1000 cells/mm^3	Generalized lymphoadenopathy
CD4/CD8 ratio >10 due to increase in CD4+ or CD3+ T-cells	Lymphoma cells in skin, lymph node, and blood
Aberrant expression of pan-T cell antigens (CD2, CD4, CD5) by flow cytometry	CD4:CD8 ratio > 10*
Increased lymphocyte count with T-cell monoclonality by PCR or Southern blot	T-cell monoclonality*
Clonal karyotypic abnormality	*Useful additional criteria

From the biologic standpoint important recent evidence suggests that signal transducer and activator of transcription 3 (STAT3) is constitutively activated in Sezary cells.[77] Eriksen and colleagues reported that STAT3 was constitutively tyrosine phosphorylated in SS cell lines and that tyrosine kinase inhibitors AG490 inhibited IL-2 induced proliferation and caused apoptosis in SS cells. In support of this is the fact that the tyrosine phosphatase SHP-1 is decreased in Sezary cells with concomitant increase in JAK3 phosphorylation.[78] This would suggest an active JAK/STAT pathway. Constitutive Stat3 may lead to constitutive expression of SOCS-3 (a negative regulator of cytokine signalling) in SS cells[79] and appears to play a role in reduced sensitivity to inteferon-α. Studies such as these suggest not only that JAK-STAT pathways are relevant in SS biology but also that novel targeted therapy against tyrosine kinases might be useful in this disease.

6. T-CELL PROLYMPHOCYTIC LEUKEMIA (T-PLL) AND T-CELL CHRONIC LYMPHOCYTIC LEUKEMIA (T-CLL)

Most of the T cell non-Hodgkin lymphomas are relatively rare compared to their B cell counterparts in the Western world, and for this reason, have been less exhaustively studied. Among these uncommon disorders are the entities referred to variously as T-PLL and T-CLL. T-PLL is a rare peripheral T-cell leukemia/lymphoma with the following characteristics: an absolute lymphocytosis typically >100 x 10^9/L with concomitant hepatosplenomegaly, anemia, and thrombocytopenia. The incidence of lymphadenopathy and cutaneous involvement is variable.[80,81] Similar to their B-cell counterpart, the cells of T-PLL are larger than resting lymphocytes, with slightly less condensed chromatin and they often contain a single nucleolus. The cells display a post-thymic phenotype and typically express CD4. Most cases are CD8 negative, although dual CD4/CD8 expression is seen in a minority of cases (particularly in the small cell variant of T-PLL—see below). There is an increased incidence of T-PLL in patients with ataxia-telangiectasia, a genetically-determined defect in DNA repair. Recurrent chromosomal abnormalities are common and often multiple, including translocations involving either TCL1 at 14q32.1 or MTCP1 at Xq28, inactivation of the ATM gene (11q22-23) by deletion and/or mutation, del 13q, and isochromosome 8.[82] In particular, the chromosomal inversion inv14(q11q32) is a frequently recurring abnormality in T-PLL/T-CLL.

Previous reports of T-cell chronic lymphocytic leukemias can be found.[29] Given the significant clinical, immunophenotypic, and genetic overlap between T-PLL and T-CLL, the disorders likely are related.[83] Because T-CLL cells appear mature relative to those of T-PLL, early reports suggested that they be classified in a fashion analogous to their supposed B-cell counterparts. However, many of these cases may have been better classified as T-cell large granular lymphocytic leukemias or adult T-cell leukemia/lymphoma.[84] An indolent clinical course might be used as an argument for the existence of T-CLL; however, it is known that some cases of T-PLL may have an initial indolent phase.[85] Similar cytogenetic abnormalities in the indolent group compared to the more aggressive group and conversion to an aggressive phase suggest that these cases can be considered within the spectrum of T-PLL. Furthermore, studies of T-cell leukemias that resemble B-CLL morphologically show a prognosis essentially identical to T-PLL.[81,83,86] In view of these findings, "T-CLL" is best categorized as a subtype of T-PLL, (small cell variant of T-PLL). Rare cases of indolent T-CLL have been reported, but it is uncertain whether a distinct category is warranted.[87] Treatment of this disease with anti-CD52 antibodies now offers hope of remissions augments treatment strategies for patients.[88,89] Monitoring of CD52 expression may be required in patients treated with this agent as loss of expression has been documented.[90]

7.   T-CELL LARGE GRANULAR LYMPHOCYTIC LEUKEMIA: (T-LGL)

T-LGL is an indolent T-cell leukemia that occurs most commonly in middle-aged patients with a median age of 55 years. It was first recognized as a syndrome of increased large granular lymphocytes and chronic neutropenia.[91] Its neoplastic nature was confirmed by demonstrating clonal cytogenetic abnormalities and careful clinicopathologic characterization defined its morphologic and immunophenotypic features.[92,93] Autoimmune disorders such as rheumatoid arthritis are commonly present and T-LGL patients usually have associated cytopenias, which are often a major causes of morbidity for patients. Other recently described clinical associations include bone marrow failure syndromes such as paroxysmal nocturnal hemoglobinuria, aplastic anemia, myelodysplasia, and red cell aplasia, suggesting an important role for immune dysregulation as part of the pathogenesis of this disease.[94]

Morphologically one sees large granular lymphocytes in blood that may only be modestly increased in number and are cytologically normal. Since the normal number of LGLs is low (less than 520/μl) this can be easily overlooked.[95] Thus, the diagnosis is often difficult to make due to the low level of circulating leukemia cells without special studies such as flow cytometry or T-cell receptor gene rearrangement studies. The most common immunophenotype is a CD3+/CD8+ $\alpha\beta$ T-cell that also expresses CD57 and cytotoxic proteins such as TIA-1 and Granzyme B. Uncommon variants are CD4+, CD4+/CD8+, or $\gamma\delta$ T-cell type (CD4-/CD8-).[93,96,97] Gene rearrangement studies, which should be done in all suspected cases, demonstrate T-cell clonality although such assays may reveal an oligoclonal pattern in the background of a dominant clone.[98]

Bone marrow findings aided by immunohistochemistry in T-LGL have only recently been described.[99,100] As in the blood, bone marrow involvement can be subtle. Bone marrow cellularity is usually increased although normocellularity or hypocellularity can be seen. A left shift in granulocytic cells is common, perhaps as a compensatory mechanism in patients with neutropenia, along with a relative increase in erythroid elements.[99,100] Megakaryocytes are normal. The lymphoid infiltrate is best seen by immunostaining. An interstitial clustering of 8 or more CD8+ or TIA1+ T-cells or 6 or more Granzyme B+ cells is characteristic of T-LGL and is not seen in other reactive conditions. A subtle intravascular/intrasinusoidal pattern is also present, again seen best with the aid of immunostains.[100]

With the availability of antibodies having specificity to many of the TCR-Vβ families, flow cytometry for specific Vβ family usage has emerged as a rapid and specific way to document skewed T-cell repertoire and thus T-cell clonality.[98,101] Lima and colleagues showed an 81% sensitivity and 100% specificity when 60% of the total CD4+ or CD8+[bright] cells used a single Vβ family.[101] Using a commercially available kit consisting of 24 Vβ family antibodies in a multicolor format, we have demonstrated good performance in variety of T-cell leukemias in blood which may obviate the need for molecular studies in many cases.[70] However, because of incomplete T-cell repertoire coverage, a negative result must be further investigated with molecular studies. Such a flow cytometric assay also has the advantage of determining the particular Vβ family used by the leukemia for potential immunologic studies and may be a useful way to monitor therapy as has been done in SS.[102]

An uncommon indolent NK-cell variant has also been described that lacks surface CD3 but expresses CD16 and CD56.[93,95,103,104] Such patients may present without symptoms or may have difficulties due to cytopenias. Rare patients have vasculitis or nephrotic syndrome. This disease should be distinguished from aggressive NK-cell leukemia, which although of a similar immunophenotype, presents in younger patients with organomegaly, B-symptoms, and lacks an association with rheumatoid arthritis.[95,105] It is uncertain whether this indolent NK cell type of leukemia is truly neoplastic due to difficulty in demonstrating monoclonality in NK cells and whether this should be considered as a variant of T-LGL or as an indolent variant of aggressive NK-cell leukemia. However, recent advances in our understanding of the biology of NK cells and their receptors may allow the determination of clonality in NK cells. A restricted pattern of CD158a and CD158b expression has been shown in NK leukemias, most often the CD158a-/CD158b- subset.[106] Evaluation of killer inhibitory and activating receptors by flow cytometry for restricted expression patterns may be a way to assess clonality in NK cells and deserves further study as reagents become available.[107]

In the area of pathogenesis with potential for influencing targeted therapy of T-LGL, recent evidence points to abnormal apoptosis regulation as a mechanism both of the leukemic cell survival and as a cause for some of the cytopenias. Despite expression of both CD95 and CD95L,[108] the leukemic LGL cells are resistant to CD95 mediated death, possibly due to abnormal STAT3 activation. LGL cells were found to contain activated STAT3 and inhibition of JAK3 with the tyrphostin AG-490 or direct inhibition with STAT3 antisense lead to apoptosis. This was associated with decreased levels of the anti-apoptotic protein Mcl-1.[109]

8.   SUMMARY

In this review, we have highlighted recent advances in chronic lymphoproliferative disorders that commonly involve the peripheral blood. As we have seen, our concepts of certain diseases are changing. Molecular genetic and immunophenotypic studies are allowing more precise characterization of CLL and defining important biologic markers that predict clinical behavior. Prolymphocytic leukemia is now more narrowly defined and its relationship to nucleolated variants of MCL is now apparent. With new reagents and techniques applied to problems such as identification of Sezary cells and T-cell monoclonality determination, our ability to diagnose, monitor, and provide prognostic information is improving. Insight into the biology of these diseases also may provide new therapeutic targets in the future.

REFERENCES

1. Oscier DG, Matutes E, Copplestone A et al. Atypical lymphocyte morphology: an adverse prognostic factor for disease progression in stage A CLL independent of trisomy 12. Br J Haematol. 1997;98:934-939

2. Matutes E, Oscier D, Garcia-Marco J et al. Trisomy 12 defines a group of CLL with atypical morphology: correlation between cytogenetic, clinical and laboratory features in 544 patients. Br J Haematol. 1996;92:382-388

3. Frater JL, McCarron KF, Hammel JP et al. Typical and atypical chronic lymphocytic leukemia differ clinically and immunophenotypically. Am J Clin Pathol. 2001;116:655-664

4. Criel A, Verhoef G, Vlietinck R et al. Further characterization of morphologically defined typical and atypical CLL: a clinical, immunophenotypic, cytogenetic and prognostic study on 390 cases. Br J Haematol. 1997;97:383-391

5. Vallespi T, Montserrat E, Sanz MA. Chronic lymphocytic leukaemia: prognostic value of lymphocyte morphological subtypes. A multivariate survival analysis in 146 patients. Br J Haematol. 1991;77:478-485

6. Cheson BD, Bennett JM, Rai KR et al. Guidlines for clincial protocols for chronic lymphocytic leukemia: recommendations of the National Cancer Institute-Sponsored Working Group. Am J Hematol. 1988;29:152-163

7. Cheson BD, Bennett JM, Grever M et al. National Cancer Institute-sponsored Working Group guidelines for chronic lymphocytic leukemia: revised guidelines for diagnosis and treatment. Blood. 1996;87:4990-4997

8. Rai KR, Sawitsky A, Cronkite EP et al. Clinical staging of chronic lymphocytic leukemia. Blood. 1975;46:219-234

9. Dohner H, Stilgenbauer S, Dohner K et al. Chromosome aberrations in B-cell chronic lymphocytic leukemia: reassessment based on molecular cytogenetic analysis. J Mol Med. 1999;77:266-281

10.   Finn WG, Thangavelu M, Yelavarthi KK et al. Karyotype correlates with peripheral blood morphology and immunophenotype in chronic lymphocytic leukemia. Am J Clin Pathol. 1996;105:458-467

11.   Dohner H, Stilgenbauer S, Benner A et al. Genomic alterrations and survival in chronic lymphocytic leukemia. N Engl J Med 2000; 343:1910-1916

12.   Damle RN, Wasil T, Fais F et al. Ig V gene mutation status and CD38 expression As novel prognostic indicators in chronic lymphocytic leukemia. Blood. 1999;94:1840-1847

13.   Hamblin TJ, Davis Z, Gardiner A et al. Unmutated Ig V(H) genes are associated with a more aggressive form of chronic lymphocytic leukemia. Blood. 1999;94:1848-1854

14.   Meeker TC, Grimaldi JC, O'Rourke R et al. Lack of detectable somatic hypermutation in the V region of the Ig H chain gene of a human chronic B lymphocytic leukemia. J Immunol. 1988;141:3994-3998

15.   Hamblin T. Chronic lymphocytic leukaemia: one disease or two? Ann Hematol. 2002;81:299-303

16.   Rosenwald A, Alizadeh AA, Widhopf G et al. Relation of gene expression phenotype to immunoglobulin mutation genotype in B cell chronic lymphocytic leukemia. J Exp Med. 2001;194:1639-1647

17.   D'Arena G, Musto P, Cascavilla N et al. CD38 expression correlates with adverse biological features and predicts poor clinical outcome in B-cell chornic lymphocytic leukemia. Leuk Lymphoma. 2001;42:109-114

18.   Ibrahim S, Keating M, Do KA et al. CD38 expression as an important prognostic factor in B-cell chronic lymphocytic leukemia. Blood. 2001;98:181-186

19.   Jelinek DF, Tschumper RC, Geyer SM et al. Analysis of clonal B-cell CD38 and immunoglobulin variable region sequence status in relation to clinical outcome for B-chronic lymphocytic leukaemia. Br J Haematol. 2001;115:854-861

20.   Krober A, Seiler T, Benner A et al. V(H) mutation status, CD38 expression level, genomic aberrations, and survival in chronic lymphocytic leukemia. Blood. 2002;100:1410-1416

21.   Hamblin TJ, Orchard JA, Ibbotson RE et al. CD38 expression and immunoglobulin variable region mutations are independent prognostic variables in chronic lymphocytic leukemia, but CD38 expression may vary during the course of the disease. Blood. 2002;99:1023-1029

22.   Lin K, Sherrington PD, Dennis M et al. Relationship between p53 dysfunction, CD38 expression, and IgV(H) mutation in chronic lymphocytic leukemia. Blood. 2002;100:1404-1409

23.   Mainou-Fowler T, Dignum H, Taylor PR et al. Quantification improves the prognostic value of CD38 expression in B-cell chronic lymphocytic leukaemia. Br J Haematol. 2002;118:755-761

24.   Hsi ED, Kopecky KJ, Appelbaum FR et al. Prognostic Significance of CD38 and CD20 Expression as Assessed by Quantitative Flow Cytometry in Chronic Lymphocytic Leukemia (CLL). Br J Haematol. 2003; 120:1017-1025

25.   Crespo M, Bosch F, Villamor N et al. ZAP-70 expression as a surrogate for immunoglobulin-variable-region mutations in chronic lymphocytic leukemia. N Engl J Med. 2003;348:1764-1775

26.   Wiestner A, Rosenwald A, Barry TS et al. ZAP-70 expression identifies a chronic lymphocytic leukemia subtype with unmutated immunoglobulin genes, inferior clinical outcome, and distinct gene expression profile. Blood. 2003

27.   Ott G, Kalla J, Hanke A et al. The cytomorphological spectrum of mantle cell lymphoma is reflected by distinct biological features. Leuk Lymphoma. 1998;32:55-63
28.   Argatoff LH, Connors JM, Klasa RJ et al. Mantle cell lymphoma: a clinicopathologic study of 80 cases. Blood. 1997;89:2067-2078
29.   Bennett JM, Catovsky D, Daniel MT et al. Proposals for the classification of chronic (mature) B and T lymphoid leukaemias. French-American-British (FAB) Cooperative Group. J Clin Pathol. 1989;42:567-584
30.   Schlette E, Bueso-Ramos C, Giles F et al. Mature B-cell leukemias with more than 55% prolymphocytes. A heterogeneous group that includes an unusual variant of mantle cell lymphoma. Am J Clin Pathol. 2001;115:571-581
31.   Dalton DAG, Goldman JM, Wiltshaw E et al. Prolymphocytic leukemia. Br J Haematol. 1974;27:7-23
32.   Jaffe ES, Harris NL, Stein H et al. Tumours of Haematopoeitic and Lymphoid Tissues. 2001; Lyon: IARC Press
33.   Matutes E, Owusu-Ankomah K, Morilla R et al. The immunological profile of B-cell disorders and proposal of a scoring system for the diagnosis of CLL. Leukemia. 1994;8:1640-1645
34.   Wong KF, So CC, Chan JK. Nucleolated variant of mantle cell lymphoma with leukemic manifestations mimicking prolymphocytic leukemia. Am J Clin Pathol. 2002;117:246-251
35.   Dunphy CH, Perkins SL. Mantle cell leukemia, prolymphocytoid type: a rarely described form. Leuk Lymphoma. 2001;41:683-687
36.   Franco V, Florena AM, Iannitto E. Splenic marginal zone lymphoma. Blood. 2003;101:2464-2472
37.   Mateo M, Mollejo M, Villuendas R et al. 7q31-32 allelic loss is a frequent finding in splenic marginal zone lymphoma. Am J Pathol. 1999;154:1583-1589
38.   Gruszka-Westwood AM, Matutes E, Coignet LJ et al. The incidence of trisomy 3 in splenic lymphoma with villous lymphocytes: a study by FISH. Br J Haematol. 1999;104:600-604
39.   Oscier DG, Matutes E, Gardiner A et al. Cytogenetic studies in splenic lymphoma with villous lymphocytes. Br J Haematol. 1993;85:487-491
40.   Hernandez JM, Garcia JL, Gutierrez NC et al. Novel genomic imbalances in B-cell splenic marginal zone lymphomas revealed by comparative genomic hybridization and cytogenetics. Am J Pathol. 2001;158:1843-1850
41.   Sole F, Salido M, Espinet B et al. Splenic marginal zone B-cell lymphomas: two cytogenetic subtypes, one with gain of 3q and the other with loss of 7q. Haematologica. 2001;86:71-77
42.   Hernandez JM, Mecucci C, Criel A et al. Cytogenetic analysis of B cell chronic lymphoid leukemias classified according to morphologic and immunophenotypic (FAB) criteria. Leukemia. 1995;9:2140-2146
43.   Gruszka-Westwood AM, Hamoudi R, Osborne L et al. Deletion mapping on the long arm of chromosome 7 in splenic lymphoma with villous lymphocytes. Genes Chromosomes Cancer. 2003;36:57-69
44.   Corcoran MM, Mould SJ, Orchard JA et al. Dysregulation of cyclin dependent kinase 6 expression in splenic marginal zone lymphoma through chromosome 7q translocations. Oncogene. 1999;18:6271-6277

45. Algara P, Mateo MS, Sanchez-Beato M et al. Analysis of the IgV(H) somatic mutations in splenic marginal zone lymphoma defines a group of unmutated cases with frequent 7q deletion and adverse clinical course. Blood. 2002;99:1299-1304

46. Bahler DW, Pindzola JA, Swerdlow SH. Splenic marginal zone lymphomas appear to originate from different B cell types. Am J Pathol. 2002;161:81-88

47. Dunn-Walters DK, Boursier L, Spencer J et al. Analysis of immunoglobulin genes in splenic marginal zone lymphoma suggests ongoing mutation. Hum Pathol. 1998;29:585-593

48. Bahler DW, Miklos JA, Swerdlow SH. Ongoing Ig gene hypermutation in salivary gland mucosa- associated lymphoid tissue-type lymphomas. Blood. 1997;89:3335-3344

49. Taswell H, Winkelmann R. Sezary syndrome - a malignant reticulemic erythroderma. JAMA. 1961;117:465-472

50. Vonderheid EC, Bernengo MG, Burg G et al. Update on erythrodermic cutaneous T-cell lymphoma: report of the International Society for Cutaneous Lymphomas. J Am Acad Dermatol. 2002;46:95-106

51. Flandrin G, Brouet JC. The Sezary cell: cytologic, cytochemical, and immunologic studies. Mayo Clin Proc. 1974;49:575-583

52. Hoppe RT, Wood GS, Abel EA. Mycosis fungoides and the Sezary syndrome: pathology, staging, and treatment. Curr Probl Cancer. 1990;14:293-371

53. Kim YH, Bishop K, Varghese A et al. Prognostic factors in erythrodermic mycosis fungoides and the Sezary syndrome. Arch Dermatol. 1995;131:1003-1008

54. Scarisbrick JJ, Whittaker S, Evans AV et al. Prognostic significance of tumor burden in the blood of patients with erythrodermic primary cutaneous T-cell lymphoma. Blood. 2001;97:624-630

55. Bunn PA, Jr., Huberman MS, Whang-Peng J et al. Prospective staging evaluation of patients with cutaneous T-cell lymphomas. Demonstration of a high frequency of extracutaneous dissemination. Ann Intern Med. 1980;93:223-230

56. Lamberg SI, Bunn PA, Jr. Cutaneous T-Cell Lymphomas: Summary of the mycosis fungoides cooperative group-national cancer institute workshop. Arch Dermatol. 1979;115:1103-1105

57. Vonderheid EC, Sobel EL, Nowell PC et al. Diagnostic and prognostic significance of Sezary cells in peripheral blood smears from patients with cutaneous T cell lymphoma. Blood. 1985;66:358-366

58. Kim YH, Bishop K, Varghese A et al. Prognostic factors in erythrodermic mycosis fungoides and the Sezary syndrome. Arch Dermatol. 1995;131:1003-1008

59. Schechter GP, Sausville EA, Fischmann AB et al. Evaluation of circulating malignant cells provides prognostic information in cutaneous T cell lymphoma. Blood. 1987;69:841-849

60. Fraser-Andrews EA, Russell-Jones R, Woolford AJ et al. Diagnostic and prognostic importance of T-cell receptor gene analysis in patients with Sezary syndrome. Cancer. 2001;92:1745-1752

61. Duncan SC, Winkelmann RK. Circulating Sezary cells in hospitalized dermatology patients. Br J Dermatol. 1978;99:171-178

62. Winkelmann RK, Diaz-Perez JL, Buechner SA. The treatment of Sezary syndrome. J Am Acad Dermatol. 1984;10:1000-1004

63. Winkelmann RK, Peters MS. Absolute number of circulatory sezary cells. Arch Dermatol. 1981;117:382

64.   Willemze R, Kerl H, Sterry W et al. EORTC classification for primary cutaneous lymphomas: a proposal from the Cutaneous Lymphoma Study Group of the European Organization for Research and Treatment of Cancer. Blood. 1997;90:354-371

65.   Bogen SA, Pelley D, Charif M et al. Immunophenotypic identification of Sezary cells in peripheral blood. Am J Clin Pathol. 1996;106:739-748

66.   Harmon CB, Witzig TE, Katzmann JA et al. Detection of circulating T cells with CD4+CD7- immunophenotype in patients with benign and malignant lymphoproliferative dermatoses. J Am Acad Dermatol. 1996;35:404-410

67.   Vonderheid EC, Bigler RD, Kotecha A et al. Variable CD7 expression on T cells in the leukemic phase of cutaneous T cell lymphoma (Sezary syndrome). J Invest Dermatol. 2001;117:654-662

68.   Bernengo MG, Novelli M, Quaglino P et al. The relevance of the CD4+ CD26- subset in the identification of circulating Sezary cells. Br J Dermatol. 2001;144:125-135

69.   Jones D, Dang NH, Duvic M et al. Absence of CD26 expression is a useful marker for diagnosis of T-cell lymphoma in peripheral blood. Am J Clin Pathol. 2001;115:885-892

70.   Beck RC, Stahl S, O'Keefe CL et al. Detection of mature T cell leukemias by flow cytometry using anti-T cell receptor Vβ antibodies. Am J Clin Pathol. 2003;In Press

71.   Ingen-Housz-Oro S, Bussel A, Flageul B et al. A prospective study on the evolution of the T-cell repertoire in patients with Sezary syndrome treated by extracorporeal photopheresis. Blood. 2002;100:2168-2174

72.   Schwab C, Willers J, Niederer E et al. The use of anti-T-cell receptor-Vbeta antibodies for the estimation of treatment success and phenotypic characterization of clonal T-cell populations in cutaneous T-cell lymphomas. Br J Haematol. 2002;118:1019-1026

73.   Washington LT, Huh YO, Powers LC et al. A stable aberrant immunophenotype characterizes nearly all cases of cutaneous T-cell lymphoma in blood and can be used to monitor response to therapy. BMC Clin Pathol. 2002;2:5

74.   Beylot-Barry M, Sibaud V, Thiebaut R et al. Evidence that an identical T cell clone in skin and peripheral blood lymphocytes is an independent prognostic factor in primary cutaneous T cell lymphomas. J Invest Dermatol. 2001;117:920-926

75.   Weinberg JM, Jaworsky C, Benoit BM et al. The clonal nature of circulating Sezary cells. Blood. 1995;86:4257-4262

76.   Muche JM, Lukowsky A, Heim J et al. Demonstration of frequent occurrence of clonal T cells in the peripheral blood but not in the skin of patients with small plaque parapsoriasis. Blood. 1999;94:1409-1417

77.   Eriksen KW, Kaltoft K, Mikkelsen G et al. Constitutive STAT3-activation in Sezary syndrome: tyrphostin AG490 inhibits STAT3-activation, interleukin-2 receptor expression and growth of leukemic Sezary cells. Leukemia. 2001;15:787-793

78.   Leon F, Cespon C, Franco A et al. SHP-1 expression in peripheral T cells from patients with Sezary syndrome and in the T cell line HUT-78: implications in JAK3-mediated signaling. Leukemia. 2002;16:1470-1477

79.   Brender C, Nielsen M, Kaltoft K et al. STAT3-mediated constitutive expression of SOCS-3 in cutaneous T-cell lymphoma. Blood. 2001;97:1056-1062

80.   Bartlett NL, Longo DL. T-small lymphocyte disorders. Semin Hematol. 1999;36:164-170

81.   Matutes E, Brito-Babapulle V, Swansbury J et al. Clinical and laboratory features of 78 cases of T-prolymphocytic leukemia. Blood. 1991;78:3269-3274

82.   Soulier J, Pierron G, Vecchione D et al. A complex pattern of recurrent chromosomal losses and gains in T-cell prolymphocytic leukemia. Genes Chromosomes Cancer. 2001;31:248-254

83.   Matutes E, Catovsky D. Similarities between T-cell chronic lymphocytic leukemia and the small-cell variant of T-prolymphocytic leukemia. Blood. 1996;87:3520-3521

84.   Berliner N. T gamma lymphocytosis and T cell chronic leukemias. Hematol Oncol Clin North Am. 1990;4:473-487

85.   Garand R, Goasguen J, Brizard A et al. Indolent course as a relatively frequent presentation in T-prolymphocytic leukaemia. Groupe Francais d'Hematologie Cellulaire. Br J Haematol. 1998;103:488-494

86.   Hoyer JD, Ross CW, Li CY et al. True T-cell chronic lymphocytic leukemia: a morphologic and immunophenotypic study of 25 cases. Blood. 1995;86:1163-1169

87.   Soma L, Cornfield DB, Prager D et al. Unusually indolent T-cell prolymphocytic leukemia associated with a complex karyotype: is this T-cell chronic lymphocytic leukemia? Am J Hematol. 2002;71:224-226

88.   Dearden CE, Matutes E, Catovsky D. Alemtuzumab in T-cell malignancies. Med Oncol. 2002;19 Suppl:S27-S32

89.   Dearden CE, Matutes E, Cazin B et al. High remission rate in T-cell prolymphocytic leukemia with CAMPATH-1H. Blood. 2001;98:1721-1726

90.   Tuset E, Matutes E, Brito-Babapulle V et al. Immunophenotype changes and loss of CD52 expression in two patients with relapsed T-cell prolymphocytic leukaemia. Leuk Lymphoma. 2001;42:1379-1383

91.   McKenna RW, Parkin J, Kersey JH et al. Chronic lymphoproliferative disorder with unusual clinical, morphologic, ultrastructural and membrane surface marker characteristics. Am J Med. 1977;62:588-596

92.   Loughran TP, Jr., Kadin ME, Starkebaum G et al. Leukemia of large granular lymphocytes: association with clonal chromosomal abnormalities and autoimmune neutropenia, thrombocytopenia, and hemolytic anemia. Ann Intern Med. 1985;102:169-175

93.   Loughran TP, Jr. Clonal diseases of large granular lymphocytes. Blood. 1993;82:1-14

94.   Karadimitris A, Li K, Notaro R et al. Association of clonal T-cell large granular lymphocyte disease and paroxysmal nocturnal haemoglobinuria (PNH): further evidence for a pathogenetic link between T cells, aplastic anaemia and PNH. Br J Haematol. 2001;115:1010-1014

95.   Lamy T, Loughran TP, Jr. Current concepts: large granular lymphocyte leukemia. Blood Rev. 1999;13:230-240

96.   Chan WC, Catovsky D, Foucar K et al. T-cell large granular lymphocyte leukemia. In: Jaffe ES, Harris NL, Stein H et al., eds. Tumours of Haematopoietic and Lymphoid TIssues.2001; Lyon: IARC Press

97.   Semenzato G, Zambello R, Starkebaum G et al. The lymphoproliferative disease of granular lymphocytes: updated criteria for diagnosis. Blood. 1997;89:256-260

98.   Langerak AW, van Den BR, Wolvers-Tettero IL et al. Molecular and flow cytometric analysis of the Vbeta repertoire for clonality assessment in mature TCRalphabeta T-cell proliferations. Blood. 2001;98:165-173

99.   Evans HL, Burks E, Viswanatha D et al. Utility of immunohistochemistry in bone marrow evaluation of T-lineage large granular lymphocyte leukemia. Hum Pathol. 2000;31:1266-1273

100. Morice WG, Kurtin PJ, Tefferi A et al. Distinct bone marrow findings in T-cell granular lymphocytic leukemia revealed by paraffin section immunoperoxidase stains for CD8, TIA-1, and granzyme B. Blood. 2002;99:268-274

101. Lima M, Almeida J, Santos AH et al. Immunophenotypic analysis of the TCR-Vbeta repertoire in 98 persistent expansions of CD3(+)/TCR-alphabeta(+) large granular lymphocytes: utility in assessing clonality and insights into the pathogenesis of the disease. Am J Pathol. 2001;159:1861-1868

102. Ingen-Housz-Oro S, Bussel A, Flageul B et al. A prospective study on the evolution of the T-cell repertoire in patients with Sezary syndrome treated by extracorporeal photopheresis. Blood. 2002;100:2168-2174

103. Rabbani GR, Phyliky RL, Tefferi A. A long-term study of patients with chronic natural killer cell lymphocytosis. Br J Haematol. 1999;106:960-966

104. Morice WG, Leibson PJ, Tefferi A. Natural killer cells and the syndrome of chronic natural killer cell lymphocytosis. Leuk Lymphoma. 2001;41:277-284

105. Imamura N, Kusunoki Y, Kawa-Ha K et al. Aggressive natural killer cell leukaemia/lymphoma: report of four cases and review of the literature. Possible existence of a new clinical entity originating from the third lineage of lymphoid cells. Br J Haematol. 1990;75:49-59

106. Zambello R, Trentin L, Ciccone E et al. Phenotypic diversity of natural killer (NK) populations in patients with NK-type lymphoproliferative disease of granular lymphocytes. Blood. 1993;81:2381-2385

107. Morice WG, Hanson CA, Tefferi A et al. Demonstration of aberrant T and NK cell antigen expression in all cases of granular lymphocytic leukemia. Mod Pathol. 2002;15:256a

108. Lamy T, Liu JH, Landowski TH et al. Dysregulation of CD95/CD95 ligand-apoptotic pathway in CD3(+) large granular lymphocyte leukemia. Blood. 1998;92:4771-4777

109. Epling-Burnette PK, Liu JH, Catlett-Falcone R et al. Inhibition of STAT3 signaling leads to apoptosis of leukemic large granular lymphocytes and decreased Mcl-1 expression. J Clin Invest. 2001;107:351-362

Chapter 7

LABORATORY HEMATOLOGY PRACTICE
Present and Future

Gerald M. Davis, Kay Lynne Lantis, William G. Finn
University of Michigan, Ann Arbor, MI

1. INTRODUCTION

Since the 1960s, the complete blood count (CBC) (the most frequently ordered test in the clinical hematology laboratory) has been performed by automated methods in most laboratories.[1] Initial analyzers were essentially less sophisticated versions of today's impedance particle counters, in which a stream of particles (blood cells) was sent through an aperture between two electrically charged electrolyte baths. Impedance of the voltage potential between the two baths would register the presence of each particle as it passed through, and the magnitude of the voltage impedance was proportional to the volume of the cell, allowing for direct measurement of mean corpuscular volume (MCV) in red cell populations and discrimination of platelets and other cells based on volume thresholds. Direct measurement of red blood cell volume also allowed for the development of a new basic red cell index, the red cell distribution width (RDW). The RDW represents the coefficient of variation of the red cell volume distribution, and provides an objective measurement of erythrocyte anisocytosis (an index previously limited to subjective interpretation from blood smear microscopy).[2]

All major automated hematology analyzers now use some combination of impedance technology combined with flow-cytometric laser optical analysis, allowing for accurate five and six-part automated leukocyte differential counts in addition to basic CBC indices.[3] Some systems rely mainly on impedance and laser light scatter (e.g. Beckman-Coulter),[4,5] and some systems additionally include cytochemical analysis (e.g. Bayer-Advia, ABX-

Pentra)[6,7] or fluorescent dye-based flow cytometric methods (e.g. Sysmex, Abbott Cell-Dyn).[7,8] All of these major manufacturers offer systems that allow for the measurement and reporting of highly accurate and precise automated differential leukocyte counts based upon the combination of these technologies.

2.   OPTIMIZING CURRENT LABORATORY HEMATOLOGY PRACTICE

Clinical practitioners currently enjoy the services of highly advanced clinical hematology laboratories that provide timely and accurate results. Despite rapid advances over the last four decades, the current practice of laboratory hematology is still based upon a sometimes awkward mixture of scientifically-derived principles, and lore passed down through tradition but not formally or scientifically validated. As a result, many laboratories maintain suboptimal practices, justified by their common usage, and by the acceptance of laboratory directors and users of laboratory services, but not always justified by scientific data. Laboratory hematology practice is optimized when automated systems are allowed to do what they do best, freeing up laboratory staff to perform only those functions that require subjective or complex human intervention.

2.1   Automated Versus Manual Blood Analysis

Major clinical laboratories perform CBCs and leukocyte differential counts by automated methods. Modern automated hematology analyzers offer rapid, high throughput analysis, low cost-per-test, high precision (due to both the high number of cells analyzed and excellent between-run reproducibility), and superb accuracy. Current automated systems are limited by an inability to quantify certain cell types (such as blasts and immature granulocyte forms), and they also require manual validation from time to time due to the presence of abnormal cell types or interference from matrix components such as cryoglobulin, icteric pigment, debris from incompletely lysed red blood cells, etc. Fortunately, all modern analyzers provide instrument warnings (or "flags") that alert users to the suspected presence of abnormal cells or analytical interference, allowing the user to make informed decisions as to which automated results require manual review or validation.

The manner in which such flagged results are further analyzed varies among different laboratories. Value is added when slide review is considered as a confirmatory test for a flagged automated result, and the manual differential count is performed only when the human eye has detected the presence of elements beyond the scope of the automated system's capabilities.[9-12] Unfortunately, however, many labs still replace automated counts with manual differential leukocyte counts solely based upon the presence of instrument flags. Such an approach raises problems. For instance, an instrument flag may be issued for suspicion of cell types not actually in the blood sample (false positives), resulting in the replacement of a perfectly valid automated differential count by the less accurate and less precise manual differential count. Indeed, previous studies have confirmed that the flagging systems in hematology analyzers tend toward false-positive flagging, with false-negative rates that are considerably lower than those seen by manual blood smear review.[5,13,14] Furthermore, manual differential counts are often performed due to the presence of solely *quantitative* abnormalities, even when individual cell identification is not in question. For instance, markedly elevated absolute lymphocyte counts in patients with known chronic lymphocytic leukemia may lead to manual differential counts, when the only real reason for manual review (aside from medical interpretation—see below) is confirmation that the cells in question are in fact lymphocytes and not another abnormal cell type such as blasts or large lymphoma cells. Clinical decision making in such cases may rely heavily upon release of precise and accurate absolute cell counts (in particular absolute neutrophil counts), which are much better assessed by automated methods.

It is useful to consider the hypothetical case of a leukemia patient with a leukocyte count of 100×10^9/L and a differential count of 98% lymphocytes and 2% neutrophils. Such a result would be flagged for further review in most laboratories. An automated 10,000-cell differential count would yield an absolute neutrophil count of $2 \pm 0.3 \times 10^9$/L (a clinically useful result), whereas a reflexively performed manual 100-cell differential count would yield an absolute neutrophil count of $2 \pm 5 \times 10^9$/L (not a clinically useful result). As noted above, manual review in such a case should be aimed at verifying that the cells counted by the instrument are indeed lymphocytes. Once such validation is made, then the automated result can be released to the patient record.

Although there is no clinical rationale for reflexively performing manual leukocyte differential counts based solely upon instrument flags, prior to a manual triage step,[12] it is important to distinguish between *validation* and *medical interpretation* in the clinical hematology lab. For example, although the manual *validation* of absolute lymphocytosis may not require performance of a manual differential count, it still may be necessary to issue a *medical interpretation* of such a case by a hematopathologist or other qualified physician regarding the nature of the circulating lymphocytes, and the likelihood of chronic lymphocytic leukemia or other leukemic lymphoproliferative disorder.

2.2   Red Blood Cell Morphology

Abnormalities of red blood cells account for a high percentage of manual blood smear reviews in the clinical hematology laboratory,[12] but properly interpreting red cell abnormalities is a deceptively difficult task.   Many clinical-morphologic correlates are well-established through decades of accumulated anecdotal experience and in vitro analysis[15] and are likely appropriate for clinical practice, but there are actually very few objective or scientific data indicating the sensitivity, specificity, or predictive value of specific red cell morphologic abnormalities for clinical decision making.

Automation is likely underutilized in the assessment of red cell morphology.[16-18] For example, many laboratories still issue subjective comments of "anisocytosis" despite the simultaneous reporting of the measured red cell distribution width (RDW)—a precise and reproducible numerical measure of anisocytosis.[19] Likewise, it appears awkward when a patient with a mean corpuscular volume of 65 fL is reported to have "occasional microcytes." Although assessment of red cell morphology on a peripheral blood smear is important, there are many clinical situations for which such an exam adds little value.   In such cases, automated red cell parameters (RBC count, hemoglobin, hematocrit, MCV, MCH, MCHC, and RDW) give an accurate representation of red cell status. For instance, an adult patient with markedly decreased hemoglobin, markedly decreased MCV, markedly elevated RDW, and no circulating nucleated red cells (as measured on a hematology analyzer) ought to be evaluated for iron deficiency anemia.   Review of the peripheral blood smear in such a case is of educational interest and could be considered a component of a complete evaluation, but adds little incremental value to the medical workup.   In contrast, the initial workup of sickle cell anemia or other morphologically distinct hemoglobinopathy may require careful manual assessment of red cell morphology on a properly prepared blood smear in order to appropriately select further procedures for diagnostic confirmation.

Previous studies have focused upon the use of red blood cell indices from automated analyzers to predict for certain types of red cell poikilocytosis,[17] or to distinguish among different causes of anemia.[16,18] In addition, hematology systems have been capable of performing automated reticulocyte counts for some time, and more recent technology allows for automated measurement of nucleated red cells, immature reticulocyte fractions, and even reticulocyte hemoglobin concentration.[20] Recent studies have applied the expanded capabilities of newer hematology analyzers, and the principles of flow cytometry to the assessment of red cell abnormalities,[21,22] and these technologies show great promise for more reproducible and clinically relevant red cell morphology analysis. Clearly, the useful application of red cell morphology reporting to clinical practice will require a fundamental reappraisal of the clinical relevance of red cell abnormalities as detected in the clinical laboratory.

2.3 Autoverification in the Clinical Hematology Laboratory

As analytical methods in automated laboratories become faster and more efficient, the rate-determining step for the release of information to the patient record is no longer the generation of data, but our ability to process and manage data. Medical technologists are responsible for numerous complex and integrated tasks in the clinical laboratory that require subjective or interpretive skill. In addition to these necessarily manual tasks, however, many of the decisions made by medical technologists involve numerical calculations, comparisons, or Boolean algorithms, which are readily adaptable (and more consistently and reliably performed) by automated methods. Therefore, one can design automated systems that exactly recapitulate decision algorithms carried out manually by technologists, and these systems can be further expanded to include decision logic that cannot be practically deployed by manual methods.[23-26] Autoverification is almost certainly underutilized in the clinical hematology laboratory community; indeed, most published information regarding autoverification appears in publications aimed at administrators and technologists. It behooves clinical pathologists and laboratory directors to become familiar with the concepts of autoverification as part of optimizing information management in the clinical laboratory.

Most laboratory information system (LIS) vendors offer autoverification software that allows for user-defined options regarding specific ranges and values acceptable for autoverification, mirroring manual verification steps that exist under the laboratory's policy. The deployment of these applications provides for the auto-release of results to the patient record in real time, if established criteria are met. Criteria are set for autoverification (see Table 7-1) based on pre-defined ranges for each parameter in the CBC, and the type of delta checking (comparison of current and previous results for the same analyte for a given patient) used for that parameter. Such a system currently results in autoverification rates between 72 and 84 percent in our laboratory.

The delta check criteria used in the set-up have become more sophisticated than most manual criteria used because computers are able to delta check previous results using standardized criteria. LIS vendors offer many sophisticated kinds of delta checking, including percentage difference from current to previous result over a user defined period, or absolute value between current and previous result, with or without proration.

The avoidance of posting errant results to the patient chart is an overriding concern with the design of autoverification systems. Strategies like the one outlined in Table 7-1 allow the autoverification of abnormal CBC results, but keep a tight delta check around the MCV and RDW. This is done so that misidentified samples can be detected. Due to the stability of the MCV and RDW within a given patient, the hematology laboratory is often the first to suspect a misidentified specimen, and is then able to alert other clinical areas that have received specimens from the same draw. Autoverification software packages offered by most LIS vendors have user designed options that suppress autoverification of results from other parameters within the blood survey when a delta fail, critical value, or out of range result is encountered. Configuration of the autoverification criteria as a strategy brings added value to the design.

Table 7-1. Typical instrument-driven criteria for autoverification of complete blood count results (not including the leukocyte differential count)

Test	Range	Delta Check Percent	Delta Check Value
WBC	2.0 to 50.0 x 10^9/L	50	NA
RBC	2.00 to 8.00 x 10^{12}/L	50	NA
HGB	8.0 to 20.0 gm/dL	NA	4.0
HCT	23.0 to 60.0%	NA	12.0
MCV	50.0 to 110.0 fL	NA	3.0
MCH	None	10	NA
MCHC	30.0 to 60.0%	NA	3.0
RDW	None	NA	2.5
PLT	20 to 1000 x 10^9/L	50	NA
MPV	None	NA	2.5

WBC=leukocyte count, RBC=erythrocyte count, HGB=hemoglobin, HCT=hematocrit, MCV=mean corpuscular volume, MCH=mean corpuscular hemoglobin, MCHC=mean corpuscular hemoglobin concentration, RDW=red cell distribution width, PLT=platelet count, MPV=mean platelet volume

The automated leukocyte differential count is usually managed differently than the CBC by autoverification software. Using instrument-level autoverification software, dependent largely upon result ranges and delta-checks, is effective for basic CBC indices (hemoglobin, hematocrit, MCV, MCH, MCHC, leukocyte count, platelet count, and MPV), but may not be sufficient for handling the complexity of leukocyte differential counts. For this purpose, *rules based systems* are more effective.[24,25] Unlike more basic autoverification systems, rules based systems employ Boolean or "if, then" type logic to assure certain requirements are met prior to release of results, and to exactly recapitulate the steps that should be taken by a human observer prior to result verification.

The rule system we use at the University of Michigan for autoverification of the automated differential count is depicted in Figure 7-1. This system is highly effective in helping to manage a high-throughput and complex patient base that includes general and specialty care services (both inpatient and outpatient) for an approximately 1000-bed medical center that generates over 1200 CBC requests per weekday. High execution rates for autoverification (about 80% of all automated hematology orders in our laboratory) shift the workflow focus from the mundane to the specialized for laboratory personnel. The resulting decrease in turnaround time changes the dynamics of the clinical hematology laboratory and enables trained professionals to use specialized skills to improve patient care.

In an autoverification algorithm like the one in Figure 7-1, the rule system is triggered as results from the automated leukocyte differential count are transmitted from the instrument to the LIS. If all criteria are met, autoverification is executed. It is impractical for realistic purposes for the LIS to capture the changing variety of instrument flagging in reference to the automated differential count. Therefore, a common strategy used by some LIS vendors is to have the ability to detect when there are no flags present in combination with the autoverified WBC. When none of the automated differential count values is flagged, autoverification is triggered to execute. Thus the rules-based system is used selectively, and only when dictated by the WBC and differential count results.

The verification of the WBC differential (automated or manual) also triggers the rule system in Figure 7-1 to order, calculate, result, and autoverify the absolute cell counts corresponding to the leukocyte differential count. The value of this complex functionality provided by the LIS should not be underestimated. Attempting to achieve the same manually, without error, would consume considerable resources, and be challenging at best. Furthermore, the general capability of a rules-based system for reflex test ordering based on prior test results has broader potential for increasing laboratory productivity.

Rule based systems in the clinical laboratory are used to close the loop on specimen result processing. They have the ability to execute a wide variety of functions such as reflexive orders, calculations, added textual comments and autoverification of results. Many LIS vendors are offering these systems as application software.

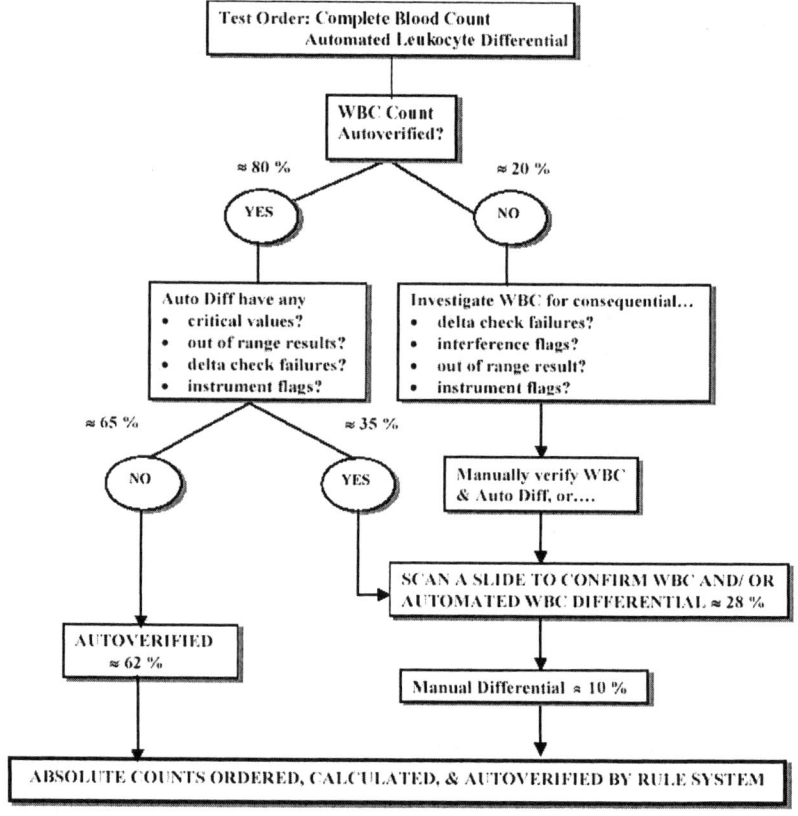

Figure 7-1. Deployment of a rules-based system for autoverification of the automated leukocyte differential count (percentage counts and absolute counts)

2.4   Laboratory Automation Systems

Total laboratory automation (TLA) systems are composed of instruments and work cells along a robotic stretch of hardware used for specimen management and transportation both within and between different clinical laboratories.[27,28] Centrifugation (when necessary), checking specimen suitability (hemolysis, clotting), decapping, aliquoting, barcode application, and routing are just some of the tasks performed by a TLA. Many TLA systems are available with a process control software component. They are intended to optimize the sorting of specimens and the throughput of samples.

TLA systems are employed to reduce labor cost, reduce operational costs, and to standardize procedures.

TLA is best suited as a front-end automation solution for a high volume environment, and in some cases may not be the best fit for the clinical hematology laboratory. The initial high capital investment, space constraints, and bottlenecks caused by batch delivery to the system are issues for many clinical laboratories. These issues have opened the door for a more modular approach to laboratory automation.

Modular laboratory automation systems (LAS) are beginning to operate in many clinical hematology laboratories. They are composed of interfaces to instrumentation, bar-coding subsystems, transport mechanisms, aliquoting robotics, and some are available with specimen storage and retrieval capabilities. This type of application exists between the LIS and the clinical hematology laboratory. The LAS parallels the LIS in basic functionality, and can be used to provide an electronic record of the instrument printout including scatter and histograms. This variety of technology eliminates the paper-tracking trail for specimens that are autoverified in real time by the LIS, and provides an electronic instrument visual on a PC workstation as accompaniment to a stained slide for scanning or performing a WBC differential. LAS are also capable of capturing instrument flags generated by the automated differential count that would not necessarily be transmitted to the LIS, but could be used as criteria for the auto release of the automated differential. In an automated clinical hematology laboratory with LAS deployment, the role of the LIS changes regarding connectivity, downloading to instruments, and uploading back to the LIS. There are several such systems available to the clinical hematology laboratory.

Acceptance of LAS on a large scale has not happened for the many reasons, including issues related to reliability, concerns of cost effectiveness and return on investment, up front cost and limited budgets in the healthcare industry, and a lack of comprehensive standards.[29] However, rising workloads, decreasing workforce, pressures to reduce cost and the continued development of standards by regulatory agencies should cause LAS and similar modular adaptations to accelerate in the near future.[27] There are many LIS vendors that have already established interface connectivity and working relationships with LAS platforms.

3.   FUTURE DEVELOPMENTS

3.1   Extended Differential Counts

Once the potential of current technologies is realized, there are several exciting developments that will be available for clinical use in the near future. Among the most imminent of these functions is the automated "extended differential count" (EDC). Currently, automated leukocyte differential counts are highly accurate and precise, but they are limited by the inability of typical analyzers to precisely quantify abnormal cell types and certain granulocyte forms (metamyelocytes, myelocytes, promyelocytes, and blasts). When instrument warnings indicate the potential presence of these cells, manual microscopic review is currently required for validation and quantitation. Using combinations of impedance and flow cytometric technologies, current generations of hematology analyzers are capable of reliably identifying and quantifying immature granulocyte forms to the extent that this category of cells has become a clinically reportable automated result for some analyzers. Analyzers have been introduced by several manufacturers that include FDA-approved nucleated red blood cell enumeration, and only recently Sysmex received FDA approval for the reporting of immature granulocytes on their XE-2100 analyzer. This instrument is also FDA approved for the reporting of hematopoietic progenitor cells as a screening tool for peripheral stem cell or bone marrow harvest for stem cell transplantation.[30]   Extended differential count capability, including instrument-derived immature granulocyte counts, will almost certainly be utilized by clinical laboratories in the near future.

The evolution of automated hematology testing to include EDCs has been hampered not by the pace of advancement in technology, but by the obsolescence of current clinical paradigms. The gold standard to which emerging technologies are held remains the antiquated and relatively imprecise NCCLS differential count standard (essentially an 800-cell manual differential count).[31] Furthermore, the widely utilized morphologic categories of immature granulocytes (metamyelocyte, myelocyte, and promyelocyte) were determined long ago based on arbitrary (and poorly reproducible) criteria. Any newly developed technology is expected to be able to recapitulate current practices of manual microscopy, despite the many shortcomings of such methods. As a result, we expect instruments to identify metamyelocytes as we currently define them, or myelocytes as we currently define them, despite a lack of evidence that these arbitrarily derived morphologic categories are sufficiently useful to justify preserving them. However, there is still no evidence-based mandate for automated systems to mirror this morphologic classification scheme.

A paradigm-shift is in order. If we open our minds to the recategorization of immature granulocyte forms using automated methods, the potential payback in terms of laboratory productivity, accuracy, precision, and speed of service is enormous. When immature granulocytes are re-classified into broader categories, correlation between manual and automated methods is excellent, and automated results are several times more precise than manual results (based on coefficients of variation of repeat analyses).[32] The field of laboratory hematology should consider changing gold standards to more precise methods, based upon flow cytometric immunophenotyping or other high-throughput technologies.

Optimum utilization of the recently acquired ability to precisely quantify low percentages of immature granulocyte forms will require an actual determination of the clinical relevance of these forms in peripheral blood samples. Such data do not currently exist. Almost every publication that seeks to determine the clinical utility of immature granulocyte quantitation focuses solely on the long-refuted "band count".[33,34] As a result, no one has established the independent value of the presence of more immature granulocytes in blood samples, and the levels at which these cells become clinically significant.

3.2 Cytomics

The sequencing of the human genome and historic advancements in information technology have brought about the age of "omics". Functional genomics ("transcriptomics"), and proteomics allow us to analyze disease patterns and physiologic states not simply by the analysis of a few select characteristics, but by broad patterns that emerge in the simultaneous analysis of thousands of expressed genes or proteins. Within each individual cell, gene expression is regulated by a complex network of mechanisms that act at the level of the gene, transcript, and protein, with innumerable feedback loops, autocrine and paracrine influences, etc. The cell itself acts as a self-contained universe with characteristic genetic, transcriptional, translational, post-translational and metabolic nuances that distinctly influence functional genomic and proteomic patterns. The term "cytomics" has emerged to describe the study of the cell as the final arbiter of these complex patterns of gene and protein expression.[35]

Current hematology analyzers offer expanded analysis capability, such as random-access assessment of CD4 and CD8-positive T-cell counts and hematopoietic progenitor cell quantitation. Differential counting of bone marrow aspirate samples may some day be an automated task.[36,37] Recent advances offer extraordinary promise for the automated or semi-automated analysis of cellular metabolic pathways, functional cell characteristics, patterns of drug resistance and innumerable other cellular properties. Such analyses will almost certainly be developed in flow cytometry laboratories before being integrated into routine hematology analyzers, but this new attitude in the development of automated analysis holds virtually limitless promise for the future of automated hematology testing.

REFERENCES

1. Ward PC. The CBC at the turn of the millennium: an overview. Clin Chem. 2000;46:1215-1220.
2. Bessman JD, Johnson RK. Erythrocyte volume distribution in normal and abnormal subjects. Blood. 1975;46:369-379.
3. Koenn ME, Kirby BA, Cook LL, Hare JL, Hall SH, Barry PM, Hissam CL, Wojcicki SB. Comparison of four automated hematology analyzers. Clin Lab Sci. 2001;14:238-242.
4. Cornbleet PJ, Myrick D, Levy R. Evaluation of the Coulter STKS five-part differential. Am J Clin Pathol. 1993;99:72-81.
5. Gulati GL, Kocher W, Schwarting R, Hyland LJ, Issa A, Arwood R, Dhanjal M. An assessment of the Coulter Gen-S automated flagging system. Lab Med. 2001;32:310-317.
6. Siekmeier R, Bierlich A, Jaross W. The white blood cell differential: three methods compared. Clin Chem Lab Med. 2001;39:432-445.
7. Van den Bossche J, Devreese K, Malfait R, Van de Vyvere M, Wauters A, Neeis H, De Schouwer P. Reference intervals for a complete blood count determined on different automated haematology analysers: Abx Pentra 120 Retic, Coulter Gen-S, Sysmex SE 9500, Abbott Cell Dyn 4000 and Bayer Advia 120. Clin Chem Lab Med. 2002;40:69-73.
8. Briggs C, Harrison P, Grant D, Staves J, MacHin SJ. New quantitative parameters on a recently introduced automated blood cell counter--the XE 2100. Clin Lab Haematol. 2000;22:345-350.
9. Arkin CF, Medeiros LJ, Pevzner LZ, Guertin BP, Kobos PJ, Phelps JW, Smith SJ. The white blood cell differential. Evaluation of rapid impression scanning versus the routine manual count. Am J Clin Pathol. 1987;87:628-632.
10. Dutcher TF. Leukocyte differentials. Are they worth the effort? Clin Lab Med. 1984;4:71-87.
11. Dutcher TF. Automated differentials: a strategy. Blood Cells. 1985;11:49-59.
12. Lantis KL, Harris RJ, Davis G, Renner N, Finn WG. Elimination of instrument-driven reflex manual differential leukocyte counts: optimization of manual blood smear review criteria in a high volume automated hematology laboratory. Am J Clin Pathol. 2003;119:656-662.
13. Koepke JA, Dotson MA, Shifman MA. A critical evaluation of the manual/visual differential leukocyte counting method. Blood Cells. 1985;11:173-186.
14. Pierre RV. Peripheral blood film review. The demise of the eyecount leukocyte differential. Clin Lab Med. 2002;22:279-297.
15. Pierre RV. Red cell morphology and the peripheral blood film. Clin Lab Med. 2002;22:25-61.
16. Bessman JD, Gilmer PR, Jr., Gardner FH. Improved classification of anemias by MCV and RDW. Am J Clin Pathol. 1983;80:322-326.
17. Bessman JD. Red blood cell fragmentation. Improved detection and identification of causes. Am J Clin Pathol. 1988;90:268-273.

18. Bessman JD, McClure S, Bates J. Distinction of microcytic disorders: comparison of expert, numerical-discriminant, and microcomputer analysis. Blood Cells. 1989;15:533-540.
19. Simel DL, DeLong ER, Feussner JR, Weinberg JB, Crawford J. Erythrocyte anisocytosis. Visual inspection of blood films vs automated analysis of red blood cell distribution width. Arch Intern Med. 1988;148:822-824.
20. Thomas C, Thomas L. Biochemical markers and hematologic indices in the diagnosis of functional iron deficiency. Clin Chem. 2002;48:1066-1076.
21. Toba K, Tsuchiyama J, Itoh H, Hashimoto S, Okazuka K, Shibazaki Y, Watanabe K, Narita M, Takahashi M, Aizawa Y. Sensitive measurement of fragmented red cell populations using flow cytometry, and its application for estimating thrombotic microangiopathy after stem cell transplantation. Cytometry (Part B). 2003;In press.
22. Scott CS, Van Zyl D, Ho E, Meyersfeld D, Ruivo L, Mendelow BV, Coetzer TL. Automated detection of malaria-associated intraleucocytic haemozoin by Cell-Dyn CD4000 depolarization analysis. Clin Lab Haematol. 2003;25:77-86.
23. Lima M, Porto B, Rodrigues M, Teixeira MA, Coutinho J, Ribeiro AC, Malheiro MI, Justica B. Cytogenetic findings in a patient presenting simultaneously with chronic lymphocytic leukemia and acute myeloid leukemia. Cancer Genetics & Cytogenetics. 1996;87:38-40.
24. Davis GM. Autoverification of the peripheral blood count. Lab Med. 1994;25:528-531.
25. Davis GM. A rule-based system for cost savings in hematology. MLO Med Lab Obs. 1994;26:44-46.
26. Smith N, Rosenfeld D, Watman R. Hematology autovalidation system. Lab Hematol. 1999;5:52-55.
27. Boyd J. Tech.Sight. Robotic laboratory automation. Science. 2002;295:517-518.
28. Markin RS, Whalen SA. Laboratory automation: trajectory, technology, and tactics. Clin Chem. 2000;46:764-771.
29. Hawker CD, Schlank MR. Development of standards for laboratory automation. Clin Chem. 2000;46:746-750.
30. Vogel W, Kopp HG, Kanz L, Einsele H. Correlations between hematopoietic progenitor cell counts as measured by Sysmex and CD34+ cell harvest yields following mobilization with different regimens. J Cancer Res Clin Oncol. 2002;128:380-384.
31. National Committee for Clinical Laboratory Standards. Reference leukocyte differential count (proportional) and evaluation of instrument methods: approved standards. NCCLS Document H20-A. Villanova, PA: NCCLS; 1992.
32. Fujimoto H, Sakata T, Hamaguchi Y, Shiga S, Tohyama K, Ichiyama S, Wang FS, Houwen B. Flow cytometric method for enumeration and classification of reactive immature granulocyte populations. Cytometry. 2000;42:371-378.
33. Cornbleet PJ. Clinical utility of the band count. Clin Lab Med. 2002;22:101-136
34. Novak RW. The beleaguered band count. Clin Lab Med. 1993;13:895-903.
35. Valet GK, Tarnok A. Cytomics in predictive medicine. Cytometry. 2003;53B:1-3
36. Shibata H, Yamane T, Yamamura R, Ohta K, Takubo T, Kamitani T, Hino M. Automatic analysis of normal bone marrow blood cells using the XE-2100 automated hematology analyzer. J Clin Lab Anal. 2003;17:12-17.
37. Yamamura R, Yamane T, Hino M, Ohta K, Shibata H, Tsuda I, Tatsumi N. Possible automatic cell classification of bone marrow aspirate using the CELL-DYN 4000 automatic blood cell analyzer. J Clin Lab Anal. 2002;16:86-90.

Chapter 8

ROLE OF FINE NEEDLE ASPIRATION IN LYMPHOMA

Aseem Lal and Ritu Nayar
Department of Pathology, Feinberg School of Medicine, Northwestern University, Chicago, IL

1.   INTRODUCTION

Fine needle aspiration biopsy (FNAB) is a minimally invasive technique utilized for rapid diagnosis of mass lesions through evaluation of cytological details of the aspirated material. This technique has been well accepted in Europe,[1-3] and barring a few countries, FNAB has seen a renaissance worldwide over the last thirty years.[4] This is especially true for lesions involving the thyroid gland, breast and salivary glands.[4] However, apart from a few select medical centers,[5] FNAB of lymph nodes is less frequently utilized in North America, and there is reluctance in rendering a diagnosis of malignant lymphoma (ML) based on this technique.[4, 6]

Until the 1980's literature on diagnosis of ML by FNAB was limited.[7] Pathologists and clinicians viewed FNAB as a screening rather than diagnostic tool.[6] Treating physicians were satisfied to know the presence or absence of lymphoma in a lymph node sample, and its main application was for recurrent or residual disease.

Application of FNAB in the primary diagnosis of ML is still somewhat controversial.[4, 8-12] Katz et al[10] have argued against the need for surgical excision to evaluate lymph node architecture in all cases of ML. Although needle tracts and other minor histopathological changes, such as, hemorrhage with organization and proliferation of spindle cells associated with prior FNAB may be observed in excised lymph nodes, significant destruction of lymph node histology such as infarction or extensive necrosis is rare.[13-15] and can be overcome using smaller needles (25 gauge or higher).

With the use of strict morphological criteria in conjunction with ancillary techniques such as immunohistochemistry, electron microscopy[11] and gene rearrangement studies,[10] diagnostic accuracy of FNAB can be enhanced. Cell yield which may be a limiting factor for supporting studies, can be enhanced by increased skill and use of fine gauge needles.[10]

On the contrary, some authors perceive this procedure as sub-optimal for the diagnosis of ML. Pinkus et al have argued against the use of radiologically guided core needle biopsies[16, 17] in the diagnosis of ML.[12] Lack of architectural details, partial involvement, interfollicular infiltrates and secondary processes associated with ML including granulomas, fibrosis, progressively transformed germinal centers in Hodgkin lymphoma (HL) maybe sources of pitfall in small needle cores assumed to be well representative of the entire lymph node.[12] In addition, difficult and unusual lesions like atypical or polymorphous lymphoid infiltrates and florid immunoblastic proliferations may prove challenging on limited biopsy material.[12]

Recent advances in the evaluation of lymphadenopathy by FNAB provide a basis for revisiting the current recommendations.[18, 19] A number of studies have documented the usefulness of FNAB, often supplemented by ancillary techniques like flow cytometry, for recognition and classification of primary and recurrent non-Hodgkin's lymphoma (NHL).[20-28] With the introduction of the revised European-American classification of lymphoid neoplasms (REAL) in 1994[29] and the WHO classification in 2001[30] there has been a transformation in evaluating malignant lymphoid proliferations. The new classification systems incorporate morphology along with immunophenotypic and genotypic characteristics. The heightened emphasis on supportive studies has opened new possibilities for cytopathologists to play a significant role in the diagnosis of ML.

The potential benefits of adopting FNAB for wider use are several. When compared to surgical biopsy, FNAB is quick, minimally invasive and by passes the requirement for anesthesia or prolonged hospital stay. It is also easier to triage the biopsy sample for culture or special stains if the initial impression is of a non-malignant disorder. This is especially true for children, an age group in which reactive lymphadenopathy is very common.[31] In patients with human immunodeficiency virus (HIV) infection who commonly have lymphadenopathy of varied etiology ranging from benign to malignant, FNAB can provide a rapid assessment.[32-35] In patients with a prior diagnosis of non-hematopoietic malignancy (i.e. carcinoma, melanoma), FNAB can document lymph node involvement by metastatic malignancy and obviate the need for further investigative procedures.[36]

2.   SPECIMEN COLLECTION

The frequently used biopsy techniques are well described in several reference texts.[1, 3, 37] Non-aspiration techniques have also utilized.[38] Superficial, palpable lymph nodes are most amenable to FNAB while deep-seated lymph nodes require radiological guidance. FNAB is best performed either by a trained cytopathologist or interventional radiologist who is aware of the clinical presentation.[1, 39, 40] Facilities for on-site adequacy assessment and preliminary interpretation, reduces concerns about inadequate sampling and allows the specimen to be triaged for additional work-up pertinent to the individual case.

The procedure is explained to the patient and a documented consent is obtained. The overlying skin is cleansed with alcohol and the mass is fixed with the non-dominant hand. We prefer FNAB without anesthesia, although topical anesthetic cream or 1% local lidocaine is utilized in many centers in America. If local anesthesia is used, its direct injection into the mass should be avoided as this may lead to sample dilution and adversely affect specimen quality and interpretation. Generally 23-25 gauge needles are optimal with a 20 ml syringe attached to a syringe holder. The needle is introduced into the lesion, at which time a negative pressure may be appreciated. Suction is applied by pulling back on the syringe and the needle is moved back and forth, each time at a different angle, into the lesion. At this point aspirated material may be observed in the hub of the needle. The negative pressure is then released and the needle is removed from the node while an assistant applies pressure over the procedure site. The syringe and the needle are removed from the holder and material smeared onto multiple slides, followed by rinsing the needle in a balanced salt solution (RPMI). The number of FNAB's is dependent on the results of initial assessment. Additional material may be required for culture or ancillary studies. In general 3 FNAB's yield adequate sample in experienced hands. Using a needle without the syringe or the syringe holder can be used to obtain a fine needle sample without aspiration.[38] This technique allows greater sensory perception of the lesion with a comparable cell yield. There is significant reduction in trauma to the lesion and surrounding tissues[38] and it may be better applicable for smaller masses.[5]

Various smear techniques have been well described by Abele et al.[41] These can be adopted to achieve the best results depending on the specimen type i.e. semi-solid, diluted or a small sample. In general the one step technique is widely applicable. Two slides are held perpendicular to each other and the specimen is placed on one slide held by the frosted end (stationary slide). The second slide (smearing slide) is held perpendicular and rotated towards the stationary slide till it comes in contact with the sample. It is then made to slide over the stationary slide, away from the frosted end such that a monolayer smear is achieved. Regardless of the technique, the intent is to achieve a thin layer such that semi-cohesivness of the cells can be maintained and pattern recognition is feasible.[41]

Smears can be fixed in alcohol and stained with Papanicolau or hematoxylin and eosin, or, air-dried and stained with either Romanowsky based stains (May-Grunwald, Wright-Geimsa or Toluidine blue) or its modifications (Diff-Quik). Alcohol fixed smears highlight nuclear details including chromatin pattern and distribution whereas Romanowsky stains better illustrate cytoplasmic features and background.

There will be instances where the underlying pathological process is not explicit based on findings of the preliminary assessment of the aspirated material. Under these circumstances, a needle core biopsy (NCB) is highly desirable. NCB is a cylindrical core of tissue obtained from the lesion under radiological guidance and is comparable to a miniature surgical biopsy. It is rapid, safe and shows preservation of architecture for evaluation in conjunction with FNAB and ability to apply immunohistochemistry (IHC). Performed as the sole procedure, it can provide accurate diagnostic information in both HL and NHL in cases with primary, progressive or recurrent disease and up to 86% of patients can be started on specific therapy based on the results of NCB.[16, 17] NCB is especially useful for deep-seated masses,[17] including mediastinum,[42] in patients unfit for surgery or anesthesia[43] and for pediatric neoplasms where a primary tumor diagnosis is achievable in 88% of cases.[44] Common problems with this procedure include inadequate specimen,[17] extensive necrosis or crush artifact. Some authors have argued against the use of NCB's for reasons of small sample size and destruction of histological architecture of subsequently excised lymph nodes.[12] The utility of NCB with FNAB is uncertain in cases of a diagnostic aspirate but maybe essential in cases of an inadequate FNAB sample, lack of facilities for flow cytometry (FC), such that IHC (essential to confirm non-hematopoietic malignancy) can be performed. Therefore, routine usage of NCB with FNAB should be avoided, exceptions being mediastinal and retroperitoneal lymph nodes where it is an accepted alternative to open biopsy.

3. PRELIMINARY EVALUATION OF FNAB SMEARS

A preliminary assessment of the nature of the aspirate at the time of FNAB is critical to guide procurement of additional material for ancillary studies. Details evaluated at low power include cellularity, architecture, necrosis and presence of lymphoglandular bodies (cytoplasmic fragments), especially prominent in ML (Table 8-1). High power cytomorphologic features include assessment of cell size, nuclear size, chromatin pattern and other, especially background features. (Table 8-2)

Table 8-1. Low-power details

Characteristic			
Cellularity	*Markedly cellular*	*Moderately cellular*	*Scant cellularity*
	Favor malignancy	Malignant (low cell	Bloody specimen
	Lymphoma	yield)	Sampling error
	Carcinoma	Lymphoma	Vascular tumor
	Melanoma	Carcinoma	
	Sarcoma (rare)	Melanoma	Non-bloody specimen
		Sarcoma (rare)	Sampling error
		Reactive	Neoplasm
			Epithelial tumor
			Vascular tumor
			Stroma rich tumor
			Cystic neoplasm
			Fibrosis
Architecture	*Cohesive*	*Diffuse*	
	Follicular lymphoma	Lymphoma	
	Reactive germinal center	Non-lymphoid	
	fragments	neoplasm	
	Epithelial tumors		
	Small cell carcinoma of		
	the lung		
	Pediatric small round blue		
	cell tumors		
	Melanoma		
	Sarcoma (rare)		
Necrosis	*Malignant*	*Benign*	
	Lymphoma	Infectious/inflammat	
	Carcinoma	ory	
	Melanoma		
	Sarcoma (rare)		

4. ANCILLARY STUDIES FOR DIAGNOSIS AND SUB-CLASSIFICATION OF ML

The WHO classification for ML [30] emphasizes the importance of clinical features combined with morphological, immunophenotypic and genotypic characteristics for diagnosis and categorization of ML and postulates a cell of origin for each neoplasm, which in many cases reflects the stage of differentiation of the malignant cell.[30]

Table 8-2. High-power details

Characteristic					
Cell size		*Nuclear details*		*Other findings*	
Small	- Chronic lymphocytic leukemia/small lymphocytic leukemia - Mantle cell lymphoma - Lymphoplasmacytic lymphoma - Follicular lymphoma - Burkitt lymphoma - Lymphblastic leukemia/ lymphoma	*Round/ clumped chromatin*	- Large cell lymphoma (immunoblastic lymphoma with prominent nucleoli) - Small lymphocytic lymphoma - Marginal zone lymphoma	*Organisms*	- Fungal organisms - Viral inclusions - Bacterial organisms

Large	- Large cell lymphoma
	- Carcinoma
	- Melanoma
	- Sarcoma (rare)
		Convoluted/ clumped chromatin	- Follicular lymphoma
			- Mantle cell lymphoma
			- Marginal zone lymphoma
				Granulomas	- Benign conditions
					- Malignant conditions
					  • Hodgkin lymphoma
					  • Large cell lymphoma

Mixed/ polymorphous	- Marginal zone lymphoma - T cell lymphoma - Hodgkin lymphoma	*Dispersed chromatin*	- Lymphoblastic lymphoma/leukemia - Myeloid leukemia	*Reed-Sternberg cells*	- Hodgkin lymphoma

Ancillary techniques, including IHC, FC, Southern blot analysis, polymerase chain reaction (PCR), conventional cytogenetics and fluorescent *in situ* hybridization (FISH), have proven beneficial for accurate diagnosis of lymphomas on FNAB. IHC, performed on formalin-fixed cell-blocks or

NCB's can be utilized for detection of lineage specific antigens (B, T cell) or oncoproteins (bcl-1, bcl-2)[45, 46] associated with chromosomal translocation in certain lymphomas. FC on fresh samples is widely used and allows characterization and quantitation of both normal and abnormal cells in suspension with fluorescent labeled antibodies directed against cell surface antigens.[47] It has the ability to analyze cells based on size, ploidy and antigenic characteristics, and allows rapid analysis of multiple antigens on cell populations of interest therefore allowing for extensive characterization of the lymphoma.[48] With complex gating strategies, small abnormal populations can be detected, which may be beyond the scope of morphological analysis alone.[47] B-cell lymphomas, which account for the majority of NHL's[49, 50] can be detected by FC by analyzing clonality based on surface immunoglobulin light chain restriction.[51-53] T-cell lymphomas are recognized by either aberrant expression of T cell antigens (or their subsets) or their abnormal distribution.[51] This technique has been successfully applied to FNAB samples[48, 54-56] and recent literature has stressed its role for accurate classification of ML.[6, 18, 20, 21, 25, 57-62]

All specimens for FC are collected in a balanced salt solution (such as RPMI) and are analyzed immediately. In case of delay, addition of fetal calf serum helps preserve viability. FC requires at least 10^6 cells for DNA and basic immunophenotypic characterization.[5, 48] The reported average cell yield has ranged from $2x10^6$ cells to $3x10^6$ cells in *in vivo* FNAB's.[55, 63-65] However the cell yield can be highly variable, and in our experience, has ranged from $<5x10^4$ to $>5x10^6$ cells. Since FNAB specimens may have a limited number of cells for analysis, a selective panel of antibodies (e.g. CD45, CD19, CD20, CD5, CD7, kappa and lambda light chain) analysis can be performed based on the preliminary morphologic impression. Washing the cell preparation may enhance separation of immunoglobulin light chain positive and negative populations, however it also can reduce cell yield, a potential problem with low cell count specimens.[48] The currently used 4-color flow cytometer allows multiparameter analysis of a wider combination of antigens.

FC aids in the distinction of ML from benign proliferations[27] and for detection of NHL. Its role is limited for aiding in the diagnosis of HL.[20, 21, 48, 58] However, absence of monoclonality, coupled with clinical and morphological features as well as immunocytochemistry help support the latter diagnosis.[27, 48] FC has also been successfully applied to T-cell lymphomas,[23, 66] where findings can be supplemented with PCR.[67] Analysis of the S-phase fraction allows delineation of aggressive lymphomas.[27]

The limitations of FC include lack of meaningful results with limited samples. It may not be definitive in surface immunoglobulin negative B-cell lymphomas[68] and many T-cell lymphomas.[69] Computerized laser scanning cytometry allows immunophenotypic analysis of specimens with cell counts as low or lower than 50, 000.[70, 71] This is a slide-based technique which allows cells to be microscopically visualized either before, during or after analysis.[72] It may be utilized for FNAB samples where cell counts are often lower than those obtained with surgical excision.[71]

In cases of surface immunoglobulin negative B-cell lymphomas or T-cell lymphomas with no definitive findings on FC, one may utilize diagnostic molecular techniques to evaluate clonality by determining immunoglobulin gene rearrangements or T-cell receptor gene rearrangement. DNA analysis for clonality or specific gene rearrangements can be performed through Southern blot analysis[73] and PCR. Recent studies have advocated the efficacy of PCR based techniques for supporting the diagnosis of both B and T-cell lymphomas.[67, 74-76] This is especially true where the boundaries between reactive lymphoid proliferations and low-grade lymphomas become indistinct. Low-grade lymphomas of thyroid and salivary gland can be difficult to differentiate from reactive lymphoid proliferations occurring in these locations (Hashimoto's thyroiditis and myoepithelial sialadenitis respectively). Demonstration of clonality leads to a conclusive diagnosis in these situations.[77-80] PCR also facilitates demonstration of clonality and lineage assignment in atypical lymphoid proliferations.[81] Molecular studies should always be correlated with morphology and other ancillary studies,[82] since occurrence of a false positive or false-negative result may lead to an erroneous diagnosis.[83] FC and PCR[60] can be utilized together in an individual case.[60] PCR can be performed prospectively on fresh samples or retrospectively by extracting DNA from formalin-fixed tissue or FNAB material on smears.

For diagnosis of ML associated with specific chromosomal aberrations, cytogenetic analysis through classic and FISH techniques can be performed on material obtained by FNA. Aneusomies of chromosomes (often associated with malignant disorders)[84] and specific chromosomal abnormalities, associated with certain subtypes of ML, as exemplified in the WHO classification,[30] can be identified through interphase FISH analysis[85, 86] or conventional cytogenetics.[87] The latter requires fresh tissue and will detect multiple chromosomal abnormalities without prior knowledge of the abnormality being sought. FISH, however, is capable of detecting a single, prospectively chosen, translocation.[6]

Morphological assessment of the specimen is very important to guide performance of these highly specialized tests. Carefully chosen and well-directed ancillary techniques help in making a precise diagnosis of ML in most instances.

5. CLASSIFICATION OF LYMPHOMAS

Cell size is a useful criteria maybe used to diagnose and sub-classify lymphomas on FNAB smears (Table 8-3).

Table 8-3 Classification of Lymphomas

Cell Size	
◆ Lymphomas with small to medium sized lymphoid cells	- Chronic lymphocytic leukemia/Small lymphocytic lymphoma - Mantle cell lymphoma - Lymphoplasmacytic lymphoma/ Waldenström macroglobulinemia - Follicular lymphoma - Burkitt lymphoma/Burkitt-like lymphoma - Lymphoblastic lymphoma/ leukemia
◆ Lymphomas with large lymphoid cells: Large cell lymphoma	- Diffuse large B cell lymphoma - Anaplastic large cell lymphoma
◆ Lymphomas with mixed large and small cells/polymorphous infiltrates	- Marginal zone lymphoma - T-cell lymphoma - Hodgkin lymphoma
◆ Others	- Plasma cell neoplasms - Histiocytic and dendritic cell malignancies - Mastocytosis

5.1 Small lymphocytic lymphoma

Small lymphocytic lymphoma (SLL) refers to the non-leukemic/tissue counterpart of chronic lymphocytic leukemia (CLL) and, together, these account for 6.7% of NHL.[30] Most patients are over 50 years of age with a male : female ratio of 2:1.[30] SLL/CLL is often disseminated at presentation with generalized lymphadenopathy, involvement of peripheral blood, bone marrow, spleen and liver.[6] Although indolent, it is incurable with the currently available therapeutic regimens.[30] 10-20% of cases may transform to large cell lymphoma/ Richter's transformation and rare transformation to Hodgkin-like or Hodgkin lymphoma has also been noted.[88-90]

5.1.1   Morphology

FNAB reveals a monotonous population of small lymphoid cells, slightly larger than small lymphocytes. The nuclear/cytoplasmic ratio is high with regular nuclear membranes and clumped chromatin. The coarse clumped chromatin observed in histological sections, "cellules grumelees" maybe observed in Papanicolau stained smears.[5] Mitoses are infrequent. The occasional presence of nuclear irregularities may suggest a diagnosis of mantle cell lymphoma.[30] However SLL is associated with a mixture of prolymphocytes (intermediate sized cells with vesicular chromatin and a small nucleolus) and paraimmunoblasts (medium-large cells with dispersed chromatin and a large prominent nucleolus), which are not observed in mantle cell lymphoma.[6, 30] Clusters of these cells correspond to proliferation centers observed in histological sections. Plasmacytoid features in SLL/CLL may suggest a diagnosis of lymphoplasmacytic lymphoma,[6] however, absence of M-protein and the lack of clinical features of Waldenström macroglobulinemia are helpful in ruling out the latter diagnosis.[6] Small cell undifferentiated carcinoma (SCUC) may be mistaken for SLL. Smears in the former are highly cellular with prominent tumor necrosis (Figure 8-1). The malignant epithelial cells in SCUC are about three times the size of normal lymphocytes with a high nuclear/cytoplasmic ratio, coarse chromatin and prominent molding.[5] Paravacuolar "blue bodies" seen adjacent to the nucleus, prominent cell streaking/ crush artifact and the absence of lymphoglandular bodies are all useful in distinguishing SCUC from lymphoma. Lymph node metastasis from squamous cell carcinoma and basal cell carcinoma can mimic SLL, however presence of molding and a cohesive architecture help rule out the latter diagnoses.[5]

5.2   Mantle cell lymphoma

Mantle cell lymphoma (MCL) commonly presents with stage III or IV disease with bone marrow involvement, generalized lymphadenopathy, and hepatosplenomegaly (often a massively enlarged spleen).[91-95] About one quarter of the cases have peripheral blood involvement and extra-nodal sites commonly include Waldeyer's ring and gastrointestinal tract.[30]

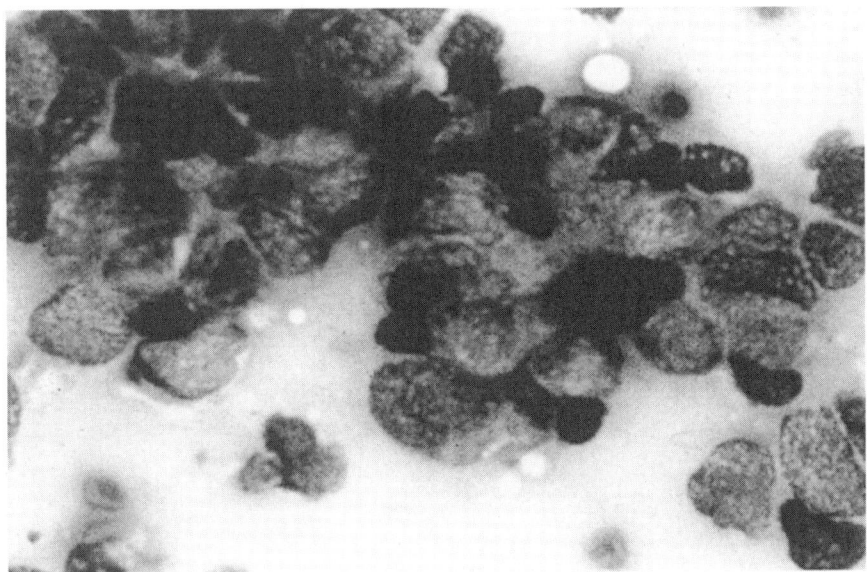

Figure 8-1. Small cell undifferentiated carcinoma of the lung. Malignant cells with high nuclear/cytoplasmic ratio, coarse chromatin and prominent molding. Paravacuolar "blue bodies" adjacent to the nucleus and absence of lymphoglandular bodies are helpful clues (x1000, Diff-Quik stain).

5.2.1　Morphology

Smears reveal small-intermediate lymphoid cells with irregular nuclear contours resembling centrocytes.[30] Chromatin is dispersed with inconspicuous nucleoli. Cells resembling prolymphocytes or paraimmunoblasts are absent. Variations in this conventional morphology may be seen with blastoid variants which include classic (cells with dispersed chromatin and active mitosis) or pleomorphic (highly variable cell morphology and prominent nucleoli) subtypes.[30] Occasionally other morphologies include cells with small round nuclei and clumped chromatin, simulating SLL or cells with abundant pale nuclei resembling marginal zone lymphoma.[30] Flow cytometric evaluation is crucial to avoid misdiagnosis as other lymphomas with a "small cell morphology" (Table 8-4).

5.2.2　Cytogenetics and molecular characteristics

A characteristic translocation t (11;14) (q13;q32) involving the immunoglobulin heavy chain and *CCND1* genes is observed in 70-75% of MCL using conventional cytogenetics or southern blot analysis.[96-99] This rearrangement can also be demonstrated by FISH techniques in almost all cases.[30] Immunohistochemical staining for cyclin D1 will demonstrate nuclear positivity and can be utilized to confirm MCL in paraffin embedded tissue.[100]

5.3   Lymphoplasmacytic lymphoma/ Waldenström macroglobulinemia

Lymphoplasmacytic lymphoma (LPL) is a rare entity accounting for approximately 2-3% of all NHL.[6] This is a disease of older adults (median age 63 years) with a slight male predominance.[101] It is a low grade B cell lymphoma with transformation to large cell lymphoma being identified in 5-10% of cases.[6] Frequently patients present with features of lymphoma (lymphadenopathy, hepatosplenomegaly and bone marrow involvement) and a monoclonal serum IgM paraprotein. They may exhibit signs of hyperviscosity, bleeding, autoimmune phenomenon or cryoglobulinemia.[102-104]

5.3.1   Morphology

Smears are characterized by an admixture of small lymphocytes, plasmacytoid lymphocytes, mature plasma cells and occasional plasmacytoid immunoblasts.[6, 30] Periodic-acid schiff (PAS) positive Dutcher bodies (intranuclear inclusions) and Russell bodies (cytoplasmic immunoglobulin) may occasionally be identified.[6] Predominance of immunoblasts may indicate an aggressive course.[88] Occasionally, the presence of epitheloid cells and mast cells may simulate morphology of a T-cell neoplasm.[105] Plasmacytoid features maybe observed in other types of ML including SLL, follicular lymphoma.[5] FC may be helpful to differentiate these entities (Table 8-4). Immunohistochemical demonstration of surface/cytoplasmic immunoglobulin can also be performed in tissue sections to confirm the diagnosis.

5.4   Follicular lymphoma

Follicular lymphoma (FL) comprises approximately 35% of adult NHL in the United States.[30] It is much less common in Europe, Asia and developing countries.[106] Patients are over 50 years of age with widespread, but asymptomatic disease commonly involving lymph nodes, spleen and bone marrow.

5.4.1   Morphology

FL's recapitulate the lymphoid constituents of a normal follicle with presence of both centrocytes (small lymphoid cells with irregular, cleaved nuclei, inconspicuous nucleoli and scarce cytoplasm) and centroblasts/ non-cleaved follicular center cells.[30] The latter can be small or large with round to oval nuclei, vesicular chromatin and one or multiple peripheral nucleoli.[30] Dendritic cells may also be identified. Monomorphic lymphoid cell aggregates and increased number of mast cells have been observed with increased frequency in FL.[107, 108] Follicular architecture may occasionally be observed in cell-blocks and can be highlighted by reticulin stains.[6] Grading of these lymphomas,[30] performed on histological sections, is not accurate on FNAB smears.[109]

FL needs to be distinguished from reactive follicular hyperplasia that displays a polymorphous population of cells including centrocytes, centroblasts, dendritic cells, plasmacytoid cells, plasma cells, immunoblasts and tingible body macrophages.[5] FC aids in ruling out hyperplasia and other mature B-cell lymphomas (Table 8-4). CD10 positivity, present in 60% of cases by immunohistochemistry and 90% of cases by FC[20, 21, 110, 111] is helpful in confirming the diagnosis of FL.[111, 112] The intensity of expression and the percentage of B-cells expressing CD10 help delineate reactive follicular hyperplasia from FL.[111] CD10 is also expressed in many cases of Burkitt lymphoma[68] and some diffuse large B cell lymphomas,[20] therefore morphological correlation is essential.

5.4.2   Cytogenetics and molecular characteristics

The most common cytogenetic abnormality in FL is t (14;18)(q32;q21) which involves re-arrangement of the *BCL2* gene.[113] Immunohistochemical staining for *BCL2*, though useful in histological sections to differentiate reactive follicular hyperplasia from follicular lymphoma, is non-productive in cell-blocks due to lack of architectural details and presence of this oncoprotein in lymphomas other than FL (Marginal zone lymphoma, SLL and Burkitt lymphoma).[6] A combined PCR analysis of IgH and *BCL2* rearrangements can be used to confirm the cytological impression of FL.[83] Automated molecular genetic DNA analysis has been applied to cytological specimens for diagnosis of FL.[114]

5.5   Burkitt lymphoma/ Burkitt-like lymphoma

Previously referred to as small non-cleaved lymphoma,[115] these are highly aggressive lymphomas that may present in a leukemic phase[116] (L3 type of acute lymphoblastic leukemia) or as an extra-nodal mass.[117, 118] The endemic form, representing the commonest childhood malignancy in equatorial Africa,[30] presents as a jaw or orbital mass,[117-119] or an extra-nodal mass with involvement of the bowel, omentum, ovaries, kidneys or breast.[117, 119, 120] Climactic factors may correspond to endemicity in these locations.[117] Sporadic forms occur worldwide, predominantly in children and young adults, often as abdominal masses.[121, 122] Immunodeficiency associated Burkitt lymphoma (BL) is often a primary manifestation of acquired immunodeficiency syndrome with EBV positivity in some cases.[123, 124] Burkitt-like lymphoma has a clinical presentation similar to sporadic BL but patients are usually older and present with lymph node involvement.[125-127]

5.5.1   Morphology

Smears reveal medium sized lymphoid cells with round nuclei, clumped chromatin and multiple basophilic nuclei (Figure 8-2). The cells have a moderate amount of deeply basophilic cytoplasm with numerous lipid vacuoles.[30] Prominent mitoses and apoptosis, attributed to a high proliferative index are characteristic. Tingible body macrophages are numerous. In tissue sections the tumor cells appear cohesive because of cytoplasmic retraction.[30] Variations of the normal morphology include Burkitt-like lymphoma and BL with plasmacytoid differentiation.[30] The former has greater variability in nuclear parameters and less prominent nucleoli. FC findings are fairly characteristic and extremely helpful in supporting the cytological diagnosis. The tumor cells reveal a mature B-cell phenotype (Table 8-4). A very high growth rate is reflected by a Ki-67 index of nearly 100%.[29]

5.5.2   Cytogenetics and molecular features

BL is associated with *MYC* translocation, t (8;14),[128] which is seen in about 80% cases or less commonly with t (8;22) or t(2;8). Thus cytogenetics is useful in confirming the diagnosis of BL.

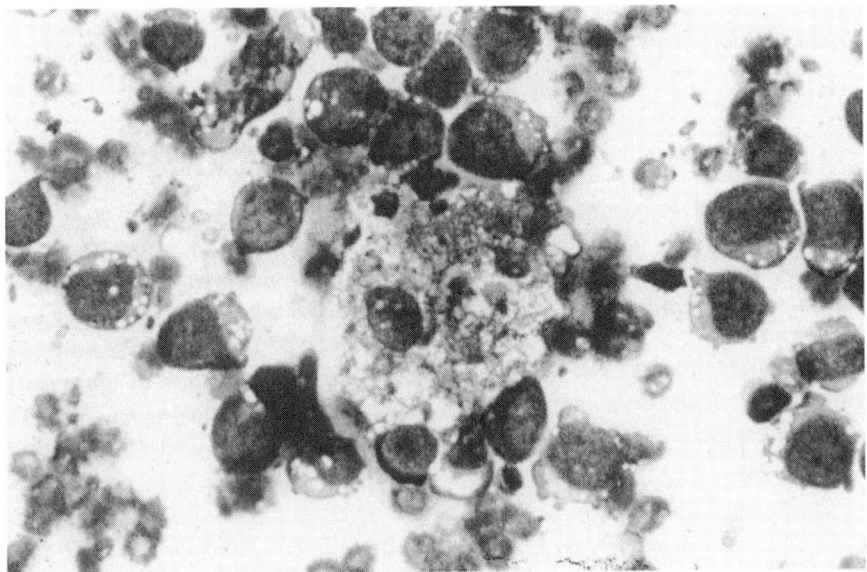

Figure 8-2. Burkitt lymphoma. Medium sized lymphoid cells with round nuclei and clumped chromatin. There is moderate basophilic cytoplasm with vacuolation. Numerous tingle body macrophages and mitotic figures are seen. (x1000, Diff-Quik stain)

Table 8-4. Immunophenotyping characteristics of CD19 positive B cell neoplasms.

	CD20	CD22	CD5	CD10	CD23	sIg	TdT
CLL/SLL	+ (dim)	–	+	–	+	+ (dim)	–
MCL	+	+	+	–	–	+	–
LPL/WM	+	+	–	–	–	+	–
FL	+	+	–	+	+/–	+ (bright)	–
MZL	+	+	–	–	–	+	–
BL	+	+	–	+	–	+	–

CLL: chronic lymphocytic leukemia, SLL: small lymphocytic lymphoma, MCL: mantle cell lymphoma, LPL: lymphoplasmacytic lymphoma, WM: waldenstrom's macroglobulinemia, FL: follicular lymphoma, MZL: marginal zone lymphoma, BL: Burkitt lymphoma.

5.6 Lymphoblastic lymphoma

Lymphoblastic lymphoma (LL) is an immature B or T cell neoplasm. B-lymphoblastic lymphoma is the nodal or extra-nodal counterpart of acute lymphoblastic leukemia.[30] It accounts for 10% of LL's with a median age of 20 years.[129] Frequently involved sites include skin, bones, lymph nodes and soft tissue.[129, 130] Peripheral blood and bone marrow involvement may be seen, but the blast percentage is low.[30] T-lymphoblastic lymphoma accounts for 90% of LL[5] and is more common in adolescent males.[120] Mediastinal mass, and pleural effusions are a common presentations,[30] and rapid growth with involvement of blood, bone marrow, central nervous system and gonadal tissue is seen.[131]

5.6.1   Morphology

FNAB smears show a monomorphic population of small to medium sized lymphoid cells with round or convoluted nuclei[6] (depending on the variant), condensed chromatin and indistinct nucleoli. Larger cells with slightly basophilic, occasionally vacuolated cytoplasm may be identified. These cells have a dispersed chromatin with multiple indistinct to prominent nucleoli.[30] Coarse granulation is seen in some cells and maybe associated with the t (9;22)(q34;q11.2) translocation.[30] Acute lymphoblastic leukemia (ALL) is divided into B-precursor ALL, pre-B ALL, B-ALL and T-ALL.[68] FC is essential for diagnosis and subclassification. B-ALL has a mature B-cell phenotype and is equivalent to the leukemic phase of Burkitt lymphoma.[68] T-cell neoplasms may lack expression of normal antigens or display aberrant combinations.[132]

LL may be mistaken for non-hematological malignancies including pediatric small blue cell tumors (Ewings sarcoma/primitive neuroectodermal tumor, embryonal rhabdomyosarcoma, neuroblastoma), small cell carcinoma, merkel cell carcinoma, extramedullary myeloid tumor, thymoma.[5, 6, 133-138] These distinctions are important especially if LL presents as an isolated lesion in an extra nodal site such as skin or bone.[139] Using a spectrum of morphological findings (single cells, rosettes, neuropil, moulding) and immunohistochemical profiles, one can confidentially differentiate pediatric small blue cell tumors from LL.[5, 140] MIC-2 has been advocated as a reliable marker in distinguishing LL from Ewing sarcoma,[141] but MIC-2 should be used with caution as it can be seen in some cases of LL. The neoplastic cells in thymoma are large with indistinct cell borders and round to slightly irregular nuclear contours with occasional small nucleoli.[138] Unlike LL, these cells are cytokeratin positive. However, entrapped thymocytes may lead to confusion with lymphoblasts, the former are small mature with clumped chromatin,[5] but with a similar immunophenotypic profile including TdT positivity.[142-144] LL may be CD45 negative[68] and therefore this marker does not always help in differentiating LL from other non-hematopoietic malignancies.[139] In difficult situations, gene-rearrangement studies are helpful and will demonstrate clonal rearrangement in LL[145, 146] as opposed to germline configuration in thymoma.[147] Extramedullary myeloid tumor has cells with more abundant cytoplasm and it may share nuclear characteristics and TdT positivity with LL. It differs in that it is positive for myeloperoxidase and CD33.[6] Hematopoietic neoplasms which need to be distinguished from LL include BL (prominent nucleoli) and the blastoid variant of MCL.[30] Positivity for TdT observed in LL, rules out these entities.[30]

5.7 Large cell lymphomas

Large cell lymphomas account for 40% of adult lymphomas[148] and one third of pediatric cases.[149] The majority of adult large cell lymphoma (LCL) are B cell in origin, whereas in children there is a near equal division of B lineage, T lineage and intermediate phenotypes.[149] CD30 positivity is frequently seen in pediatric LCL's.[149]

5.7.1 Diffuse large B cell lymphoma

Diffuse large B-cell lymphoma accounts for about 30-40% of adult NHL in the western hemisphere.[30] The age range is wide with cases reported in children.[92, 149] Although aggressive, they respond well to chemotherapy.[150] Both nodal and extra-nodal presentations have been reported, the latter primarily include the gastrointestinal tract, but any organ maybe involved.[30]

5.7.1.1 Morphology

Sheets of large lymphoid cells, three times or greater than the size of a small lymphocyte are occasionally admixed with a small percentage of mature lymphocytes[5] (Figure 8-3). Nuclei are large (in comparison to the nucleus of an endothelial or histiocytic cell) but may have diverse morphological features depending on the variant. Centroblastic lymphoma appears either polymorphic or monomorphic with vesicular nuclei, fine chromatin and two or more peripheral nucleoli.[30] Multilobated cells may also be seen. The immunoblastic variant has large nuclei with a central prominent nucleolus and abundant cytoplasm.[30] In the T-cell/ histiocyte rich variant,[30] there are numerous benign T cells that may mask the large neoplastic cells and the overall picture can resemble Hodgkin lymphoma.[5] The anaplastic variant[30] has bizarre, pleomorphic cells resembling Reed-Sternberg cells or even carcinoma and is unrelated to anaplastic large cell lymphoma of the T or null cell lineage.[151] Rare variants include the plasmablastic type, which are morphologically similar to immunoblastic lymphoma, but are negative for CD20/CD45 in majority of the cases and express the plasma cell markers CD38 and CD138.[30] Sheets of large cells on cell-block sections are very suggestive of large cell lymphoma.[6]

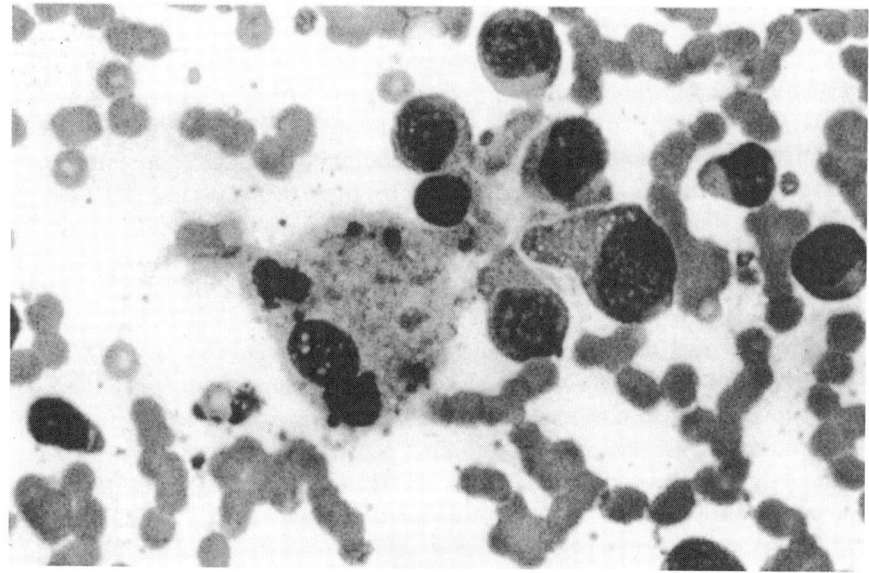

Figure 8-3. Large cell lymphoma. Clusters of large lymphoid cells with large nuclei and a few lymphocytes are seen in the background. A tingible body macrophage is seen in the center. (x1000, Diff-Quik stain).

FC is helpful in confirming the diagnosis and ruling out other non-lymphoid neoplasms. The majority of B cell lymphomas are positive for CD19, CD20 and CD45.[6] CD10 positivity, if identified indicates follicular center cell origin.[20] However the extreme fragility of the tumor cells make lead to false negative result on FC[68] and we routinely obtain needle core biopsies in these cases and perform IHC if FC is unsuccessful. Another source of difficulty is the frequent surface immunoglobulin negativity of the tumor cells, especially mediastinal B-cell lymphomas.[152] The presence of B-lineage markers CD19, CD20 and CD22 is supportive of the diagnosis, even in the face of negative surface immunoglobulin staining.[68]

5.7.1.2   Cytogenetics and molecular features

BCL6 gene is frequently rearranged and associated with a B cell phenotype and better prognosis.[148, 153] BCL-1 gene rearrangement is not present and is thus helpful in ruling out a blastic variant of MCL.[6]

5.7.2   Anaplastic Large Cell Lymphoma

Anaplastic large cell lymphoma is a T-cell lymphoma that accounts for 3% of adult NHL's and about 10-30% of pediatric lymphomas.[154] Primary systemic anaplastic large cell lymphoma (ALCL) needs to be differentiated from primary cutaneous ALCL with which it shares some features.

5.7.2.1   Morphology

The smears show large cells with abundant cytoplasm and irregular, horse-shoe shaped nuclei and a distinct eosinophilic paranuclear region ("hallmark cells") in the common/ classic variant.[155] The majority of the cases are positive for anaplastic large cell lymphoma kinase protein (ALK).[30] The morphology can be highly variable; with the histiocytic variant in which the tumor cells are overshadowed by a predominant population of histiocytes and plasma cells[30, 155] and the small cell variant where the neoplastic cells are small to medium with irregular nuclei admixed with more characteristic cells that are centered around blood vessels.[30, 155] The latter feature may not be observed on FNAB smears and confusion with a T cell lymphoma is likely. ALCL with predominance of giant cells, signet ring cells, neutrophils and sarcoma-like features have also been observed.[30, 155] Owing to the diverse morphological features, many differential diagnoses need to be entertained and ruled out with close correlation of ancillary data. These include HL, peripheral T-cell lymphoma, diffuse large B cell lymphoma (DLBCL) and non-hematopoietic neoplasms including carcinoma, melanoma and even germ cell tumors.[5] An immunohistochemical panel of antibodies is helpful in ruling out the majority of these differential diagnoses and thus for confirmation the diagnosis, a core biopsy is highly desirable. ALCL cells are positive for CD30 (membranous and golgi staining)[30] and ALK protein expression is identified in 50-80% of cases.[5] Staining may be cytoplasmic and nuclear, in cases of t(2;5)(p23;q35), or only cytoplasmic in cases where variant translocations induce ALK protein expression.[155] The expression of ALK is fairly specific for ALCL, since it is negative in most other lymphomas, including HL,[156] and non-lymphoid neoplasms with the rare exception of a few DLBCL's[157] and inflammatory myofibroblastic tumors.[158] Other important markers include epithelial membrane antigen (EMA), which is positive in most cases.[155] ALCL is typically CD45+, CD15- (up to 20-25% of cases may show a reverse pattern)[5] and most cases express one or more T cell markers,[155] with CD2 and CD4 being positive in majority of the cases.[30] Even with the apparent "null cell" phenotype, there is evidence of clonal rearrangement of the T cell receptor at the molecular level.[159] These tumors also express cytotoxic granule proteins including TIA-1, granzyme B and perforin indicating their cytotoxic potential.[159, 160] Immunohistochemical stains may be performed as a panel to distinguish classic Hodgkin lymphoma (CD15+/CD30+/CD45-/EMA-) and B cell lymphomas (evidence of B lineage differentiation) from ALCL.

5.7.2.2   Molecular and cytogenetic features

90% of cases show T cell gene rearrangement at the molecular level[30] with t (2;5)(p23;35) seen in majority of the cases. These alterations can be demonstrated by PCR to confirm diagnosis.

5.8   Marginal Zone Lymphoma

Marginal zone lymphoma (MZL) represents a subgroup of NHL comprised of low-grade B cell lymphomas occurring in nodal (monocytoid B-cell lymphoma), splenic (splenic marginal zone lymphoma) and extra nodal (low grade lymphomas of mucosa associated lymphoid tissue, MALT) locations.[24] Although most commonly a disease of adults,[161] recent reports document its occurrence in younger individuals.[162] It is an indolent lymphoma with a tendency to remain localized for a prolonged period of time.[163, 164] The gastrointestinal tract is most common location for MALT lymphomas.[165]   Autoimmune   disorders   (Sjogren's   syndrome   and Hashimoto's thyroidits) confer a greater risk for development of MZL.[30] Involvement of multiple extra nodal sites, seen in a small percentage of cases doesn't represent true dissemination.[30] Nodal MZL are rare,[92, 161] with most patients presenting with peripheral, localized or systemic lymph node enlargement.[30]

5.8.1   Morphology

MZL can be a difficult diagnosis on FNAB smears since it is comprised of a heterogeneous population of cells including small lymphocytes, centrocyte-like cells, transformed cells, plasmacytoid lymphocytes, plasma cells and pale staining cells (monocytoid B cells), which may be presumed to be "reactive".[20, 24] The presence of this infiltrate in an extra nodal location is very suggestive of lymphoma, however similar findings in a lymph node overlap with reactive processes[24] (Figure 8-4). Therefore ancillary studies including FC should be utilized. MZL lack a specific immunophentype and may be difficult to classify.[20] In general, the majority express surface immunoglobulin,[6] and cytoplasmic immunoglobulin, if present, can be demonstrated in paraffin sections.[166] MZL needs to be differentiated from other small B cell lymphomas including FL, MCL, SLL/CLL, with which it may have some overlapping morphological features. CD5, CD10 and CD23 are useful antibodies since they are usually negative in MZL and expressed in different combinations in the other small B cell lymphomas.[6] (Table 8-4) If the diagnosis cannot be confirmed, an excisional biopsy should be suggested.[24]

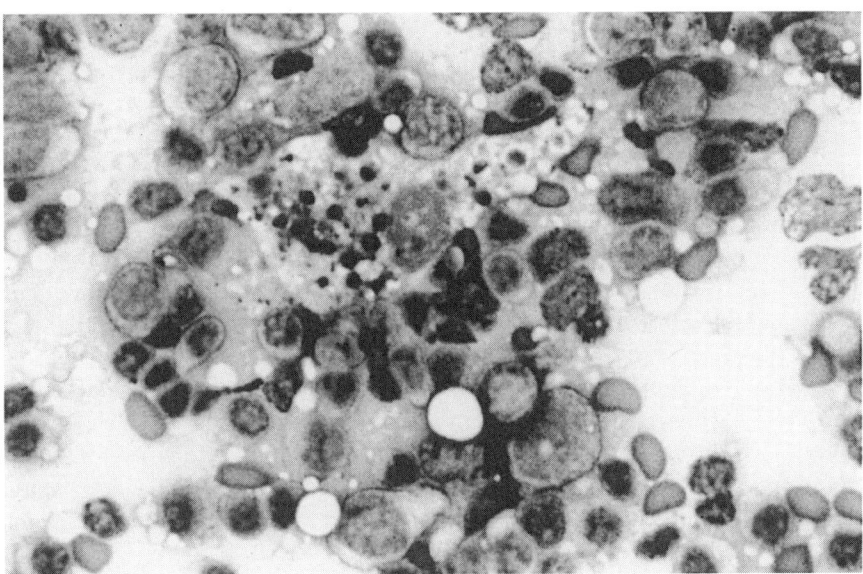

Figure 8-4. Reactive lymph node comprised of a heterogeneous population of lymphoid cells including small lymphocytes, transformed cells and tingible body macrophages (x1000, Diff-Quik stain).

5.8.2   Cytogenetics and molecular features

Trisomy 3 and t (11;18)(q21;q21) are demonstrated in a variable number of MALT lymphomas[167, 168] may support the diagnosis.

5.9   T-cell lymphoma

T-cell lymphomas comprise a heterogeneous group of neoplasms and have been divided into immature (precursor T-lymphoblastic leukemia/lymphoma) and mature phenotypes (mature T-cell and NK-cell neoplasms) in the recent WHO classification.[30] These neoplasms account for approximately 10% of NHL in North America but are found with increased frequency in Asian countries.[5] T-cell lymphoma is a difficult diagnosis by FNAB.[67] A specific sub-classification of the mature subtypes is not possible based on FNAB, since the precise classification of these neoplasms relies heavily on the clinical features, morphology and thorough immunophenotypic analysis with an extended antibody panel that usually requires a larger sample. Peripheral T-cell lymphoma, unspecified, does not fall into the well-defined groups of T-cell lymphomas.[30] Nodal presentation with extra nodal involvement during the course of the disease, including skin, bone marrow, liver and spleen is not uncommon.[169-172]

5.9.1   Morphology

Peripheral T-cell lymphomas encompass a broad morphological spectrum with medium to large cells having irregular nuclear outlines, pleomorphic nuclei with hyperchromatic or vesicular chromatin, prominent nucleoli and active mitosis.[30] Clear cell features[6] and Reed Sternberg like cells may be identified.[173] There is a variable admixture of non-neoplastic inflammatory cells including eosinophils, lymphocytes, plasma cells, neutrophils and histiocytes.[5] This overlap with reactive and other lymphoid neoplasms (Hodgkin lymphoma, B cell lymphoma) may make the diagnosis of T-cell lymphoma difficult and therefore the morphologic impression should be correlated with ancillary studies. Immunohistochemistry on the cell-block or core biopsy will reveal T cell antigen expression in the malignant cells and absence of B cell phenotype.[6] FC reveals tumor cells with expression of one or more pan T-cell antigens (CD2, CD3, CD5 and CD7) and not uncommonly an aberrant phenotype with loss of one or more of these markers.[172] The majority have a CD4+ helper phenotype,[172] however loss of CD4 and CD8 or their co-expression may also be observed.[174] Difficult cases may require T-cell receptor gene rearrangement studies, (identified in 80-90% of cases),[6] however absence of a re-arrangement does not necessarily exclude this diagnosis.[175] The highly aggressive nature of these neoplasms requires their accurate diagnosis and in equivocal cases an excisional biopsy is necessary.

5.10   Hodgkin Lymphoma

Approximately 30% of all lymphomas fall into this category[30] and have been divided in to (1) Nodular lymphocyte predominant HL (2) Classical HL with further subtypes including (a) Nodular sclerosis, (b) Mixed cellularity, (c) Lymphocyte-rich and (d) Lymphocyte-depleted in the WHO classification.[30] Features common to all subtypes include preferential involvement of cervical lymph nodes, predominance in the younger age group and the presence of characteristic large tumor cells designated as Reed Sternberg (RS) cells.[30]

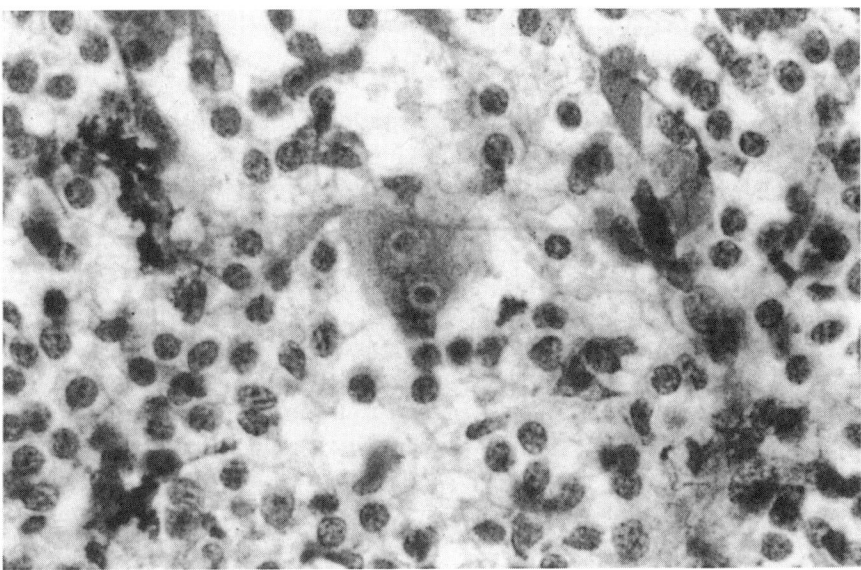

Figure 8-5. Classic "owl-eye" Reed-Sternberg cell in a case of Hodgkin Lymphoma. These are large binucleate cells with abundant cytoplasm and a central prominent eosinophilic nucleolus (x1000, Papanicolau stain).

5.10.1 Morphology

Cytology plays a role in the initial diagnosis of Hodgkin lymphoma (HL) and in the recognition of recurrent disease.[6, 176, 177] The broad spectrum of morphological features and the associated background findings result in overlap with a vast range of lymphoid and non-lymphoid tumors, at times making HL a difficult diagnosis on FNAB. Therefore, a clear understanding of the differential diagnosis, including cytological mimickers of RS cells is essential. HL smears are comprised of a polymorphous population of cells including neutrophils, eosinophils, lymphocytes, plasma cells, with or without fibrosis, necrosis, and a granulomatous response. Due to smaller numbers, the classic tumor cells (RS cells) may or may not be identified and therefore their absence does not exclude this diagnosis on FNAB smears.[5] Classic RS cells are large with abundant cytoplasm and at least two nuclei each with a central prominent eosinophilic nucleolus (Figure 8-5).[30] Variant forms of RS cells are identified in the various subtypes of HL and include lacunar cells (an artifact of formalin fixation and therefore not recognized on FNAB smears), mummified cells (cells with a hyperchromatic nucleus), and "popcorn cells" (cells with polylobated nuclei) seen in the nodular lymphocyte predominant type of HL. While recognition of HL is certainly possible based on morphology and IHC, accurate sub-classification of HL is not always possible on FNAB smears.[5] HL needs to be differentiated from other B and T cell lymphomas including ALCL. Abundance of Reed Sternberg cells may give a false impression of a non-lymphoid malignancy including carcinoma, melanoma or sarcoma. IHC on a cell-block or core-biopsy is essential to prevent misdiagnosis. The tumor cells in nodular lymphocyte predominant HL are CD45+, CD15-, CD30-/+ (occasional), EMA+/- (positivity in about 50% cases),[178] CD20+ and CD3-.[30] Classical HL, on the other hand, reveals a different immunophenotype with CD45-, CD15+/-, CD30+, EMA-, CD20-/+ and CD3-.[5] Antibodies to cytokeratin, or S-100 may be helpful to rule out non-lymphoid malignancies. HL also needs to be distinguished from benign conditions like suppurative lymphadenitis, since neutrophilic infiltrates and necrosis are not uncommonly seen in HL especially nodular sclerosis.[179] Granulomatous inflammation, seen in HL is also observed in both infectious/inflammatory and other malignant disorders (lymphoid and non lymphoid neoplasms) including large cell lymphoma, squamous cell carcinoma, anaplastic carcinoma of thyroid, lymphoepithelial carcinoma.[180] Discrete epitheloid cells have been note in approximately 70% of HL in one study and are a soft pointer for the diagnosis in the absence of other diagnostic features.[181] Immunoblasts, commonly observed in reactive conditions may mimic RS cells and may lead to a misinterpretation of HL.[5] FC is unhelpful in HL with most cases revealing a non-specific reactive pattern[68] and if our on-site evaluation of the FNAB is suggestive of HL, we obtain a NCB only and do not send the specimen for FC. Therefore in cases of primary presentation, failure to make an unequivocal diagnosis of HL should be followed by an excisional biopsy. However, if FNAB is diagnostic in recurrent disease, a tissue confirmation is not required.

5.11   Plasma cell neoplasms

Plasma cell neoplasms diagnosed by FNAB include bony[182, 183] and extramedullary plasmacytoma. The latter may involve virtually any organ including larynx,[184] soft tissue, scalp, oral and nasal mucosa,[185] skin, liver, spleen, lymph nodes,[186] breast,[187] thyroid, parotid[188] and pancreas.[189]

5.11.1   Morphology

Smears demonstrate dispersed sheets of mature or immature plasma cells. The former reveal an eccentric nucleus with "clock face" chromatin, paranuclear halo (corresponding to the golgi apparatus) and abundant basophilic cytoplasm. Binucleate and multinucleate forms are common.

Immature plasma cells have a larger nucleus with dispersed chromatin, a high nuclear/cytoplasmic ratio and prominent nucleolus. The latter findings are associated with a poor prognosis.[190, 191] Occasionally, plasma cells may show multilobated or pleomorphic features, or so called "anaplastic" morphology[190, 192] (Figure 8-6). The differential diagnosis includes inflammatory pseudotumor (has inflammatory and mesenchymal cell types and fibrosis), and medullary thyroid cancer (has other cell shapes/ sizes, neuroendocrine chromatin and calcitonin positivity). Occasionally the tumor cells in plasma cell neoplasms and medullary thyroid carcinoma may be associated with amyloid[188, 193, 194] which appears as amorphous clumps of extracellular eosinophilic material admixed with giant cells. Amyloid maybe confused with pleomorphic adenoma in the parotid gland[188] and plasma cells in the pancreas may lead to confusion with islet cell tumor.[189]

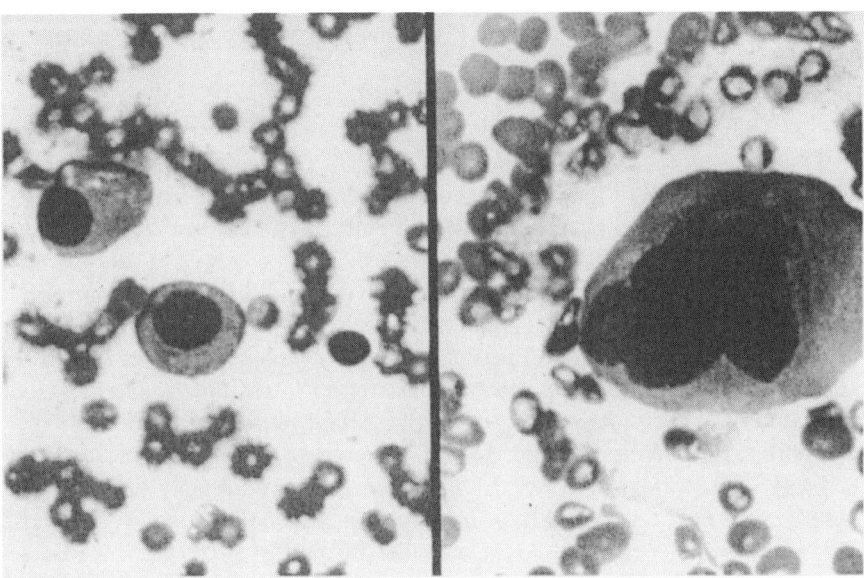

Figure 8-6. Plasma cell neoplasm. Left: reveals plasma cells with eccentric nuclei and abundant cytoplasm. Right: pleomorphic plasma cells in a case of multiple myeloma involving the liver (x1000, Diff-Quik stain).

5.11.2   Ancillary Studies

Mature plasma cells in a plasmacytoma may be interpreted as a reactive process. In such cases, IHC for *kappa* and *lambda* will aid in excluding exuberant reactive proliferations that will be polyclonal by IHC. The presence of amyloid can be confirmed with a Congo red stain (on cell block or NCB) or demonstrated by electron microscopy, if additional material is available.

Abdominal fat pad FNAB to assess the presence of amyloid by Congo red staining is used routinely at our institution. A fat pad aspirate for amyloid is obtained as a baseline test during the workup of patients with monoclonal gammopathy of undetermined significance/multiple myeloma and in established cases with a recent deterioration in cardiac or renal function. The interpretation of amyloid should be done cautiously to avoid false negatives and false positives.

The terminology used to report a plasma cell neoplasm on FNAB should be generic, i.e. plasma cell neoplasm and the extent of disease, plasmacytoma versus multiple myeloma, should be left to clinical judgment based on the evaluation of results of blood, urine monoclonal proteins, bone marrow biopsy and skeletal survey.

6.   LIMITATIONS

FNAB is not free of limitations. Sampling issues, either because of inadequate material or a non-representative sample, may be sources of error. The former may occur because of extensive necrosis, hemorrhage, fibrosis or dilution with blood.[21] The latter involves the inability to definitively ascertain whether the sample is representative of the lesion being sampled.[8] Composite lymphoma,[195] concomitant lymphoma and carcinoma,[196] focal large cell transformation,[8] and partial nodal involvement[12] may lead to errors in diagnosis because of lack of representation in the sample. False negative or misinterpreted results related to sampling issues have been reported.[28, 197-199] Discordance of morphology and FC (negative FC with cytomorphology favoring ML and vice versa,[8, 21] surface immunoglobulin negative lymphoma[6]) may require further investigation. Some diagnosis, such as HL and peripheral T-cell lymphoma, can be difficult even in the face of an adequate FNAB sample. The former may be confused with reactive hyperplasia with prominent immunoblasts, NHL with abundant immunoblasts or a peripheral T-cell lymphoma.[21] IHC on centrifuged specimens or cell-blocks is often helpful in these cases.[21] If the material is insufficient for ancillary studies, a repeat procedure, either FNAB or excisional biopsy, is necessary for an accurate diagnosis.

7. CONCLUSION

FNAB has an important role to play in the diagnosis of potential hematopoietic neoplasms. Although surgical biopsy may be more accepted than FNAB in many institutions, it is not always the best approach in every patient. Lack of superficial lymph nodes, extremely ill patients and the need for a rapid diagnosis (i.e. highly proliferative tumors like BL) make the availability of a good FNAB service crucial. To achieve the greatest accuracy in diagnosis, FNAB should combine skilled aspiration and triage techniques to obtain representative material, morphological evaluation of the sample by an experienced cytopathologist, and availability of ancillary techniques, such as flow cytometric immunophenotyping, IHC and molecular analysis.

REFERENCES

1. Soderstrom, N., Fine-needle aspiration biopsy used as a direct adjunct in clinical diagnostic work. 1966, New York: Grune & Stratton.
2. Zajicek, J., Cytology of supradiaphragmatic organs. Vol. 4. 1974: Basel:Karger.
3. Zajicek, J., Cytology of infradiaphragmatic organs. Monographs in clinical cytology: aspiration biopsy cytology. Vol. 7. 1979: Basel: Karger.
4. Wakely, P.E., Jr. Aspiration cytopathology of malignant lymphoma: coming of age. Cancer, 1999. 87(6): p. 322-4.
5. Wakely, P.E., Jr. Aspiration Cytopathology of Lymph Nodes. in United States and Canadian Academy of Pathology. 2002. Chicago, Illinois.
6. Young, N.A. and Al-Saleem, T. Diagnosis of lymphoma by fine-needle aspiration cytology using the revised European-American classification of lymphoid neoplasms. Cancer, 1999. 87(6): p. 325-45.
7. Koo, C.H., Rappaport, H., Sheibani, K., Pangalis, G.A., Nathwani, B.N., and Winberg, C.D. Imprint cytology of non-Hodgkin's lymphomas based on a study of 212 immunologically characterized cases: correlation of touch imprints with tissue sections. Hum Pathol, 1989. 20(12 Suppl 1): p. 1-137.
8. Sandhaus, L.M. Fine-needle aspiration cytology in the diagnosis of lymphoma. The next step. Am J Clin Pathol, 2000. 113(5): p. 623-7.
9. Young, N.A. and Al-Saleem, T. Hematopathologists and cytopathologists: enemies or allies? Diagn Cytopathol, 1999. 21(5): p. 305-6.
10. Katz, R.L. and Caraway, N.P. FNA lymphoproliferative diseases: myths and legends. Diagn Cytopathol, 1995. 12(2): p. 99-100.
11. Leong, A.S. and Stevens, M. Fine-needle aspiration biopsy for the diagnosis of lymphoma: a perspective. Diagn Cytopathol, 1996. 15(4): p. 352-7.
12. Pinkus, G.S. Needle biopsy in malignant lymphoma. J Clin Oncol, 1996. 14(9): p. 2415-6.

13. Dekmezian, R.H., Sneige, N., and Katz, R.L. The effect of fine needle aspiration on lymph node morphology in lymphoproliferative disorders. Acta Cytol, 1989. 33: p. 732-33.

14. Behm, F.G., O'Dowd, G.J., and Frable, W.J. Fine-needle aspiration effects on benign lymph node histology. Am J Clin Pathol, 1984. 82(2): p. 195-8.

15. Tsang, W.Y. and Chan, J.K. Spectrum of morphologic changes in lymph nodes attributable to fine needle aspiration. Hum Pathol, 1992. 23(5): p. 562-5.

16. Ben-Yehuda, D., Polliack, A., Okon, E., Sherman, Y., Fields, S., Lebenshart, P., Lotan, H., and Libson, E. Image-guided core-needle biopsy in malignant lymphoma: experience with 100 patients that suggests the technique is reliable. J Clin Oncol, 1996. 14(9): p. 2431-4.

17. Pappa, V.I., Hussain, H.K., Reznek, R.H., Whelan, J., Norton, A.J., Wilson, A.M., Love, S., Lister, T.A., and Rohatiner, A.Z. Role of image-guided core-needle biopsy in the management of patients with lymphoma. J Clin Oncol, 1996. 14(9): p. 2427-30.

18. Saboorian, M.H. and Ashfaq, R. The use of fine needle aspiration biopsy in the evaluation of lymphadenopathy. Semin Diagn Pathol, 2001. 18(2): p. 110-23.

19. Jaffer, S. and Zakowski, M. Fine-needle aspiration biopsy of axillary lymph nodes. Diagn Cytopathol, 2002. 26(2): p. 69-74.

20. Dong, H.Y., Harris, N.L., Preffer, F.I., and Pitman, M.B. Fine-needle aspiration biopsy in the diagnosis and classification of primary and recurrent lymphoma: a retrospective analysis of the utility of cytomorphology and flow cytometry. Mod Pathol, 2001. 14(5): p. 472-81.

21. Meda, B.A., Buss, D.H., Woodruff, R.D., Cappellari, J.O., Rainer, R.O., Powell, B.L., and Geisinger, K.R. Diagnosis and subclassification of primary and recurrent lymphoma. The usefulness and limitations of combined fine-needle aspiration cytomorphology and flow cytometry. Am J Clin Pathol, 2000. 113(5): p. 688-99.

22. Chhieng, D.C., Cohen, J.M., and Cangiarella, J.F. Cytology and immunophenotyping of low- and intermediate-grade B-cell non-Hodgkin's lymphomas with a predominant small-cell component: a study of 56 cases. Diagn Cytopathol, 2001. 24(2): p. 90-7.

23. Yao, J.L., Cangiarella, J.F., Cohen, J.M., and Chhieng, D.C. Fine-needle aspiration biopsy of peripheral T-cell lymphomas. A cytologic and immunophenotypic study of 33 cases. Cancer, 2001. 93(2): p. 151-9.

24. Matsushima, A.Y., Hamele-Bena, D., and Osborne, B.M. Fine-needle aspiration biopsy findings in marginal zone B cell lymphoma. Diagn Cytopathol, 1999. 20(4): p. 190-8.

25. Young, N.A., Al-Saleem, T.I., Ehya, H., and Smith, M.R. Utilization of fine-needle aspiration cytology and flow cytometry in the diagnosis and subclassification of primary and recurrent lymphoma. Cancer, 1998. 84(4): p. 252-61.

26. Jeffers, M.D., Milton, J., Herriot, R., and McKean, M. Fine needle aspiration cytology in the investigation on non-Hodgkin's lymphoma. Journal of Clinical Pathology, 1998. 51(3): p. 189-96.

27. Tarantino, D.R., McHenry, C.R., Strickland, T., and Khiyami, A. The role of fine-needle aspiration biopsy and flow cytometry in the evaluation of persistent neck adenopathy. Am J Surg, 1998. 176(5): p. 413-7.

28. Stewart, C.J., Duncan, J.A., Farquharson, M., and Richmond, J. Fine needle aspiration cytology diagnosis of malignant lymphoma and reactive lymphoid hyperplasia. J Clin Pathol, 1998. 51(3): p. 197-203.
29. Harris, N.L., Jaffe, E.S., Stein, H., Banks, P.M., Chan, J.K., Cleary, M.L., Delsol, G., De Wolf-Peeters, C., Falini, B., and Gatter, K.C. A revised European-American classification of lymphoid neoplasms: a proposal from the International Lymphoma Study Group. Blood, 1994. 84(5): p. 1361-92.
30. Jaffe, E.S., Harris, N.L., Stein, H., and Vardiman, J.W., World Health Organization Classification of Tumours. Pathology and Genetics of Tumours of Haematopoietic and Lymphoid Tissues. 2001.
31. Buchino, J.J. and Jones, V.F. Fine needle aspiration in the evaluation of children with lymphadenopathy. Arch Pediatr Adolesc Med, 1994. 148(12): p. 1327-30.
32. Martin-Bates, E., Tanner, A., Suvarna, S.K., Glazer, G., and Coleman, D.V. Use of fine needle aspiration cytology for investigating lymphadenopathy in HIV positive patients. Journal of Clinical Pathology, 1993. 46(6): p. 564-6.
33. Oertel, J., Oertel, B., Lobeck, H., and Huhn, D. Immunocytochemical analysis of lymph node aspirates in patients with human immunodeficiency virus infection. Journal of Clinical Pathology, 1990. 43(10): p. 844-6.
34. Shapiro, A.L. and Pincus, R.L. Fine-needle aspiration of diffuse cervical lymphadenopathy in patients with acquired immunodeficiency syndrome. Otolaryngol Head Neck Surg, 1991. 105(3): p. 419-21.
35. Saikia, U.N., Dey, P., Jindal, B., and Saikia, B. Fine needle aspiration cytology in lymphadenopathy of HIV-positive cases. Acta Cytol, 2001. 45(4): p. 589-92.
36. Schultenover, S.J., Ramzy, I., Page, C.P., LeFebre, S.M., and Cruz, A.B., Jr. Needle aspiration biopsy: role and limitations in surgical decision making. Am J Clin Pathol, 1984. 82(4): p. 405-10.
37. Frable, W.J. Thin-needle aspiration biopsy. A personal experience with 469 cases. Am J Clin Pathol, 1976. 65(2): p. 168-82.
38. Zajdela, A., Zillhardt, P., and Voillemot, N. Cytological diagnosis by fine needle sampling without aspiration. Cancer, 1987. 59(6): p. 1201-5.
39. Christopherson, W.M. Lucy Wortham James Award. Cytologic detection and diagnosis of cancer. Its contributions and limitations. Cancer, 1983. 51(7): p. 1201-8.
40. Koss, L.G. Thin needle aspiration biopsy. Acta Cytol, 1980. 24(1): p. 1-3.
41. Abele, J.S., Miller, T.R., King, E.B., and Lowhagen, T. Smearing techniques for the concentration of particles from fine needle aspiration biopsy. Diagn Cytopathol, 1985. 1(1): p. 59-65.
42. Sklair-Levy, M., Polliack, A., Shaham, D., Applbaum, Y.H., Gillis, S., Ben-Yehuda, D., Sherman, Y., and Libson, E. CT-guided core-needle biopsy in the diagnosis of mediastinal lymphoma. Eur Radiol, 2000. 10(5): p. 714-8.
43. Wotherspoon, A.C., Norton, A.J., Lees, W.R., Shaw, P., and Isaacson, P.G. Diagnostic fine needle core biopsy of deep lymph nodes for the diagnosis of lymphoma in patients unfit for surgery. J Pathol, 1989. 158(2): p. 115-21.
44. Willman, J.H., White, K., and Coffin, C.M. Pediatric Core Needle Biopsy: Strengths and Limitations in Evaluation of Masses. Pediatr Dev Pathol, 2001. 3(4): p. 46-52.

45. Hughes, J.H., Caraway, N.P., and Katz, R.L. Blastic variant of mantle-cell lymphoma: cytomorphologic, immunocytochemical, and molecular genetic features of tissue obtained by fine-needle aspiration biopsy. Diagn Cytopathol, 1998. 19(1): p. 59-62.

46. Ngan, B.Y., Chen-Levy, Z., Weiss, L.M., Warnke, R.A., and Cleary, M.L. Expression in non-Hodgkin's lymphoma of the bcl-2 protein associated with the t(14;18) chromosomal translocation. N Engl J Med, 1988. 318(25): p. 1638-44.

47. Peterson, L.C. and Goolsby, C. Flow cytometric immunophenotyping of hematologic malignancies involving the blood and bone marrow. Curr Diagn Pathol, 1997. 4: p. 187-95.

48. Zander, D.S., Iturraspe, J.A., Everett, E.T., Massey, J.K., and Braylan, R.C. Flow cytometry. In vitro assessment of its potential application for diagnosis and classification of lymphoid processes in cytologic preparations from fine-needle aspirates. Am J Clin Pathol, 1994. 101(5): p. 577-86.

49. Pinkus, G.S. and Said, J.W. Characterization of non-Hodgkin's lymphomas using multiple cell markers. Immunologic, morphologic, and cytochemical studies of 72 cases. Am J Pathol, 1979. 94(2): p. 349-80.

50. Filippa, D.A., Lieberman, P.H., Erlandson, R.A., Koziner, B., Siegal, F.P., Turnbull, A., Zimring, A., and Good, R.A. A study of malignant lymphomas using light and ultramicroscopic, cytochemical and immunologic technics: correlation with clinical features. Am J Med, 1978. 64(2): p. 259-68.

51. Picker, L.J., Weiss, L.M., Medeiros, L.J., Wood, G.S., and Warnke, R.A. Immunophenotypic criteria for the diagnosis of non-Hodgkin's lymphoma. Am J Pathol, 1987. 128(1): p. 181-201.

52. Gajl-Peczalska, K.J., Bloomfield, C.D., Coccia, P.F., Sosin, H., Brunning, R.D., and Kersey, J.H. B and T cell lymphomas. Analysis of blood and lymph nodes in 87 patients. Am J Med, 1975. 59(5): p. 674-85.

53. Aisenberg, A.C., Wilkes, B.M., and Harris, N.L. Monoclonal antibody studies in non-Hodgkin's lymphoma. Blood, 1983. 61(3): p. 469-75.

54. Chernoff, W.G., Lampe, H.B., Cramer, H., and Banerjee, D. The potential clinical impact of the fine needle aspiration/flow cytometric diagnosis of malignant lymphoma. J Otolaryngol, 1992. 21(Suppl 1): p. 1-15.

55. Johnson, A., Akerman, M., and Cavallin-Stahl, E. Flow cytometric detection of B-clonal excess in fine needle aspirates for enhanced diagnostic accuracy in non-Hodgkin's lymphoma in adults. Histopathology, 1987. 11(6): p. 581-90.

56. Ketai, L., Chauncey, J., and Duque, R. Combination of flow cytometry and transbronchial needle aspiration in the diagnosis of mediastinal lymphoma. Chest, 1985. 88(6): p. 936.

57. Cannon, C.R. and Richardson, L.D. Value of flow cytometry in the evaluation of head and neck fine-needle lymphoid aspirates: a 3-year retrospective review of a community-based practice. Otolaryngol Head Neck Surg, 2001. 124(5): p. 544-8.

58. Liu, K., Stern, R.C., Rogers, R.T., Dodd, L.G., and Mann, K.P. Diagnosis of hematopoietic processes by fine-needle aspiration in conjunction with flow cytometry: A review of 127 cases. Diagn Cytopathol, 2001. 24(1): p. 1-10.

59. Cannon, C.R. and Richardson, D. Value of flow cytometry with fine needle aspiration biopsy in patients with head and neck lymphoma. Otolaryngol Head Neck Surg, 2000. 123(6): p. 696-9.

60. Davidson, B., Risberg, B., Berner, A., Smeland, E.B., and Torlakovic, E. Evaluation of lymphoid cell populations in cytology specimens using flow cytometry and polymerase chain reaction. Diagn Mol Pathol, 1999. 8(4): p. 183-8.

61. Ravinsky, E., Morales, C., Kutryk, E., Chrobak, A., and Paraskevas, F. Cytodiagnosis of lymphoid proliferations by fine needle aspiration biopsy. Adjunctive value of flow cytometry. Acta Cytol, 1999. 43(6): p. 1070-8.

62. Zardawi, I.M., Jain, S., and Bennett, G. Flow-cytometric algorithm on fine-needle aspirates for the clinical workup of patients with lymphadenopathy. Diagn Cytopathol, 1998. 19(4): p. 274-8.

63. Shabb, N., Katz, R., Ordonez, N., Goodacre, A., Hirsch-Ginsberg, C., and el-Naggar, A. Fine-needle aspiration evaluation of lymphoproliferative lesions in human immunodeficiency virus-positive patients. A multiparameter approach. Cancer, 1991. 67(4): p. 1008-18.

64. Katz, R.L., Gritsman, A., Cabanillas, F., Fanning, C.V., Dekmezian, R., Ordonez, N.G., Barlogie, B., and Butler, J.J. Fine-needle aspiration cytology of peripheral T-cell lymphoma. A cytologic, immunologic, and cytometric study. Am J Clin Pathol, 1989. 91(2): p. 120-31.

65. Dunphy, C.H., Katz, R.L., Fanning, C.V., and Dalton, W.T., Jr. Leukemic lymphadenopathy: diagnosis by fine needle aspiration. Hematol Pathol, 1989. 3(1): p. 35-44.

66. Al Omran, S.M.W.A.A.M.A. gamma/delta Peripheral T-cell lymphoma of the breast diagnosed by fine-needle aspiration biopsy. Diagn Cytopathol, 2002. 26(3): p. 170-3.

67. Al Shanqeety, O. and Mourad, W.A. Diagnosis of peripheral T-cell lymphoma by fine-needle aspiration biopsy: a cytomorphologic and immunophenotypic approach. Diagn Cytopathol, 2000. 23(6): p. 375-9.

68. Jennings, C.D. and Foon, K.A. Recent advances in flow cytometry: application to the diagnosis of hematologic malignancy. Blood, 1997. 90(8): p. 2863-92.

69. Katz, R.L. Pitfalls in the diagnosis of fine-needle aspiration of lymph nodes. Monogr Pathol, 1997(39): p. 118-33.

70. Clatch, R.J. Immunophenotyping of hematological malignancies by laser scanning cytometry. Methods Cell Biol, 2001. 64: p. 313-42.

71. Clatch, R.J., Foreman, J.R., and Walloch, J.L. Simplified immunophenotypic analysis by laser scanning cytometry. Cytometry, 1998. 34(1): p. 3-16.

72. Clatch, R.J., Walloch, J.L., Zutter, M.M., and Kamentsky, L.A. Immunophenotypic analysis of hematologic malignancy by laser scanning cytometry. Am J Clin Pathol, 1996. 105(6): p. 744-55.

73. Williams, M.E., Frierson, H.F., Jr., Tabbarah, S., and Ennis, P.S. Fine-needle aspiration of non-Hodgkin's lymphoma. Southern blot analysis for antigen receptor, bcl-2, and c-myc gene rearrangements. Am J Clin Pathol, 1990. 93(6): p. 754-9.

74. Movilia, A., De Servi, B., and Assi, A. [Application of PCR in the diagnosis of B-type non-Hodgkin's lymphomas in cytological specimens from fine-needle aspiration]. Pathologica, 2000. 92(3): p. 172-6.

75. Grosso, L.E. and Collins, B.T. DNA polymerase chain reaction using fine needle aspiration biopsy smears to evaluate non-Hodgkin's lymphoma. Acta Cytol, 1999. 43(5): p. 837-41.

76. Vianello, F., Tison, T., Radossi, P., Poletti, A., Galligioni, A., Giacon, C., Girolami, A., and Dazzi, F. Detection of B-cell monoclonality in fine needle aspiration by PCR analysis. Leukemia & Lymphoma, 1998. 29(1-2): p. 179-85.

77. Takashima, S., Takayama, F., Saito, A., Wang, Q., Hidaka, K., and Sone, S. Primary thyroid lymphoma: diagnosis of immunoglobulin heavy chain gene rearrangement with polymerase chain reaction in ultrasound-guided fine-needle aspiration. Thyroid, 2000. 10(6): p. 507-10.

78. Takano, T., Miyauchi, A., Matsuzuka, F., Yoshida, H., Kuma, K., and Amino, N. Diagnosis of thyroid malignant lymphoma by reverse transcription-polymerase chain reaction detecting the monoclonality of immunoglobulin heavy chain messenger ribonucleic acid. J Clin Endocrinol Metab, 2000. 85(2): p. 671-5.

79. Lovchik, J., Lane, M.A., and Clark, D.P. Polymerase chain reaction-based detection of B-cell clonality in the fine needle aspiration biopsy of a thyroid mucosa-associated lymphoid tissue (MALT) lymphoma. Hum Pathol, 1997. 28(8): p. 989-92.

80. Ruschenburg, I., Korabiowska, M., Schlott, T., Kubitz, A., and Droese, M. The value of PCR technique in fine needle aspiration biopsy of salivary gland for diagnosis of low-grade B-cell lymphoma. Int J Mol Med, 1998. 2(3): p. 339-41.

81. Katz, R.L., Hirsch-Ginsberg, C., Childs, C., Dekmezian, R., Fanning, T., Ordonez, N., Cabanillis, F., and Sneige, N. The role of gene rearrangements for antigen receptors in the diagnosis of lymphoma obtained by fine-needle aspiration. A study of 63 cases with concomitant immunophenotyping. Am J Clin Pathol, 1991. 96(4): p. 479-90.

82. Jeffers, M.D., McCorriston, J., Farquharson, M.A., Stewart, C.J., and Mutch, A.F. Analysis of clonality in cytologic material using the polymerase chain reaction (PCR). Cytopathology, 1997. 8(2): p. 114-21.

83. Aiello, A., Delia, D., Giardini, R., Alasio, L., Bartoli, C., Pierotti, M.A., and Pilotti, S. PCR analysis of IgH and BCL2 gene rearrangement in the diagnosis of follicular lymphoma in lymph node fine-needle aspiration. A critical appraisal. Diagn Mol Pathol, 1997. 6(3): p. 154-60.

84. Chen, Z., Wang, D.D., Peier, A., Stone, J.F., and Sandberg, A.A. FISH in the evaluation of pleural and ascitic fluids. Cancer Genet Cytogenet, 1995. 84(2): p. 116-9.

85. Katz, R.L., Caraway, N.P., Gu, J., Jiang, F., Pasco-Miller, L.A., Glassman, A.B., Luthra, R., Hayes, K.J., Romaguera, J.E., Cabanillas, F.F., and Medeiros, L.J. Detection of chromosome 11q13 breakpoints by interphase fluorescence in situ hybridization. A useful ancillary method for the diagnosis of mantle cell lymphoma. Am J Clin Pathol, 2000. 114(2): p. 248-57.

86. Younes, A., Pugh, W., Goodacre, A., Katz, R., Rodriguez, M.A., Hill, D., Cabanillas, F., and Andreeff, M. Polysomy of chromosome 12 in 60 patients with non-Hodgkin's lymphoma assessed by fluorescence in situ hybridization: differences between follicular and diffuse large cell lymphoma. Genes Chromosomes Cancer, 1994. 9(3): p. 161-7.

87. Anastasi, J. Interphase cytogenetic analysis in the diagnosis and study of neoplastic disorders. Am J Clin Pathol, 1991. 95(4 Suppl 1): p. S22-8.

88. Berger, F., Felman, P., Sonet, A., Salles, G., Bastion, Y., Bryon, P.A., and Coiffier, B. Nonfollicular small B-cell lymphomas: a heterogeneous group of patients with distinct clinical features and outcome. Blood, 1994. 83(10): p. 2829-35.

89. Brecher, M. and Banks, P.M. Hodgkin's disease variant of Richter's syndrome. Report of eight cases. Am J Clin Pathol, 1990. 93(3): p. 333-9.

90. Momose, H., Jaffe, E.S., Shin, S.S., Chen, Y.Y., and Weiss, L.M. Chronic lymphocytic leukemia/small lymphocytic lymphoma with Reed-Sternberg-like cells and possible transformation to Hodgkin's disease. Mediation by Epstein-Barr virus. Am J Surg Pathol, 1992. 16(9): p. 859-67.

91. Campo, E., Raffeld, M., and Jaffe, E.S. Mantle-cell lymphoma. Semin Hematol, 1999. 36(2): p. 115-27.

92. Armitage, J.O. and Weisenburger, D.D. New approach to classifying non-Hodgkin's lymphomas: clinical features of the major histologic subtypes. Non-Hodgkin's Lymphoma Classification Project. J Clin Oncol, 1998. 16(8): p. 2780-95.

93. Bosch, F., Lopez-Guillermo, A., Campo, E., Ribera, J.M., Conde, E., Piris, M.A., Vallespi, T., Woessner, S., and Montserrat, E. Mantle cell lymphoma: presenting features, response to therapy, and prognostic factors. Cancer, 1998. 82(3): p. 567-75.

94. Norton, A.J., Matthews, J., Pappa, V., Shamash, J., Love, S., Rohatiner, A.Z., and Lister, T.A. Mantle cell lymphoma: natural history defined in a serially biopsied population over a 20-year period. Ann Oncol, 1995. 6(3): p. 249-56.

95. Velders, G.A., Kluin-Nelemans, J.C., De Boer, C.J., Hermans, J., Noordijk, E.M., Schuuring, E., Kramer, M.H., Van Deijk, W.A., Rahder, J.B., Kluin, P.M., and Van Krieken, J.H. Mantle-cell lymphoma: a population-based clinical study. J Clin Oncol, 1996. 14(4): p. 1269-74.

96. Rosenberg, C.L., Wong, E., Petty, E.M., Bale, A.E., Tsujimoto, Y., Harris, N.L., and Arnold, A. PRAD1, a candidate BCL1 oncogene: mapping and expression in centrocytic lymphoma. Proc Natl Acad Sci U S A, 1991. 88(21): p. 9638-42.

97. Williams, M.E., Westermann, C.D., and Swerdlow, S.H. Genotypic characterization of centrocytic lymphoma: frequent rearrangement of the chromosome 11 bcl-1 locus. Blood, 1990. 76(7): p. 1387-91.

98. Williams, M.E., Swerdlow, S.H., Rosenberg, C.L., and Arnold, A. Chromosome 11 translocation breakpoints at the PRAD1/cyclin D1 gene locus in centrocytic lymphoma. Leukemia, 1993. 7(2): p. 241-5.

99. Vandenberghe, E., De Wolf-Peeters, C., van den Oord, J., Wlodarska, I., Delabie, J., Stul, M., Thomas, J., Michaux, J.L., Mecucci, C., and Cassiman, J.J. Translocation (11;14): a cytogenetic anomaly associated with B-cell lymphomas of non-follicle centre cell lineage. J Pathol, 1991. 163(1): p. 13-8.

100. Zukerberg, L.R., Yang, W.I., Arnold, A., and Harris, N.L. Cyclin D1 expression in non-Hodgkin's lymphomas. Detection by immunohistochemistry. Am J Clin Pathol, 1995. 103(6): p. 756-60.

101. Dimopoulos, M.A., Panayiotidis, P., Moulopoulos, L.A., Sfikakis, P., and Dalakas, M. Waldenstrom's macroglobulinemia: clinical features, complications, and management. J Clin Oncol, 2000. 18(1): p. 214-26.

102. Waldenstrom, J. Macroglobulinemia. Adv Metab Disord, 1965. 2: p. 115-58.

103. Krajny, M. and Pruzanski, W. Waldenstrom's macroglobulinemia: review of 45 cases. CMAJ, 1976. 114(10): p. 899-900, 02, 05.

104. Stein, R.S., Ellman, L., and Bloch, K.J. The clinical correlates of IgM M-components: an analysis of thirty-four patients. Am J Med Sci, 1975. 269(2): p. 209-16.

105. Patsouris, E., Noel, H., and Lennert, K. Lymphoplasmacytic/lymphoplasmacytoid immunocytoma with a high content of epithelioid cells. Histologic and immunohistochemical findings. Am J Surg Pathol, 1990. 14(7): p. 660-70.

106. Anderson, J.R., Armitage, J.O., and Weisenburger, D.D. Epidemiology of the non-Hodgkin's lymphomas: distributions of the major subtypes differ by geographic locations. Non-Hodgkin's Lymphoma Classification Project. Ann Oncol, 1998. 9(7): p. 717-20.

107. Saikia, U.N.D.P.S.B.D.A. Fine-needle aspiration biopsy in diagnosis of follicular lymphoma: Cytomorphologic and immunohistochemical analysis. Diagn Cytopathol, 2002. 26(4): p. 251-6.

108. Suh, Y.K., Shabaik, A., Meurer, W.T., and Shin, S.S. Lymphoid cell aggregates: a useful clue in the fine-needle aspiration diagnosis of follicular lymphomas. Diagn Cytopathol, 1997. 17(6): p. 467-71.

109. Young, N.A., Al-Saleem, T.I., Al-Saleem, Z., Ehya, H., and Smith, M.R. The value of transformed lymphocyte count in subclassification of non-Hodgkin's lymphoma by fine-needle aspiration. Am J Clin Pathol, 1997. 108(2): p. 143-51.

110. Chu, P.G., Chang, K.L., Arber, D.A., and Weiss, L.M. Immunophenotyping of hematopoietic neoplasms. Semin Diagn Pathol, 2000. 17(3): p. 236-56.

111. Almasri, N.M., Iturraspe, J.A., and Braylan, R.C. CD10 expression in follicular lymphoma and large cell lymphoma is different from that of reactive lymph node follicles. Arch Pathol Lab Med, 1998. 122(6): p. 539-44.

112. Xu, Y., McKenna, R.W., and Kroft, S.H. Assessment of CD10 in the diagnosis of small B-cell lymphomas: a multiparameter flow cytometric study. Am J Clin Pathol, 2002. 117(2): p. 291-300.

113. Rowley, J.D. Chromosome studies in the non-Hodgkin's lymphomas: the role of the 14;18 translocation. J Clin Oncol, 1988. 6(5): p. 919-25.

114. Ruschenburg, I., Schlott, T., Linke, B., Reimer, S., and Droese, M. Automated molecular genetic DNA analysis for detecting B-cell non-Hodgkin's lymphoma in cytologic specimens. Analytical & Quantitative Cytology & Histology, 1997. 19(3): p. 255-63.

115. Committee, T.N.-H.s.L.P.C.P. National Cancer Institute sponsored study of classifications of non-Hodgkin's lymphomas: summary and description of a working formulation for clinical usage. The Non-Hodgkin's Lymphoma Pathologic Classification Project. Cancer, 1982. 49(10): p. 2112-35.

116. Soussain, C., Patte, C., Ostronoff, M., Delmer, A., Rigal-Huguet, F., Cambier, N., Leprise, P.Y., Francois, S., Cony-Makhoul, P., and Harousseau, J.L. Small noncleaved cell lymphoma and leukemia in adults. A retrospective study of 65 adults treated with the LMB pediatric protocols. Blood, 1995. 85(3): p. 664-74.

117. Burkitt, D.P., General features and facial tumors, in Burkitt's lymphoma, D.P. Burkitt and D.H. Wright, Editors. 1970, Livingstone: Edinburgh.

118. Burkitt, D.P. A sarcoma involving the jaws in African children. Br J Surg, 1958. 46: p. 218.

119. Wright, D.H., Burkitt's lymphoma: a review of the pathology, immunology and possible etiological factors. 1971, Appleton-Century-Crofts: New York. p. 337-63.

120. Warnke, R.A., Weiss, L.M., Chan, J.K.C., Cleary, M.L., and Dorfman, R.F., Tumors of the lymph nodes and spleen. Atlas of tumor pathology. 1995, Washington, D.C.: Armed Forces Institute of Pathology.

121. Divine, M., Casassus, P., Koscielny, S., Bosq, J., Moullet, L., Lemaignan, C., Stamberg, J., Dupriez, B., Najman, A., and Pico, J. Small non-cleaved cell lymphoma. A prospective multicenter study of 51 adults treated with the LMB pediatric protocol. Blood, 1999. 10(Suppl 1): p. 523a.

122. Magrath, I.T. and Sariban, E. Clinical features of Burkitt's lymphoma in the USA. IARC Sci Publ, 1985(60): p. 119-27.

123. Hamilton-Dutoit, S.J., Raphael, M., Audouin, J., Diebold, J., Lisse, I., Pedersen, C., Oksenhendler, E., Marelle, L., and Pallesen, G. In situ demonstration of Epstein-Barr virus small RNAs (EBER 1) in acquired immunodeficiency syndrome-related lymphomas: correlation with tumor morphology and primary site. Blood, 1993. 82(2): p. 619-24.

124. Raphael, M., Gentilhomme, O., Tulliez, M., Byron, P.A., and Diebold, J. Histopathologic features of high-grade non-Hodgkin's lymphomas in acquired immunodeficiency syndrome. The French Study Group of Pathology for Human Immunodeficiency Virus-Associated Tumors. Arch Pathol Lab Med, 1991. 115(1): p. 15-20.

125. Grogan, T.M., Warnke, R.A., and Kaplan, H.S. A comparative study of Burkitt's and non-Burkitt's "undifferentiated" malignant lymphoma: immunologic, cytochemical, ultrastructural, cytologic, histopathologic, clinical and cell culture features. Cancer, 1982. 49(9): p. 1817-28.

126. Levine, A.M., Pavlova, Z., Pockros, A.W., Parker, J.W., Teitelbaum, A.H., Paganini-Hill, A., Powars, D.R., Lukes, R.J., and Feinstein, D.I. Small noncleaved follicular center cell (FCC) lymphoma: Burkitt and non-Burkitt variants in the United States. I. Clinical features. Cancer, 1983. 52(6): p. 1073-9.

127. Miliauskas, J.R., Berard, C.W., Young, R.C., Garvin, A.J., Edwards, B.K., and DeVita, V.T., Jr. Undifferentiated non-Hodgkin's lymphomas (Burkitt's and non-Burkitt's types). The relevance of making this histologic distinction. Cancer, 1982. 50(10): p. 2115-21.

128. Zech, L., Haglund, U., Nilsson, K., and Klein, G. Characteristic chromosomal abnormalities in biopsies and lymphoid-cell lines from patients with Burkitt and non-Burkitt lymphomas. Int J Cancer, 1976. 17(1): p. 47-56.

129. Lin, P., Jones, D., Dorfman, D.M., and Medeiros, L.J. Precursor B-cell lymphoblastic lymphoma: a predominantly extranodal tumor with low propensity for leukemic involvement. Am J Surg Pathol, 2000. 24(11): p. 1480-90.

130. Maitra, A., McKenna, R.W., Weinberg, A.G., Schneider, N.R., and Kroft, S.H. Precursor B-cell lymphoblastic lymphoma. A study of nine cases lacking blood and bone marrow involvement and review of the literature. Am J Clin Pathol, 2001. 115(6): p. 868-75.

131. Nathwani, B.N., Diamond, L.W., Winberg, C.D., Kim, H., Bearman, R.M., Glick, J.H., Jones, S.E., Gams, R.A., Nissen, N.I., and Rappaport, H. Lymphoblastic lymphoma: a clinicopathologic study of 95 patients. Cancer, 1981. 48(11): p. 2347-57.

132. Traweek, S.T. Immunophenotypic analysis of acute leukemia. Am J Clin Pathol, 1993. 99(4): p. 504-12.

133. Furman, W.L., Fitch, S., Hustu, H.O., Callihan, T., and Murphy, S.B. Primary lymphoma of bone in children. J Clin Oncol, 1989. 7(9): p. 1275-80.

134. Yunis, E.J. Ewing's sarcoma and related small round cell neoplasms in children. Am J Surg Pathol, 1986. 10(Suppl 1): p. 54-62.

135. Battifora, H. and Silva, E.G. The use of antikeratin antibodies in the immunohistochemical distinction between neuroendocrine (Merkel cell) carcinoma of the skin, lymphoma, and oat cell carcinoma. Cancer, 1986. 58(5): p. 1040-6.

136. Visscher, D., Cooper, P.H., Zarbo, R.J., and Crissman, J.D. Cutaneous neuroendocrine (Merkel cell) carcinoma: an immunophenotypic, clinicopathologic, and flow cytometric study. Mod Pathol, 1989. 2(4): p. 331-8.

137. Kant, J.A. and Hicks, D.J., Interpretation of non-lymphoid elements in lymph node biopsy specimens, in Surgical pathology of the ymph nodes and related organs, E. Jaffe, Editor. 1995, W B Saunders: Philadelphia. p. 594-623.

138. Rosai, J. and Levine, G.D., Tumors of the thymus, in Atlas of tumor pathology. 1976, Armed Forces Institute of Pathology: Washington, DC.

139. Knowles, D.M., Lymphoblastic Lymphoma, in Neoplastic Hematopathology, D.M. Knowles, Editor. 2001, Lippincott Williams & Wilkins: Philadelphia. p. 915-51.

140. Akhtar, M., Iqbal, M.A., Mourad, W., and Ali, M.A. Fine-needle aspiration biopsy diagnosis of small round cell tumors of childhood: A comprehensive approach. Diagn Cytopathol, 1999. 21(2): p. 81-91.

141. Halliday, B.E., Slagel, D.D., Elsheikh, T.E., and Silverman, J.F. Diagnostic utility of MIC-2 immunocytochemical staining in the differential diagnosis of small blue cell tumors. Diagn Cytopathol, 1998. 19(6): p. 410-6.

142. Ichikawa, Y., Shimizu, H., Yoshida, M., and Arimori, S. Two-color flow cytometric analysis of thymic lymphocytes from patients with myasthenia gravis and/or thymoma. Clinical Immunology & Immunopathology, 1992. 62(1 Pt 1): p. 91-6.

143. Mokhtar, N., Hsu, S.M., Lad, R.P., Haynes, B.F., and Jaffe, E.S. Thymoma: lymphoid and epithelial components mirror the phenotype of normal thymus. Hum Pathol, 1984. 15(4): p. 378-84.

144. Borowitz, M.J. and Falletta, J.M. Leukemias and lymphomas of thymic differentiation. Clin Lab Med, 1988. 8(1): p. 119-34.

145. Flug, F., Pelicci, P.G., Bonetti, F., Knowles, D.M., 2nd, and Dalla-Favera, R. T-cell receptor gene rearrangements as markers of lineage and clonality in T-cell neoplasms. Proc Natl Acad Sci U S A, 1985. 82(10): p. 3460-4.

146. Waldmann, T.A. The arrangement of immunoglobulin and T cell receptor genes in human lymphoproliferative disorders. Adv Immunol, 1987. 40: p. 247-321.

147. Katzin, W.E., Fishleder, A.J., Linden, M.D., and Tubbs, R.R. Immunoglobulin and T-cell receptor genes in thymomas: genotypic evidence supporting the nonneoplastic nature of the lymphocytic component. Hum Pathol, 1988. 19(3): p. 323-8.

148. Offit, K., Lo Coco, F., Louie, D.C., Parsa, N.Z., Leung, D., Portlock, C., Ye, B.H., Lista, F., Filippa, D.A., and Rosenbaum, A. Rearrangement of the bcl-6 gene as a prognostic marker in diffuse large-cell lymphoma. N Engl J Med, 1994. 331(2): p. 74-80.

149. Hutchison, R.E., Berard, C.W., Shuster, J.J., Link, M.P., Pick, T.E., and Murphy, S.B. B-cell lineage confers a favorable outcome among children and adolescents with large-cell lymphoma: a Pediatric Oncology Group study. J Clin Oncol, 1995. 13(8): p. 2023-32.

150. Anagnostopoulos, I., Dallenbach, F., and Stein, H., Diffuse Large Cell Lymphomas, in Neoplastic Hematopathology, D.M. Knowles, Editor. 2001, Lippincott Williams & Wilkins: Philadelphia. p. 855-913.

151. Haralambieva, E., Pulford, K.A., Lamant, L., Pileri, S., Roncador, G., Gatter, K.C., Delsol, G., and Mason, D.Y. Anaplastic large-cell lymphomas of B-cell phenotype are anaplastic lymphoma kinase (ALK) negative and belong to the spectrum of diffuse large B-cell lymphomas. Br J Haematol, 2000. 109(3): p. 584-91.

152. Lazzarino, M., Orlandi, E., Paulli, M., Boveri, E., Morra, E., Brusamolino, E., Kindl, S., Rosso, R., Astori, C., and Buonanno, M.C. Primary mediastinal B-cell lymphoma with sclerosis: an aggressive tumor with distinctive clinical and pathologic features. J Clin Oncol, 1993. 11(12): p. 2306-13.

153. Bastard, C., Deweindt, C., Kerckaert, J.P., Lenormand, B., Rossi, A., Pezzella, F., Fruchart, C., Duval, C., Monconduit, M., and Tilly, H. LAZ3 rearrangements in non-Hodgkin's lymphoma: correlation with histology, immunophenotype, karyotype, and clinical outcome in 217 patients. Blood, 1994. 83(9): p. 2423-7.

154. Stein, H., Mason, D.Y., Gerdes, J., O'Connor, N., Wainscoat, J., Pallesen, G., Gatter, K., Falini, B., Delsol, G., and Lemke, H. The expression of the Hodgkin's disease associated antigen Ki-1 in reactive and neoplastic lymphoid tissue: evidence that Reed-Sternberg cells and histiocytic malignancies are derived from activated lymphoid cells. Blood, 1985. 66(4): p. 848-58.

155. Benharroch, D., Meguerian-Bedoyan, Z., Lamant, L., Amin, C., Brugieres, L., Terrier-Lacombe, M.J., Haralambieva, E., Pulford, K., Pileri, S., Morris, S.W., Mason, D.Y., and Delsol, G. ALK-positive lymphoma: a single disease with a broad spectrum of morphology. Blood, 1998. 91(6): p. 2076-84.

156. Herling, M., Rassidakis, G.Z., Viviani, S., Bonfante, V., Giardini, R., Gianni, M., Morris, S.W., Cabanillas, F., Medeiros, L.J., and Sarris, A.H. Anaplastic lymphoma kinase (ALK) is not expressed in Hodgkin's disease: results with ALK-11 antibody in 327 untreated patients. Leukemia & Lymphoma, 2001. 42(5): p. 969-79.

157. Delsol, G., Lamant, L., Mariame, B., Pulford, K., Dastugue, N., Brousset, P., Rigal-Huguet, F., al Saati, T., Cerretti, D.P., Morris, S.W., and Mason, D.Y. A new subtype of large B-cell lymphoma expressing the ALK kinase and lacking the 2; 5 translocation. Blood, 1997. 89(5): p. 1483-90.

158. Cook, J.R., Dehner, L.P., Collins, M.H., Ma, Z., Morris, S.W., Coffin, C.M., and Hill, D.A. Anaplastic lymphoma kinase (ALK) expression in the inflammatory myofibroblastic tumor: a comparative immunohistochemical study. Am J Surg Pathol, 2001. 25(11): p. 1364-71.

159. Foss, H.D., Anagnostopoulos, I., Araujo, I., Assaf, C., Demel, G., Kummer, J.A., Hummel, M., and Stein, H. Anaplastic large-cell lymphomas of T-cell and null-cell phenotype express cytotoxic molecules. Blood, 1996. 88(10): p. 4005-11.

160. Krenacs, L., Wellmann, A., Sorbara, L., Himmelmann, A.W., Bagdi, E., Jaffe, E.S., and Raffeld, M. Cytotoxic cell antigen expression in anaplastic large cell lymphomas of T-and null-cell type and Hodgkin's disease: evidence for distinct cellular origin. Blood, 1997. 89(3): p. 980-9.

161. Anonymous. A clinical evaluation of the International Lymphoma Study Group classification of non-Hodgkin's lymphoma. The Non-Hodgkin's Lymphoma Classification Project. Blood, 1997. 89(11): p. 3909-18.

162. Elenitoba-Johnson, K.S., Kumar, S., Lim, M.S., Kingma, D.W., Raffeld, M., and Jaffe, E.S. Marginal zone B-cell lymphoma with monocytoid B-cell lymphocytes in pediatric patients without immunodeficiency. A report of two cases. Am J Clin Pathol, 1997. 107(1): p. 92-8.

163. Zinzani, P.L., Magagnoli, M., Ascani, S., Ricci, P., Poletti, V., Gherlinzoni, F., Frezza, G., Bendandi, M., Stefanetti, C., Merla, E., Pileri, S., and Tura, S. Nongastrointestinal mucosa-associated lymphoid tissue (MALT) lymphomas: clinical and therapeutic features of 24 localized patients. Ann Oncol, 1997. 8(9): p. 883-6.

164. Thieblemont, C., Bastion, Y., Berger, F., Rieux, C., Salles, G., Dumontet, C., Felman, P., and Coiffier, B. Mucosa-associated lymphoid tissue gastrointestinal and nongastrointestinal lymphoma behavior: analysis of 108 patients. J Clin Oncol, 1997. 15(4): p. 1624-30.

165. Radaszkiewicz, T., Dragosics, B., and Bauer, P. Gastrointestinal malignant lymphomas of the mucosa-associated lymphoid tissue: factors relevant to prognosis. Gastroenterology, 1992. 102(5): p. 1628-38.

166. Weiss, L., Arber, D., and Chang, K., Lymph nodes and spleen, in Principles and practice of surgical pathology, S. Silverberg, R. DeLellis, and W. Frable, Editors. 1997, Churchill Livingstone: New York. p. 675-772.

167. Ott, G., Katzenberger, T., Greiner, A., Kalla, J., Rosenwald, A., Heinrich, U., Ott, M.M., and Muller-Hermelink, H.K. The t(11;18)(q21;q21) chromosome translocation is a frequent and specific aberration in low-grade but not high-grade malignant non-Hodgkin's lymphomas of the mucosa-associated lymphoid tissue (MALT-) type. Cancer Res, 1997. 57(18): p. 3944-8.

168. Wotherspoon, A.C., Finn, T.M., and Isaacson, P.G. Trisomy 3 in low-grade B-cell lymphomas of mucosa-associated lymphoid tissue. Blood, 1995. 85(8): p. 2000-4.

169. Ascani, S., Zinzani, P.L., Gherlinzoni, F., Sabattini, E., Briskomatis, A., de Vivo, A., Piccioli, M., Fraternali Orcioni, G., Pieri, F., Goldoni, A., Piccaluga, P.P., Zallocco, D., Burnelli, R., Leoncini, L., Falini, B., Tura, S., and Pileri, S.A. Peripheral T-cell lymphomas. Clinico-pathologic study of 168 cases diagnosed according to the R.E.A.L. Classification. Ann Oncol, 1997. 8(6): p. 583-92.

170. Gisselbrecht, C., Gaulard, P., Lepage, E., Coiffier, B., Briere, J., Haioun, C., Cazals-Hatem, D., Bosly, A., Xerri, L., Tilly, H., Berger, F., Bouhabdallah, R., and Diebold, J. Prognostic significance of T-cell phenotype in aggressive non-Hodgkin's lymphomas. Groupe d'Etudes des Lymphomes de l'Adulte (GELA). Blood, 1998. 92(1): p. 76-82.

171. Lopez-Guillermo, A., Cid, J., Salar, A., Lopez, A., Montalban, C., Castrillo, J.M., Gonzalez, M., Ribera, J.M., Brunet, S., Garcia-Conde, J., Fernandez de Sevilla, A., Bosch, F., and Montserrat, E. Peripheral T-cell lymphomas: initial features, natural history, and prognostic factors in a series of 174 patients diagnosed according to the R.E.A.L. Classification. Ann Oncol, 1998. 9(8): p. 849-55.

172. Pinkus, G.S., O'Hara, C.J., and Said, J.W. Peripheral/post-thymic T-cell lymphomas: a spectrum of disease. Clinical, pathologic, and immunologic features of 78 cases. Cancer, 1990. 65(4): p. 971-98.

173. Quintanilla-Martinez, L., Fend, F., Moguel, L.R., Spilove, L., Beaty, M.W., Kingma, D.W., Raffeld, M., and Jaffe, E.S. Peripheral T-cell lymphoma with Reed-Sternberg-like cells of B-cell phenotype and genotype associated with Epstein-Barr virus infection. Am J Surg Pathol, 1999. 23(10): p. 1233-40.

174. Hastrup, N., Ralfkiaer, E., and Pallesen, G. Aberrant phenotypes in peripheral T cell lymphomas. Journal of Clinical Pathology, 1989. 42(4): p. 398-402.

175. Weiss, L.M., Picker, L.J., Grogan, T.M., Warnke, R.A., and Sklar, J. Absence of clonal beta and gamma T-cell receptor gene rearrangements in a subset of peripheral T-cell lymphomas. Am J Pathol, 1988. 130(3): p. 436-42.

176. Jimenez-Heffernan, J.A., Vicandi, B., Lopez-Ferrer, P., Hardisson, D., and Viguer, J.M. Value of fine needle aspiration cytology in the initial diagnosis of Hodgkin's disease. Analysis of 188 cases with an emphasis on diagnostic pitfalls. Acta Cytol, 2001. 45(3): p. 300-6.

177. Fulciniti, F., Vetrani, A., Zeppa, P., Giordano, G., Marino, M., De Rosa, G., and Palombini, L. Hodgkin's disease: diagnostic accuracy of fine needle aspiration; a report based on 62 consecutive cases. Cytopathology, 1994. 5(4): p. 226-33.

178. Anagnostopoulos, I., Hansmann, M.L., Franssila, K., Harris, M., Harris, N.L., Jaffe, E.S., Han, J., van Krieken, J.M., Poppema, S., Marafioti, T., Franklin, J., Sextro, M., Diehl, V., and Stein, H. European Task Force on Lymphoma project on lymphocyte predominance Hodgkin disease: histologic and immunohistologic analysis of submitted cases reveals 2 types of Hodgkin disease with a nodular growth pattern and abundant lymphocytes. Blood, 2000. 96(5): p. 1889-99.

179. Vicandi, B., Jimenez-Heffernan, J.A., Lopez-Ferrer, P., Gamallo, C., and Viguer, J.M. Hodgkin's disease mimicking suppurative lymphadenitis: a fine-needle aspiration report of five cases. Diagn Cytopathol, 1999. 20(5): p. 302-6.

180. Khurana, K.K., Stanley, M.W., Powers, C.N., and Pitman, M.B. Aspiration cytology of malignant neoplasms associated with granulomas and granuloma-like features: diagnostic dilemmas. Cancer, 1998. 84(2): p. 84-91.

181. Iyengar, K.R.M.S. Discrete epithelioid cells: Useful clue to Hodgkin's disease cytodiagnosis. Diagn Cytopathol, 2002. 26(3): p. 142-4.

182. Soderlund, V., Tani, E., Skoog, L., Bauer, H.C., and Kreicbergs, A. Diagnosis of skeletal lymphoma and myeloma by radiology and fine needle aspiration cytology. Cytopathology, 2001. 12(3): p. 157-67.

183. Phadke, D.M., Lucas, D.R., and Madan, S. Fine-needle aspiration biopsy of vertebral and intervertebral disc lesions: specimen adequacy, diagnostic utility, and pitfalls. Archives of Pathology & Laboratory Medicine, 2001. 125(11): p. 1463-8.

184. Saad, R., Raab, S., Liu, Y., Pollice, P., and Silverman, J.F. Plasmacytoma of the larynx diagnosed by fine-needle aspiration cytology: a case report. Diagnostic Cytopathology, 2001. 24(6): p. 408-11.

185. Tani, E., Santos, G.C., Svedmyr, E., and Skoog, L. Fine-needle aspiration cytology and immunocytochemistry of soft-tissue extramedullary plasma-cell neoplasms. Diagnostic Cytopathology, 1999. 20(3): p. 120-4.

186. Bangerter, M., Hildebrand, A., Waidmann, O., and Griesshammer, M. Fine needle aspiration cytology in extramedullary plasmacytoma. Acta Cytol, 2000. 44(3): p. 287-91.

187. Cangiarella, J., Waisman, J., Cohen, J.M., Chhieng, D., Symmans, W.F., and Goldenberg, A. Plasmacytoma of the breast. A report of two cases diagnosed by aspiration biopsy. Acta Cytol, 2000. 44(1): p. 91-4.

188. Ustun, M.O., Ekinci, N., and Payzin, B. Extramedullary plasmacytoma of the parotid gland. Report of a case with extensive amyloid deposition masking the cytologic and histopathologic picture. Acta Cytol, 2001.·45(3): p. 449-53.

189. Dodd, L.G., Evans, D.B., Symmans, F., and Katz, R.L. Fine-needle aspiration of pancreatic extramedullary plasmacytoma: possible confusion with islet cell tumor. Diagnostic Cytopathology, 1994. 10(4): p. 371-4; discussion 74-5.

190. Bartl, R., Frisch, B., Burkhardt, R., Fateh-Moghadam, A., Mahl, G., Gierster, P., Sund, M., and Kettner, G. Bone marrow histology in myeloma: its importance in diagnosis, prognosis, classification and staging. Br J Haematol, 1982. 51(3): p. 361-75.

191. Greipp, P.R., Leong, T., Bennett, J.M., Gaillard, J.P., Klein, B., Stewart, J.A., Oken, M.M., Kay, N.E., Van Ness, B., and Kyle, R.A. Plasmablastic morphology--an independent prognostic factor with clinical and laboratory correlates: Eastern Cooperative Oncology Group (ECOG) myeloma trial E9486 report by the ECOG Myeloma Laboratory Group. Blood, 1998. 91(7): p. 2501-7.

192. Grogan, T.M. and Spier, C.M., B-Cell Immunoproliferative Disorders, Including Multiple Myeloma and Amyloidosis, in Neoplastic Hematopathology, D.M. Knowles, Editor. 2001, Lippincott Williams & Wilkins: Philadelphia. p. 1557-87.

193. Arnesen, M. and Manivel, J.C. Plasmacytoma of the thoracic spine with intracellular amyloid and massive extracellular amyloid deposition. Ultrastruct Pathol, 1993. 17(3-4): p. 447-53.

194. Yakulis, R., Dawson, R.R., Wang, S.E., and Kennerdell, J.S. Fine needle aspiration diagnosis of orbital plasmacytoma with amyloidosis. A case report. Acta Cytol, 1995. 39(1): p. 104-10.

195. Kim, H., Hendrickson, R., and Dorfman, R.F. Composite lymphoma. Cancer, 1977. 40(3): p. 959-76.

196. Caraway, N.P., Wojcik, E.M., Saboorian, H.M., and Katz, R.L. Concomitant lymphoma and metastatic carcinoma in a lymph node: diagnosis by fine-needle aspiration biopsy in two cases. Diagnostic Cytopathology, 1997. 17(4): p. 287-91.

197. Sangalli, G., Serio, G., Zampatti, C., Lomuscio, G., and Colombo, L. Fine needle aspiration cytology of primary lymphoma of the thyroid: a report of 17 cases. Cytopathology, 2001. 12(4): p. 257-63.

198. Guo, Z., Kurtycz, D.F., De Las Casas, L.E., and Hoerl, H.D. Radiologically guided percutaneous fine-needle aspiration biopsy of pelvic and retroperitoneal masses: a retrospective study of 68 cases. Diagnostic Cytopathology, 2001. 25(1): p. 43-9.

199. Cafferty, L.L., Katz, R.L., Ordonez, N.G., Carrasco, C.H., and Cabanillas, F.R. Fine needle aspiration diagnosis of intraabdominal and retroperitoneal lymphomas by a morphologic and immunocytochemical approach. Cancer, 1990. 65(1): p. 72-7.

Chapter 9

ANGIOGENESIS IN LEUKEMIA AND LYMPHOMA

Ameet R. Kini
Cardinal Bernardin Cancer Center & Stritch School of Medicine, Loyola University Chicago, Maywood, IL

1. INTRODUCTION

Increased bone marrow blood flow in hematologic malignancies was described about 50 years ago.[1] However, it was only after the publication in 1997 of a study by Judah Folkman's group, demonstrating increased angiogenesis in acute lymphoblastic leukemia,[2] that the field received a major fillip, and attracted a lot of attention. Since then, as in any nascent field, the number of publications has grown exponentially, and there are now over 300 publications on this subject. The purpose of this review is to describe the progress in this field and to explain the significance of angiogenesis in leukemia and lymphoma.

2. A BRIEF OVERVIEW OF TUMOR ANGIOGENESIS

The hypothesis that tumor growth is angiogenesis-dependent was first proposed in 1971.[3] Many lines of evidence indicate that growth of tumors beyond a diameter of 2-3 mm requires formation of new blood vessels.[4-6] These blood vessels supply oxygen and nutrients to the growing tumor, and also promote metastasis.[5] Specific anti-angiogenesis agents such as endostatin[7-9] and anti-VEGF antibodies[10] suppress tumors in animal models, providing strong support for the hypothesis that tumors are angiogenesis-dependent.

There are numerous inducers of angiogenesis including vascular endothelial growth factor (VEGF), basic fibroblast growth factor (bFGF), hepatocyte growth factor (HGF), the ephrins, and the angiopoietins.[5, 11] VEGF is the best-characterized vascular growth factor, and is critical for blood vessel formation. Deletion of a single allele in knockout mice results in embryonic lethality.[12] Apart from VEGF, the VEGF family also includes VEGF-B, VEGF-C, VEGF-D, VEGF-E, and placental growth factor (PlGF).[13, 14] VEGF itself has multiple splice isoforms, encoding (most commonly) polypeptides composed of 121, 165, 189 and 206 amino acids.[14] The actions of VEGF are mediated by its receptors, including VEGFR-1 (also known as flt-1), VEGFR-2 (KDR, flk-1), VEGFR-3 (flt-4), and neuropilin. Deletion of the flt-1 gene[15] or flk-1 gene[16] results in lack of organized vascular channels, and embryonic lethality, illustrating the importance of the VEGF system in the formation of blood vessels.

There are also many endogenous inhibitors of angiogenesis, including thrombospondin-1, prolactin, angiostatin and endostatin.[5, 6] Angiogenesis is a tightly regulated process, and is triggered by an "angiogenic switch", i.e. a shift in the balance between the inducers and inhibitors of angiogenesis.[5, 6] There is now considerable evidence for a genetic basis of regulation for this angiogenic switch, based on the actions of tumor suppressor genes and oncogenes.[6, 17-19]

For a more detailed overview of angiogenesis, readers are referred to reviews on the subject by Folkman,[5] Zetter,[20] and Kerbel,[6] and to reviews on VEGF and its receptors by Ferrara[14] and Dvorak.[13] A historic account of the progress in angiogenesis research was recently published by Ferrara.[21]

3.   ANGIOGENESIS IN MYELODYSPLASTIC SYNDROME (MDS) AND ACUTE MYELOID LEUKEMIA (AML)

Numerous groups have documented increased vascularity in bone marrow biopsies of patients with AML[22-29] and MDS,[23, 29-31] as compared to normal control bone marrow biopsies. In our study[26] we specifically looked at angiogenesis in acute promyelocytic leukemia (APL), which is a subtype of AML. We showed that bone marrow angiogenesis is increased in APL, and is decreased after treatment with all-*trans* retinoic acid. A similar decrease in angiogenesis, after therapy, has been seen in other subtypes of AML.[25]

The main mediator of angiogenesis in AML and MDS appears to be VEGF. Many studies have demonstrated expression of VEGF in AML blasts.[24, 26-28, 32] Other angiogenic factors such as bFGF[24, 38-40] and angiogenin[39, 41, 42] have also been demonstrated in AML and MDS. However, the relative contribution of these other growth factors to the angiogenic phenotype is not clear. In our studies,[26] we have shown that neutralizing antibodies to VEGF completely inhibit endothelial cell migration induced by APL cells, demonstrating that VEGF is the most important (and possibly the only) mediator of the angiogenic phenotype in APL. AML cells express the VEGF receptors VEGFR-1, VEGFR-2 and VEGFR-3[32, 37, 43] (in various combinations) suggesting the possibility of paracrine or autocrine loops. VEGF also appears to be involved in leukemia progenitor self-renewal in MDS, by acting in an autocrine fashion.[35] Another VEGF family member, VEGF-C, has been shown to promote proliferation, survival and resistance to chemotherapy in AML cell lines and primary AML cells, by acting through VEGFR-3.[44] This raises the possibility that VEGF-C, produced by endothelial cells, is involved in a paracrine angiogenic loop in VEGFR-3-positive leukemias.[44]

The downstream pathways of VEGF signaling in AML are not well-characterized and may vary depending on the biologic subtype of AML. In the HL-60 myelomonocytic cell line, VEGF prevents apoptosis through induction of bcl-2, possibly mediated by heat shock protein 90.[45] In the OCI/AML-2 cell line, VEGF promotes cell growth and survival by acting on VEGFR-2 and producing nitric oxide through the PI3kinase/Akt pathway.[46]

Animal models have been used to study the functional relevance of angiogenesis in AML. Injection of a neutralizing antibody to VEGFR-2 in a non-obese diabetic immunocompromised (NOD-SCID) mouse model for primary leukemic cells and AML cell lines, results in increased survival.[47] It was further shown that inhibition of both the autocrine and paracrine VEGF/VEGFR-2 angiogenic loops is required to achieve long-term remission in this mouse model of AML.[48] Addition of VEGF results in increased tumor growth in a murine chloroma model, whereas addition of the VEGF antagonist, soluble neuropilin-1,[49] causes suppression of tumor growth. In a systemic mouse model of leukemia, injection of adenovirus encoding for soluble neuropilin-1 results in increased survival.[49] Treatment with the angiogenic inhibitors, endostatin and PI-88, significantly decreases leukemic cell mass in rat models of juvenile myelomonocytic leukemia and AML.[50]

Patients with AML and MDS were shown to have increased plasma[38] and serum[41] levels of VEGF. Elevated VEGF levels correlated with shorter complete remission (CR) rates and overall survival in AML patients, but not in MDS.[38] Similarly, increased cellular VEGF levels were detected in bone marrow samples from MDS[51] and AML[33] patients, and increasing VEGF levels were associated with decreased survival. AML patients had elevated plasma bFGF levels, but there was no correlation with CR rates or survival.[38]

Anti-angiogenic drugs have been used in clinical trials for AML. The VEGF receptor inhibitor SU5416 had partial activity in a small subset of patients with refractory AML and MDS,[52] although SU5416 may be acting through other receptor tyrosine kinases such as c-kit.[52, 53] Treatment of AML with thalidomide resulted in partial response in a subset of patients and was accompanied by a decrease in bone marrow microvascular density and plasma levels of bFGF.[40] While this suggests an anti-angiogenic effect, thalidomide has diverse effects, and the relative contribution of the anti-angiogenic effect is not clear.[40] Randomized controlled trials are necessary to validate these early promising results.

4.   ANGIOGENESIS IN ACUTE LYMPHOBLASTIC LEUKEMIA (ALL)

Perez-Atayde *et al.*[2] showed that microvessel density in bone marrow biopsies obtained from children with ALL was significantly higher than normal control bone marrow biopsies. The microvessels in ALL bone marrows were tortuous and arborizing, while microvessels in normal bone marrows were straight and with no branching.[2] Urine levels of bFGF were higher in ALL patients, compared to age-matched controls.[2] Urine bFGF levels and bone marrow microvessel density were decreased after therapy, but these differences were not statistically significant.[2] Aguayo *et al.*[54] also found higher bone marrow microvessel density in ALL patients, and an increase in plasma bFGF levels. Pule *et al.*[55] showed increased microvessel density in ALL bone marrows, with a significant decrease in remission. However microvessel density was not associated with prognosis. Koomagi *et al.*[56] used real-time PCR to show that VEGF levels were higher in bone marrow samples from patients with recurrent ALL compared to newly diagnosed ALL. The patients with high VEGF levels at diagnosis had lower relapse-free and overall survival compared to patients with low VEGF levels; however, these differences were not significant.

5. ANGIOGENESIS IN MYELOPROLIFERATIVE DISORDERS

Increased blood flow in myeloproliferative disorders was noted over 30 years ago.[57] Subsequent studies have documented increased bone marrow vascularity or blood flow in myelofibrosis,[58-65] chronic myelogenous leukemia (CML),[22, 58, 63, 66, 67] essential thrombocythemia (64) and polycythemia vera.[64]

The mediators of angiogenesis in myeloproliferative disorders appear to be VEGF and bFGF. In myelofibrosis, megakaryocytic cells have been shown to express increased levels of bFGF,[65, 68, 69] and bFGF may be involved in promoting increased angiogenesis as well as fibrosis. Elevated serum levels of VEGF have also been demonstrated in patients with myelofibrosis.[70, 71] In polycythemia vera, serum[72, 73] and plasma[74] levels of VEGF are elevated, and appear to be associated with splenomegaly[72] and thrombotic complications.[73, 74] High plasma[66, 74] and serum[71] levels of VEGF, and plasma bFGF[75] have been demonstrated in patients with CML. Bone marrow samples from CML patients were shown to have higher levels of cellular VEGF, and high VEGF levels correlated with shorter survival.[76] Increased bone marrow expression of VEGFR-2 was also associated with shorter survival in CML.[77]

The regulation of angiogenesis in CML is particularly interesting. *BCR-ABL*-positive K562 cells produce VEGF.[34, 78] Treatment of these cells with the *BCR-ABL* tyrosine kinase inhibitor, STI-571 (imatinib mesylate, Gleevec®) results in decreased expression of VEGF.[78] Transfection of *BCR-ABL* into murine myeloid,[78] murine B-cell,[79, 80] and human megakaryocytic cell lines[78] (which do not express endogenous *BCR-ABL*) leads to increased VEGF production. In the murine Ba/F3 B-cell line, transfection of *BCR-ABL* induces the expression of hypoxia inducible factor-1α,[79] which is a major inducer of VEGF expression. STI-571-resistant murine Baf/*BCR-ABL*-r1 cells produce increased amounts of VEGF, and this increased VEGF production can be inhibited by higher concentrations of STI-571.[78] Taken together, these results suggest that *BCR-ABL* drives VEGF expression, and STI-571 may be partly mediating its actions through an anti-angiogenesis mechanism.

6.   ANGIOGENESIS IN CHRONIC LYMPHOCYTIC LEUKEMIA (CLL)

We have shown that there is increased microvessel density in bone marrow biopsies from patients with CLL, compared to normal control biopsies.[81] There was a positive correlation between microvessel density and Rai clinical stage.[81] We also showed that urine levels of bFGF were significantly higher in CLL patients as compared to healthy controls.[81] Urine levels of VEGF were also shown to be higher in CLL patients, but the difference was not statistically significant.[81] Molica *et al.*[82] also found increased microvessel area and counts in CLL bone marrow biopsies. They showed that high microvessel area was associated with increased risk of disease progression in early stage CLL. Serum VEGF levels were elevated in CLL patients, and high VEGF levels also predicted disease progression in early stage CLL.[82, 83] In contrast, high cellular VEGF levels were shown to be associated with better prognosis in early stage CLL patients.[84] Aguayo *et al.*[85] demonstrated increased plasma levels of bFGF and VEGF in CLL patients, but no increase in bone marrow vascularity. Chen *et al.*[86] showed increased microvessel density in lymph nodes with CLL involvement compared to normal nodes. They also showed that CLL cells produce functionally active VEGF.

In addition to pro-angiogenic molecules such as bFGF[87-93] and VEGF,[84, 86, 88, 90, 92, 94] CLL cells also express anti-angiogenic molecules including thrombospondin-1.[92] This suggests that, similar to solid tumors, the angiogenic phenotype in CLL may depend on the relative balance between pro and anti-angiogenic factors. CLL cells have been shown to express angiogenic receptors including VEGFR-1[92, 95] and VEGFR-2[92, 96] and tie1,[95] suggesting a possible autocrine pathway.

Higher levels of VEGFR-2[96] and tie1[95] were associated with poor prognosis in early stage CLL. Intracellular levels of bFGF in CLL were positively correlated with stage, and were associated with resistance to fludarabine.[87] This resistance appears to be mediated through the upregulation of the anti-apoptotic molecule bcl-2 by bFGF.[97] These results suggest that angiogenic factors such as VEGF and bFGF are involved in promoting cell survival, apart from stimulating angiogenesis.

7.   ANGIOGENESIS IN LYMPHOMA

In an insightful article from 1975, Wolf *et al*[98] described angiogenesis in a cutaneous lymphoma (classified as "malignant lymphoma, undifferentiated, non-Burkitt type"). They showed that lymphoma fragments stimulated angiogenesis in a hamster cheek pouch model, even when separated by a Millipore membrane.[98] This observation led the authors to conclude that "a diffusable tumour angiogenic factor may play a vital role in tumour survival and portends a therapeutic potential."[98] Experiments using a chick chorioallantoic membrane (CAM) model also demonstrated that lymphomas induce neovascularization.[99, 100]

In 1985 Reilly *et al.* demonstrated increased vascularity in nodular sclerosis Hodgkin's disease.[101] Subsequently, Ribatti *et al.*[102] showed increased microvessel density in non-Hodgkin's lymphoma (NHL). High grade lymphomas had higher counts than intermediate grade lymphomas, which in turn had higher counts than low-grade lymphomas, suggesting that angiogenesis may be involved in disease progression.[102] Arias *et al.*[103] found a similar difference between low grade and high grade NHL, but not between intermediate and high grade NHL, or between follicular hyperplasia and follicular lymphoma. Schaerer *et al.*[104] found higher microvessel density in primary cutaneous lymphomas compared to reactive lymphoid infiltrates, although assessment of microvessel density was not useful as a diagnostic tool. Vacca *et al.*[105] documented higher microvessel density in mycosis fungoides lesions compared to normal skin, with an increase in microvessel density with disease progression.

Foss *et al.*[106] used in situ hybridization to show that VEGF is expressed in Hodgkin's disease and T-cell lymphomas, but this expression was confined to stromal cells including fibroblasts. Subsequently, a number of groups have shown that NHL cells themselves express VEGF.[34, 107-110] In Hodgkin's disease bFGF has been shown to be expressed by the Reed-Sternberg cells and by the stromal cells.[111] bFGF expression was highest in nodular sclerosis Hodgkin's disease, suggesting that bFGF in involved in angiogenesis as well as fibrosis.[111] VEGF expression has also been demonstrated in the Reed-Sternberg cells.[112]

In primary effusion lymphomas (PEL), the lymphoma cells secrete VEGF.[113] In HHV-8 infected PEL cell lines, VEGF secretion appears to be induced by virally derived macrophage inflammatory protein 1A and IL-6.[114] Injection of a neutralizing anti-VEGF antibody prevents development of ascites in a mouse model of PEL, indicating an important role for VEGF in the pathogenesis of these lymphomas.[113]

Folkman's group found high urine bFGF levels in patients with a number of malignancies including lymphoma and leukemia, with lower survival in lymphoma patients with high urine bFGF.[115] A high level of serum VEGF was shown to be associated with poorer remission rates and lower survival in NHL.[116, 117] Similarly, high serum bFGF levels were associated with poor prognosis in NHL.[118] Remarkably, in multivariate analysis, serum bFGF levels were shown to have higher predictive value than the traditional parameters, serum lactate dehydrogenase and number of extranodal sites.[118] Simultaneous elevation of both serum VEGF and serum bFGF was associated with a particularly poor outcome in NHL.[119] Similarly, high plasma VEGF and bFGF levels were associated with a worse outcome.[120]

Animal models have been used to assess the importance of angiogenesis in lymphoma. In a mouse model of Burkitt's lymphoma, vasostatin (a fragment of calreticulin) suppresses angiogenesis and tumor growth.[121, 122] The anti-angiogenic drug, endostatin, prevents tumor growth after treatment with chemotherapy or Rituximab (anti-CD20 antibody) in a NOD/SCID mouse model of Burkitt's lymphoma,[123] suggesting that anti-angiogenic agents may be a useful addition to current lymphoma therapies.

8.   PERSPECTIVE

There are now numerous reports showing increased angiogenesis and increased production of various angiogenic factors (most notably VEGF) in hematologic malignancies. Two questions remain to be clarified, and are undergoing active investigation by many groups. First, what is the basis of regulation of angiogenesis? All indications are that, similar to solid tumors, angiogenesis in hematologic malignancies is regulated by a complex interplay between pro-angiogenic factors and anti-angiogenic factors. Transcriptional regulation of angiogenic factors is mediated by tumor suppressor genes and oncogenes in solid tumors,[6, 17, 19] and there could be a similar mode of regulation in hematologic malignancies. A second mode of regulation is through the production of alternatively spliced isoforms that have differing functions. For example, different splice isoforms of VEGF mediate diverse functions.[13, 14] Similarly, VEGF receptors have splice isoforms that have distinct functions. For example, VEGFR-1 is produced as a soluble isoform that sequesters VEGF and suppresses angiogenesis,[124] in contradistinction to the full-length isoform that promotes VEGF-mediated actions.

Second, is angiogenesis essential for the progression of hematologic malignancies or is it largely an epiphenomenon? Numerous clinical studies have shown that the degree of angiogenesis or the levels of angiogenic factors are correlated with the extent or stage of disease, prognosis or response to therapy. These studies support a role for angiogenesis in pathogenesis, but do not provide direct evidence of causality. However, recently, anti-angiogenic agents have been shown to be effective in animal models of leukemia and lymphoma, bolstering the case for an essential role for angiogenesis in hematologic malignancies.

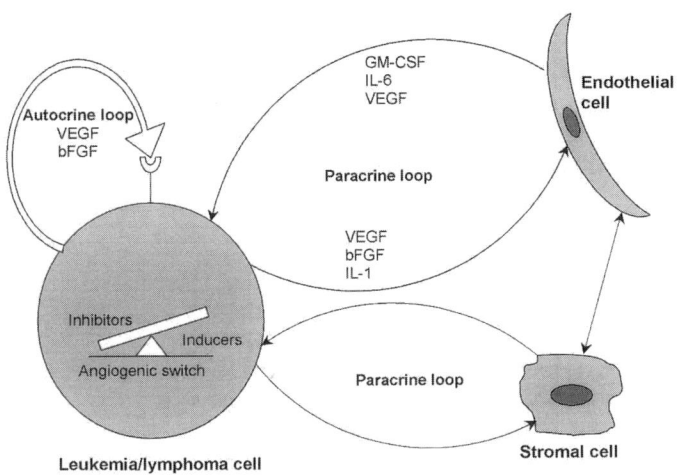

Figure 9-1. Putative mechanism of angiogenesis in leukemia and lymphoma

As has been discussed earlier, there are many putative mechanisms by which angiogenesis is involved in pathogenesis of these diseases (See Figure 9-1). Increased microvessels density in bone marrow and lymph nodes may be important in providing oxygen and nutrients to the malignant cells, as is the case in solid tumors. The relevance of this mechanism in hematologic malignancies is not clear, and we favor a limited role for this mechanism. It may, however, be possible that the increased endothelial cell mass is relevant by producing cytokines and growth factors that act on the malignant cells in paracrine fashion, promoting proliferation or survival. Stromal elements in bone marrow and other tissues may also be involved in such paracrine interactions. Since the malignant cells produce angiogenic factors and express receptors for these factors, functional autocrine loops may also be important in hematologic malignancies.

Assessment of angiogenic parameters, such as microvessel density and expression of angiogenic growth factors, has provided a new perspective and insight into the pathogenesis of hematologic malignancies. However, measurement of these angiogenic parameters appears to have limited value in the diagnosis of these diseases, and is unlikely to supplant or even supplement the present modalities of morphology, immunophenotyping, cytogenetics and molecular analysis. While angiogenic parameters are significantly increased in hematologic malignancies, there is often overlap with normal values, and these angiogenic parameters do not have a good predictive value in individual cases. However, in the future, angiogenic parameters may be useful in selecting patients for anti-angiogenic therapy, similar to the assessment of HER-2/neu expression in breast cancer patients receiving Herceptin®.

Angiogenic parameters show far greater promise in the assessment of prognosis. A number of studies have shown an association between angiogenic factors and prognosis. Most promising are easily performed tests such as measurement of urine, serum or plasma levels of angiogenic factors including bFGF and VEGF. In most cases a high level of an angiogenic factor is associated with poor prognosis, and this has been consistently and reproducibly shown in certain hematologic malignancies such as non-Hodgkin's lymphoma.[116, 118-120]

In clinical trials thus far, anti-angiogenic agents appear to have some activity in a subset of hematologic malignancies, although in many cases the drugs have multiple modalities of action and it is difficult to discern the specific contribution of an anti-angiogenic effect. Because of the complex nature of angiogenesis, a cocktail of drugs that act at different phases of the angiogenic cycle may be required for effectiveness and to forestall resistance.[9] A single anti-angiogenic agent is unlikely to act as a magic bullet for the treatment of hematologic malignancies. The anti-angiogenic cocktails may have to be used in concert with conventional therapeutic modalities. The challenge in the next few years is to characterize and comprehend the complex interactions and regulatory mechanisms that modulate angiogenesis in hematologic malignancies, so as to design effective therapeutic strategies to counteract these diseases.

REFERENCES

1. Petrakis NL, Masouredis SP, Miller P. The local blood flow in human bone marrow in leukemia and neoplastic diseases as determined by the clearance rate of radioiodine (I-131). J Clin Invest 1953; 32:952-963.
2. Perez-Atayde AR, Sallan SE, Tedrow U, Connors S, Allred E, Folkman J. Spectrum of tumor angiogenesis in the bone marrow of children with acute lymphoblastic leukemia. Am J Pathol 1997; 150(3):815-821.
3. Folkman J. Tumor angiogenesis: therapeutic implications. N Engl J Med 1971; 285(21):1182-1186.
4. Folkman J. What is the evidence that tumors are angiogenesis dependent? J Natl Cancer Inst 1990; 82(1):4-6.

5. Folkman J. Clinical applications of research on angiogenesis. N Engl J Med 1995; 333(26):1757-1763.
6. Kerbel RS. Tumor angiogenesis: past, present and the near future. Carcinogenesis 2000; 21(3):505-515.
7. Boehm T, Folkman J, Browder T, O'Reilly MS. Antiangiogenic therapy of experimental cancer does not induce acquired drug resistance. Nature 1997; 390(6658):404-407.
8. O'Reilly MS, Boehm T, Shing Y et al. Endostatin: an endogenous inhibitor of angiogenesis and tumor growth. Cell 1997; 88(2):277-285.
9. Bergers G, Javaherian K, Lo KM, Folkman J, Hanahan D. Effects of angiogenesis inhibitors on multistage carcinogenesis in mice. Science 1999; 284(5415):808-812.
10. Kim KJ, Li B, Winer J et al. Inhibition of vascular endothelial growth factor-induced angiogenesis suppresses tumour growth in vivo. Nature 1993; 362(6423):841-844.
11. Yancopoulos GD, Davis S, Gale NW, Rudge JS, Wiegand SJ, Holash J. Vascular-specific growth factors and blood vessel formation. Nature 2000; 407(6801):242-248.
12. Ferrara N, Carver-Moore K, Chen H et al. Heterozygous embryonic lethality induced by targeted inactivation of the VEGF gene. Nature 1996; 380(6573):439-442.
13. Dvorak HF. Vascular permeability factor/vascular endothelial growth factor: a critical cytokine in tumor angiogenesis and a potential target for diagnosis and therapy. J Clin Oncol 2002; 20(21):4368-4380.
14. Ferrara N, Gerber HP, LeCouter J. The biology of VEGF and its receptors. Nat Med 2003; 9(6):669-676.
15. Fong GH, Rossant J, Gertsenstein M, Breitman ML. Role of the Flt-1 receptor tyrosine kinase in regulating the assembly of vascular endothelium. Nature 1995; 376(6535):66-70.
16. Shalaby F, Rossant J, Yamaguchi TP et al. Failure of blood-island formation and vasculogenesis in Flk-1-deficient mice. Nature 1995; 376(6535):62-66.
17. Bouck N. Tumor angiogenesis: the role of oncogenes and tumor suppressor genes. Cancer Cells 1990; 2(6):179-185.
18. Dameron KM, Volpert OV, Tainsky MA, Bouck N. Control of angiogenesis in fibroblasts by p53 regulation of thrombospondin-1. Science 1994; 265(5178):1582-1584.
19. Hanahan D, Folkman J. Patterns and emerging mechanisms of the angiogenic switch during tumorigenesis. Cell 1996; 86(3):353-364.
20. Zetter BR. Angiogenesis and tumor metastasis. Annu Rev Med 1998; 49:407-424.
21. Ferrara N. VEGF and the quest for tumour angiogenesis factors. Nat Rev Cancer 2002; 2(10):795-803.
22. Dilly SA, Jagger CJ. Bone marrow stromal cell changes in haematological malignancies. J Clin Pathol 1990; 43(11):942-946.
23. Aguayo A, Kantarjian H, Manshouri T et al. Angiogenesis in acute and chronic leukemias and myelodysplastic syndromes. Blood 2000; 96(6):2240-2245.
24. Hussong JW, Rodgers GM, Shami PJ. Evidence of increased angiogenesis in patients with acute myeloid leukemia. Blood 2000; 95(1):309-313.
25. Padro T, Ruiz S, Bieker R et al. Increased angiogenesis in the bone marrow of patients with acute myeloid leukemia. Blood 2000; 95(8):2637-2644.

26. Kini AR, Peterson LA, Tallman MS, Lingen MW. Angiogenesis in acute promyelocytic leukemia: induction by vascular endothelial growth factor and inhibition by all-trans retinoic acid. Blood 2001; 97(12):3919-3924.

27. Lee JJ, Chung IJ, Park MR, Ryang DW, Park CS, Kim HJ. Increased angiogenesis and Fas-ligand expression are independent processes in acute myeloid leukemia. Leuk Res 2001; 25(12):1067-1073.

28. Litwin C, Leong KG, Zapf R, Sutherland H, Naiman SC, Karsan A. Role of the microenvironment in promoting angiogenesis in acute myeloid leukemia. Am J Hematol 2002; 70(1):22-30.

29. Korkolopoulou P, Apostolidou E, Pavlopoulos PM et al. Prognostic evaluation of the microvascular network in myelodysplastic syndromes. Leukemia 2001; 15(9):1369-1376.

30. Pruneri G, Bertolini F, Soligo D et al. Angiogenesis in myelodysplastic syndromes. Br J Cancer 1999; 81(8):1398-1401.

31. Ribatti D, Polimeno G, Vacca A et al. Correlation of bone marrow angiogenesis and mast cells with tryptase activity in myelodysplastic syndromes. Leukemia 2002; 16(9):1680-1684.

32. Fiedler W, Graeven U, Ergun S et al. Vascular endothelial growth factor, a possible paracrine growth factor in human acute myeloid leukemia. Blood 1997; 89(6):1870-1875.

33. Aguayo A, Estey E, Kantarjian H et al. Cellular vascular endothelial growth factor is a predictor of outcome in patients with acute myeloid leukemia. Blood 1999; 94(11):3717-3721.

34. Bellamy WT, Richter L, Frutiger Y, Grogan TM. Expression of vascular endothelial growth factor and its receptors in hematopoietic malignancies. Cancer Res 1999; 59(3):728-733.

35. Bellamy WT, Richter L, Sirjani D et al. Vascular endothelial cell growth factor is an autocrine promoter of abnormal localized immature myeloid precursors and leukemia progenitor formation in myelodysplastic syndromes. Blood 2001; 97(5):1427-1434.

36. de Bont ES, Rosati S, Jacobs S, Kamps WA, Vellenga E. Increased bone marrow vascularization in patients with acute myeloid leukaemia: a possible role for vascular endothelial growth factor. Br J Haematol 2001; 113(2):296-304.

37. Padro T, Bieker R, Ruiz S et al. Overexpression of vascular endothelial growth factor (VEGF) and its cellular receptor KDR (VEGFR-2) in the bone marrow of patients with acute myeloid leukemia. Leukemia 2002; 16(7):1302-1310.

38. Aguayo A, Kantarjian HM, Estey EH et al. Plasma vascular endothelial growth factor levels have prognostic significance in patients with acute myeloid leukemia but not in patients with myelodysplastic syndromes. Cancer 2002; 95(9):1923-1930.

39. Glenjen N, Mosevoll KA, Bruserud O. Serum levels of angiogenin, basic fibroblast growth factor and endostatin in patients receiving intensive chemotherapy for acute myelogenous leukemia. Int J Cancer 2002; 101(1):86-94.

40. Steins MB, Padro T, Bieker R et al. Efficacy and safety of thalidomide in patients with acute myeloid leukemia. Blood 2002; 99(3):834-839.

41. Brunner B, Gunsilius E, Schumacher P, Zwierzina H, Gastl G, Stauder R. Blood levels of angiogenin and vascular endothelial growth factor are elevated in myelodysplastic syndromes and in acute myeloid leukemia. J Hematother Stem Cell Res 2002; 11(1):119-125.

42. Verstovsek S, Kantarjian H, Aguayo A et al. Significance of angiogenin plasma concentrations in patients with acute myeloid leukaemia and advanced myelodysplastic syndrome. Br J Haematol 2001; 114(2):290-295.

43. Fielder W, Graeven U, Ergun S et al. Expression of FLT4 and its ligand VEGF-C in acute myeloid leukemia. Leukemia 1997; 11(8):1234-1237.

44. Dias S, Choy M, Alitalo K, Rafii S. Vascular endothelial growth factor (VEGF)-C signaling through FLT-4 (VEGFR-3) mediates leukemic cell proliferation, survival, and resistance to chemotherapy. Blood 2002; 99(6):2179-2184.

45. Dias S, Shmelkov SV, Lam G, Rafii S. VEGF(165) promotes survival of leukemic cells by Hsp90-mediated induction of Bcl-2 expression and apoptosis inhibition. Blood 2002; 99(7):2532-2540.

46. Koistinen P, Siitonen T, Mantymaa P et al. Regulation of the acute myeloid leukemia cell line OCI/AML-2 by endothelial nitric oxide synthase under the control of a vascular endothelial growth factor signaling system. Leukemia 2001; 15(9):1433-1441.

47. Dias S, Hattori K, Zhu Z et al. Autocrine stimulation of VEGFR-2 activates human leukemic cell growth and migration. J Clin Invest 2000; 106(4):511-521.

48. Dias S, Hattori K, Heissig B et al. Inhibition of both paracrine and autocrine VEGF/VEGFR-2 signaling pathways is essential to induce long-term remission of xenotransplanted human leukemias. Proc Natl Acad Sci U S A 2001; 98(19):10857-10862.

49. Schuch G, Machluf M, Bartsch G, Jr. et al. In vivo administration of vascular endothelial growth factor (VEGF) and its antagonist, soluble neuropilin-1, predicts a role of VEGF in the progression of acute myeloid leukemia in vivo. Blood 2002; 100(13):4622-4628.

50. Iversen PO, Sorensen DR, Benestad HB. Inhibitors of angiogenesis selectively reduce the malignant cell load in rodent models of human myeloid leukemias. Leukemia 2002; 16(3):376-381.

51. Verstovsek S, Estey E, Manshouri T et al. Clinical relevance of vascular endothelial growth factor receptors 1 and 2 in acute myeloid leukaemia and myelodysplastic syndrome. Br J Haematol 2002; 118(1):151-156.

52. Giles FJ, Stopeck AT, Silverman LR et al. SU5416, a small molecule tyrosine kinase receptor inhibitor, has biologic activity in patients with refractory acute myeloid leukemia or myelodysplastic syndromes. Blood 2003.

53. Spiekermann K, Faber F, Voswinckel R, Hiddemann W. The protein tyrosine kinase inhibitor SU5614 inhibits VEGF-induced endothelial cell sprouting and induces growth arrest and apoptosis by inhibition of c-kit in AML cells. Exp Hematol 2002; 30(7):767-773.

54. Aguayo A, Kantarjian H, Manshouri T et al. Angiogenesis in acute and chronic leukemias and myelodysplastic syndromes. Blood 2000; 96(6):2240-2245.

55. Pule MA, Gullmann C, Dennis D, McMahon C, Jeffers M, Smith OP. Increased angiogenesis in bone marrow of children with acute lymphoblastic leukaemia has no prognostic significance. Br J Haematol 2002; 118(4):991-998.

56. Koomagi R, Zintl F, Sauerbrey A, Volm M. Vascular endothelial growth factor in newly diagnosed and recurrent childhood acute lymphoblastic leukemia as measured by real-time quantitative polymerase chain reaction. Clin Cancer Res 2001; 7(11):3381-3384.

57. Van Dyke D, Parker H, Anger HO et al. Markedly increased bone blood flow in myelofibrosis. Journal of Nuclear Medicine 1971; 12(7):506-12.

58. Lahtinen R, Lahtinen T, Romppanen T. Bone and bone-marrow blood flow in chronic granulocytic leukemia and primary myelofibrosis. J Nucl Med 1982; 23(3):218-224.
59. Reilly JT, Nash JR, Mackie MJ, McVerry BA. Endothelial cell proliferation in myelofibrosis. Br J Haematol 1985; 60(4):625-630.
60. Hasselbalch H. On the pathogenesis of angiogenesis in idiopathic myelofibrosis. Am J Hematol 1990; 33(2):151.
61. Baglin TP, Crocker J, Timmins A, Chandler S, Boughton BJ. Bone marrow hypervascularity in patients with myelofibrosis identified by infra-red thermography. Clin Lab Haematol 1991; 13(4):341-348.
62. Thiele J, Rompcik V, Wagner S, Fischer R. Vascular architecture and collagen type IV in primary myelofibrosis and polycythaemia vera: an immunomorphometric study on trephine biopsies of the bone marrow. Br J Haematol 1992; 80(2):227-234.
63. Lundberg LG, Lerner R, Sundelin P, Rogers R, Folkman J, Palmblad J. Bone marrow in polycythemia vera, chronic myelocytic leukemia, and myelofibrosis has an increased vascularity. Am J Pathol 2000; 157(1):15-19.
64. Mesa RA, Hanson CA, Rajkumar SV, Schroeder G, Tefferi A. Evaluation and clinical correlations of bone marrow angiogenesis in myelofibrosis with myeloid metaplasia. Blood 2000; 96(10):3374-3380.
65. Chou JM, Li CY, Tefferi A. Bone marrow immunohistochemical studies of angiogenic cytokines and their receptors in myelofibrosis with myeloid metaplasia. Leuk Res 2003; 27(6):499-504.
66. Aguayo A, Kantarjian H, Manshouri T et al. Angiogenesis in acute and chronic leukemias and myelodysplastic syndromes. Blood 2000; 96(6):2240-2245.
67. Korkolopoulou P, Viniou N, Kavantzas N et al. Clinicopathologic correlations of bone marrow angiogenesis in chronic myeloid leukemia: a morphometric study. Leukemia 2003; 17(1):89-97.
68. Martyre MC, Bousse-Kerdiles MC, Romquin N et al. Elevated levels of basic fibroblast growth factor in megakaryocytes and platelets from patients with idiopathic myelofibrosis. Br J Haematol 1997; 97(2):441-448.
69. Bousse-Kerdiles MC, Martyre MC. Involvement of the fibrogenic cytokines, TGF-beta and bFGF, in the pathogenesis of idiopathic myelofibrosis. Pathol Biol (Paris) 2001; 49(2):153-157.
70. Di Raimondo F, Azzaro MP, Palumbo GA et al. Elevated vascular endothelial growth factor (VEGF) serum levels in idiopathic myelofibrosis. Leukemia 2001; 15(6):976-980.
71. Molica S, Santoro R, Iuliano F, Di Raimondo F, Fichera E, Giustolisi R. Serum levels of vascular endothelial growth factor in chronic leukemias. A comparative study with emphasis on myeloproliferative disorders. Haematologica 2001; 86(7):771.
72. Murphy P, Ahmed N, Hassan HT. Increased serum levels of vascular endothelial growth factor correlate with splenomegaly in polycythemia vera. Leuk Res 2002; 26(11):1007-1010.
73. Cacciola RR, Di Francesco E, Giustolisi R, Cacciola E. Elevated serum vascular endothelial growth factor levels in patients with polycythemia vera and thrombotic complications. Haematologica 2002; 87(7):774-775.
74. Musolino C, Calabro' L, Bellomo G et al. Soluble angiogenic factors: implications for chronic myeloproliferative disorders. Am J Hematol 2002; 69(3):159-163.

75. Krejci P, Dvorakova D, Krahulcova E et al. FGF-2 abnormalities in B cell chronic lymphocytic and chronic myeloid leukemias. Leukemia 2001; 15(2):228-237.
76. Verstovsek S, Kantarjian H, Manshouri T et al. Prognostic significance of cellular vascular endothelial growth factor expression in chronic phase chronic myeloid leukemia. Blood 2002; 99(6):2265-2267.
77. Verstovsek S, Lunin S, Kantarjian H et al. Clinical relevance of VEGF receptors 1 and 2 in patients with chronic myelogenous leukemia. Leuk Res 2003; 27(7):661-669.
78. Ebos JM, Tran J, Master Z et al. Imatinib mesylate (STI-571) reduces Bcr-Abl-mediated vascular endothelial growth factor secretion in chronic myelogenous leukemia. Mol Cancer Res 2002; 1(2):89-95.
79. Mayerhofer M, Valent P, Sperr WR, Griffin JD, Sillaber C. BCR/ABL induces expression of vascular endothelial growth factor and its transcriptional activator, hypoxia inducible factor-1alpha, through a pathway involving phosphoinositide 3-kinase and the mammalian target of rapamycin. Blood 2002; 100(10):3767-3775.
80. Janowska-Wieczorek A, Majka M, Marquez-Curtis L, Wertheim JA, Turner AR, Ratajczak MZ. Bcr-abl-positive cells secrete angiogenic factors including matrix metalloproteinases and stimulate angiogenesis in vivo in Matrigel implants. Leukemia 2002; 16(6):1160-1166.
81. Kini AR, Kay NE, Peterson LC. Increased bone marrow angiogenesis in B cell chronic lymphocytic leukemia. Leukemia 2000; 14(8):1414-1418.
82. Molica S, Vacca A, Ribatti D et al. Prognostic value of enhanced bone marrow angiogenesis in early B-cell chronic lymphocytic leukemia. Blood 2002; 100(9):3344-3351.
83. Molica S, Vitelli G, Levato D, Gandolfo GM, Liso V. Increased serum levels of vascular endothelial growth factor predict risk of progression in early B-cell chronic lymphocytic leukaemia. Br J Haematol 1999; 107(3):605-610.
84. Aguayo A, O'Brien S, Keating M et al. Clinical relevance of intracellular vascular endothelial growth factor levels in B-cell chronic lymphocytic leukemia. Blood 2000; 96(2):768-770.
85. Aguayo A, Kantarjian H, Manshouri T et al. Angiogenesis in acute and chronic leukemias and myelodysplastic syndromes. Blood 2000; 96(6):2240-2245.
86. Chen H, Treweeke AT, West DC et al. In vitro and in vivo production of vascular endothelial growth factor by chronic lymphocytic leukemia cells. Blood 2000; 96(9):3181-3187.
87. Menzel T, Rahman Z, Calleja E et al. Elevated intracellular level of basic fibroblast growth factor correlates with stage of chronic lymphocytic leukemia and is associated with resistance to fludarabine. Blood 1996; 87(3):1056-1063.
88. Bairey O, Zimra Y, Shaklai M, Rabizadeh E. Bcl-2 expression correlates positively with serum basic fibroblast growth factor (bFGF) and negatively with cellular vascular endothelial growth factor (VEGF) in patients with chronic lymphocytic leukaemia. Br J Haematol 2001; 113(2):400-406.
89. Krejci P, Dvorakova D, Krahulcova E et al. FGF-2 abnormalities in B cell chronic lymphocytic and chronic myeloid leukemias. Leukemia 2001; 15(2):228-237.
90. Bauvois B, Dumont J, Mathiot C, Kolb JP. Production of matrix metalloproteinase-9 in early stage B-CLL: suppression by interferons. Leukemia 2002; 16(5):791-798.
91. Gora-Tybor J, Blonski JZ, Robak T. Cladribine decreases the level of angiogenic factors in patients with chronic lymphocytic leukemia. Neoplasma 2002; 49(3):145-148.

92. Kay NE, Bone ND, Tschumper RC et al. B-CLL cells are capable of synthesis and secretion of both pro- and anti-angiogenic molecules. Leukemia 2002; 16(5):911-919.

93. Rimsza L, Pastos K, Massey K, Braylan R. Endothelial stimulation by small lymphocytic lymphoma correlates with secreted levels of basic fibroblastic growth factor. Br J Haematol 2003; 120(5):753-758.

94. Molica S, Santoro R, Digiesi G, Dattilo A, Levato D, Muleo G. Vascular endothelial growth factor isoforms 121 and 165 are expressed on B-chronic lymphocytic leukemia cells. Haematologica 2000; 85(10):1106-1108.

95. Aguayo A, Manshouri T, O'Brien S et al. Clinical relevance of Flt1 and Tie1 angiogenesis receptors expression in B-cell chronic lymphocytic leukemia (CLL). Leuk Res 2001; 25(4):279-285.

96. Ferrajoli A, Manshouri T, Estrov Z et al. High levels of vascular endothelial growth factor receptor-2 correlate with shortened survival in chronic lymphocytic leukemia. Clin Cancer Res 2001; 7(4):795-799.

97. Konig A, Menzel T, Lynen S et al. Basic fibroblast growth factor (bFGF) upregulates the expression of bcl-2 in B cell chronic lymphocytic leukemia cell lines resulting in delaying apoptosis. Leukemia 1997; 11(2):258-265.

98. Wolf JE, Hubler WR. Tumour angiogenic factor associated with subcutaneous lymphoma. Br J Dermatol 1975; 92(3):273-277.

99. Mostafa LK, Jones DB, Wright DH. Mechanism of the induction of angiogenesis by human neoplastic lymphoid tissue: studies on the chorioallantoic membrane (CAM) of the chick embryo. J Pathol 1980; 132(3):191-205.

100. Ribatti D, Vacca A, Bertossi M, De Benedictis G, Roncali L, Dammacco F. Angiogenesis induced by B-cell non-Hodgkin's lymphomas. Lack of correlation with tumor malignancy and immunologic phenotype. Anticancer Res 1990; 10(2A):401-406.

101. Reilly JT, Nash JR, Mackie MJ, McVerry BA. Distribution of fibronectin and laminin in normal and pathological lymphoid tissue. J Clin Pathol 1985; 38(8):849-854.

102. Ribatti D, Vacca A, Nico B, Fanelli M, Roncali L, Dammacco F. Angiogenesis spectrum in the stroma of B-cell non-Hodgkin's lymphomas. An immunohistochemical and ultrastructural study. Eur J Haematol 1996; 56(1-2):45-53.

103. Arias V, Soares FA. Vascular density (tumor angiogenesis) in non-Hodgkin's lymphomas and florid follicular hyperplasia: a morphometric study. Leuk Lymphoma 2000; 40(1-2):157-166.

104. Schaerer L, Schmid MH, Mueller B, Dummer RG, Burg G, Kempf W. Angiogenesis in cutaneous lymphoproliferative disorders: microvessel density discriminates between cutaneous B-cell lymphomas and B-cell pseudolymphomas. Am J Dermatopathol 2000; 22(2):140-143.

105. Vacca A, Moretti S, Ribatti D et al. Progression of mycosis fungoides is associated with changes in angiogenesis and expression of the matrix metalloproteinases 2 and 9. Eur J Cancer 1997; 33(10):1685-1692.

106. Foss HD, Araujo I, Demel G, Klotzbach H, Hummel M, Stein H. Expression of vascular endothelial growth factor in lymphomas and Castleman's disease. J Pathol 1997; 183(1):44-50.

107. Ho CL, Sheu LF, Li CY. Immunohistochemical expression of basic fibroblast growth factor, vascular endothelial growth factor, and their receptors in stage IV

non-Hodgkin lymphoma. Appl Immunohistochem Mol Morphol 2002; 10(4):316-321.

108. Potti A, Ganti AK, Kargas S, Koch M. Immunohistochemical detection of C-kit (CD117) and vascular endothelial growth factor (VEGF) overexpression in mantle cell lymphoma. Anticancer Res 2002; 22(5):2899-2901.

109. Stewart M, Talks K, Leek R et al. Expression of angiogenic factors and hypoxia inducible factors HIF 1, HIF 2 and CA IX in non-Hodgkin's lymphoma. Histopathology 2002; 40(3):253-260.

110. Ho CL, Sheu LF, Li CY. Immunohistochemical expression of angiogenic cytokines and their receptors in reactive benign lymph nodes and non-Hodgkin lymphoma. Ann Diagn Pathol 2003; 7(1):1-8.

111. Ohshima K, Sugihara M, Suzumiya J et al. Basic fibroblast growth factor and fibrosis in Hodgkin's disease. Pathol Res Pract 1999; 195(3):149-155.

112. Doussis-Anagnostopoulou IA, Talks KL, Turley H et al. Vascular endothelial growth factor (VEGF) is expressed by neoplastic Hodgkin-Reed-Sternberg cells in Hodgkin's disease. J Pathol 2002; 197(5):677-683.

113. Aoki Y, Tosato G. Role of vascular endothelial growth factor/vascular permeability factor in the pathogenesis of Kaposi's sarcoma-associated herpesvirus-infected primary effusion lymphomas. Blood 1999; 94(12):4247-4254.

114. Liu C, Okruzhnov Y, Li H, Nicholas J. Human herpesvirus 8 (HHV-8)-encoded cytokines induce expression of and autocrine signaling by vascular endothelial growth factor (VEGF) in HHV-8-infected primary-effusion lymphoma cell lines and mediate VEGF-independent antiapoptotic effects. J Virol 2001; 75(22):10933-10940.

115. Nguyen M, Watanabe H, Budson AE, Richie JP, Hayes DF, Folkman J. Elevated levels of an angiogenic peptide, basic fibroblast growth factor, in the urine of patients with a wide spectrum of cancers [see comments]. Journal of the National Cancer Institute 1994; 86(5):356-61.

116. Salven P, Teerenhovi L, Joensuu H. A high pretreatment serum vascular endothelial growth factor concentration is associated with poor outcome in non-Hodgkin's lymphoma. Blood 1997; 90(8):3167-3172.

117. Niitsu N, Okamato M, Nakamine H et al. Simultaneous elevation of the serum concentrations of vascular endothelial growth factor and interleukin-6 as independent predictors of prognosis in aggressive non-Hodgkin's lymphoma. Eur J Haematol 2002; 68(2):91-100.

118. Salven P, Teerenhovi L, Joensuu H. A high pretreatment serum basic fibroblast growth factor concentration is an independent predictor of poor prognosis in non-Hodgkin's lymphoma. Blood 1999; 94(10):3334-3339.

119. Salven P, Orpana A, Teerenhovi L, Joensuu H. Simultaneous elevation in the serum concentrations of the angiogenic growth factors VEGF and bFGF is an independent predictor of poor prognosis in non-Hodgkin lymphoma: a single-institution study of 200 patients. Blood 2000; 96(12):3712-3718.

120. Bertolini F, Paolucci M, Peccatori F et al. Angiogenic growth factors and endostatin in non-Hodgkin's lymphoma. Br J Haematol 1999; 106(2):504-509.

121. Pike SE, Yao L, Jones KD et al. Vasostatin, a calreticulin fragment, inhibits angiogenesis and suppresses tumor growth. J Exp Med 1998; 188(12):2349-2356.

122. Pike SE, Yao L, Setsuda J et al. Calreticulin and calreticulin fragments are endothelial cell inhibitors that suppress tumor growth. Blood 1999; 94(7):2461-2468.

123. Bertolini F, Fusetti L, Mancuso P et al. Endostatin, an antiangiogenic drug, induces tumor stabilization after chemotherapy or anti-CD20 therapy in a NOD/SCID mouse model of human high-grade non-Hodgkin lymphoma. Blood 2000; 96(1):282-287.

124. Kendall RL, Thomas KA. Inhibition of vascular endothelial cell growth factor activity by an endogenously encoded soluble receptor. Proc Natl Acad Sci U S A 1993; 90(22):10705-10709.

Chapter 10

CLINICAL FLOW CYTOMETRY
A Transition in Utilization

Charles L. Goolsby, Mary Paniagua, Laura Marszalek
Department of Pathology (CLG), Robert H. Lurie Comprehensive Cancer Center (CLG and MP), Northwestern University Feinberg School of Medicine, and Northwestern Memorial Hospital (LM), Chicago, Illinois

1. INTRODUCTION

Over the last 25 years, flow cytometry analysis of hematopoietic malignancies has evolved dramatically. In the early days, single color analysis, or one antigen at a time, on ficoll-hypaque separated cells was the standard approach. Thus, co-expression of antigens on cells, a hallmark of current practice, could only be inferred by comparing numbers of cells positive for each antigen. Density gradient preparation of the cells carried with it the potential for either loss or enrichment of specific cell populations that was variable from sample to sample. These technical limitations limited the sensitivity and specificity of leukemia/lymphoma immunophenotyping in those early days. Certainly, even with these limitations, however, these data were still very useful as an adjunct to diagnosis, although at the time, seldom were they integrated into the primary diagnostic package. Most frequently, the immunophenotypic results were issued as a separate document, frequently days after the primary diagnostic pathology report.

In the intervening years since those early beginnings, there has been steady development of reagents and instrumentation. We have seen not only dramatic increases in the numbers of highly specific monoclonal antibodies but, particularly recently, in the numbers of fluorescent dyes available as well. The standard of practice is now routine four color immunophenotyping with many laboratories moving to five, six, seven or more colors. For the most part, density gradient preparation of cells for these analyses is a thing of the past. These changes have dramatically increased the sensitivity and specificity of these assays. The analyses have become the preferred method of lineage determination in acute leukemias when morphology or special stains are unable to make that assessment.[1,2] Sub-classification of the B cell chronic lymphoproliferative disorders now depends heavily on immunophenotypic data,[2] and cytometric analyses provide a sensitive method of detection of clonal B cell populations.[2] Routinely, laboratories can detect malignant cell populations at significantly less than 1% of the total cells (frequently less than 0.1%) and in some cases can approach RT-PCR levels of sensitivity. In addition, it is now accepted that careful and thorough correlation of these data with other pathology findings, cytogenetics, and molecular analyses is critical for correct interpretation and maximizing the appropriate utilization of these data.[1,2] As a result, in most institutions, immunphenotyping has become part of the primary diagnostic work-up, ideally incorporated into the primary diagnostic reports. In addition, to continuing to serve an increasingly important adjunctive role in diagnosis, in some instances, immunophenotyping provides important prognostic information as well, for example CD38 expression in HIV,[3] CD38 expression in B-CLL,[4-6] or Zap70 expression levels in B-CLL.[7] Although not the topic of this chapter, the reader is referred to any of a number of excellent reviews on the diagnostic and prognostic uses of these data for more details.[1,2] It is worth noting that the role as an adjunct to diagnosis continues to evolve with new AML sub-classifications based on signal pathway responses to growth factors being proposed.[8] This is a very attractive concept in that these measurements will most likely reflect at the functional level abnormalities that are the result of disease characteristic translocations and genetic abnormalities. Perhaps most exciting is that they may then directly tie to new, and emerging, "targeted" therapies directed at these abnormal signaling events that in many instances have lead to the dysregulated proliferation and/or apoptosis that drive the disease process.

2.   HISTORICAL PERSPECTIVE

In addition to its utility as an adjunct to diagnosis, exciting new horizons for clinical cytometry are rapidly emerging, and developing, as tools in the therapeutic management of leukemia and lymphoma patients. Increasingly flow cytometric analyses are becoming key in therapeutic decisions and in therapeutic monitoring of patients. The explosion of antigen and ligand directed therapies for a range of hematopoietic malignancies, including anti-CD20,[9-12] anti-CD22,[13] anti-CD52,[11,12,14] anti-CD30,[15] anti-CD33,[11,12,16-18] anti-CD45,[11,17,18] and IL-2,[19] are having a significant impact on most clinical flow cytometry laboratories. Determining whether the malignant cells express the relevant antigen or ligand receptor is key in determining patient eligibility for a given therapy. Further, monitoring to see if the therapeutic reagent has bound and whether that has resulted in cell death of both the relevant malignant cells as well as normal cells is key in therapeutic monitoring.[9] The first major foray of flow cytometry into the arena of therapeutic monitoring of an antibody treatment was in the setting of OKT3 immunosuppressive therapy in solid organ transplant patients.[20-24] OKT3, an anti-CD3 directed antibody, bound to the T cells leading to death of the T cells and reductions or loss of cell mediated immune responses in these transplant patients. Flow cytometric analyses employing a panel of antibodies reacting with T cell antigens were used to determine if the drug (OKT3 antibody) had bound to the T cells. Detection of T cells using fluorescently labeled antibodies directed against either CD3 epitopes independent of the OKT3 binding site, TCR, or other T cell associated antigens such as CD2, CD5, or CD7 were employed along with a fluorescently labeled OKT3 antibody. This allowed one to first, determine on the T cells present (detected based on TCR, CD2, CD5, or CD7 staining) whether the unlabeled OKT3 drug had bound since it would block binding of the labeled OKT3 reagent being used. Further, it facilitated determination of therapeutic efficacy by enumerating either, or both, the relative or absolute numbers of T cells indicating whether the drug had successfully eliminated the T cells. Flow cytometric bead based assays were also used to monitor circulating levels of the OKT3 drug[21] and to determine if the patient was producing antibodies directed against the treatment OKT3 antibody[23,24] which might potentially be responsible for immunosuppressive treatment failure. In addition, examination of T cells and T cell subsets was useful in assessing T cell immune status following reduction or modulation of immunosuppressive therapy.

3. CURRENT ROLE IN PATIENT THERAPEUTIC MANAGEMENT

As noted above, the use of flow cytometric immunophenotyping as a tool in therapeutic monitoring is growing, at least initially, primarily due to the rapidly expanding numbers of antigen, or receptor, directed therapies that are now options for treatment of a number of hematopoietic malignancies.[9-19] The first impact of immunophenotyping is in determining whether a patient is eligible for a specific targeted therapy through assessment of the relevant therapeutic target (antigen(s) or receptor(s)) expression specifically on the malignant cells. Many clinical flow cytometry laboratories now routinely catalogue the expression of a number of potential therapeutically relevant antigens on the malignant cells (CD20, CD22, CD25, CD52, CD30 for example) for every relevant diagnostic specimen. In many instances, this permits alternative treatment decisions to be made at a later time, potentially without the need to re-biopsy the patient. In addition, as with OKT3 immunosuppressive therapy, flow cytometric immunphenotyping can be useful in monitoring therapy by determining if the drug has bound and if that has lead to reductions or loss of the malignant cells. Importantly, the effect of drug on the patient's normal cells expressing the same therapeutic target (antigen or receptor) can also be assessed.

As an example, monitoring of rituximab (anti-CD20) therapy in patients with a B cell malignancy is now routine and can play an important role in monitoring of these patients.[9] In a like manner to monitoring of OKT3 therapy described above, a panel of antibodies directed against B cell related antigens including CD20, CD19, CD79b, kappa, and lambda, allows one to determine if the anti-CD20 therapeutic has bound and whether the B cells, more specifically the clonal B cells, have been eliminated in that patient. With initiation of rituximab therapy, typically, a loss of peripheral B cells is seen over 1-3 weeks.[9,25,26] However, in some patients, one can see binding of the drug but no loss of the clonal B cells.[9] An example of this demonstrating successful binding of the anti-CD20 therapeutic without loss of the clonal B cells in a rituximab treated B cell lymphoma patient is shown in Figure 1.

Flow cytometric analyses can also provide a sensitive tool for monitoring of recurrence in these patients, a not always clear picture as morphologic assessment of post-treatment bone marrows following rituximab therapy can be complex. Immunophenotypic analyses can be a significant adjunct in differentiating reactive responses from residual or recurrent disease in these patients.[9] In addition, it is worth noting that, although rare, recurrence of true CD20 negative B cells of the same clone as the pre-treatment malignancy have also been reported. Further, flow cytometric analyses provide a highly sensitive detection of residual disease cells in the setting of antibody mediated therapies.[27] Although at present it is not always clear how to interpret the finding of a small (<0.1%) clonal population, the potential for detecting, and understanding, emergence of resistance in this setting remains. This sensitivity may also prove useful in selecting and assessing the effectiveness of additional, or co-, therapies. Again, although the potential impact of small B cell clones may not be clear, screening of patients prior to stem cell collection, or of collected stem cell products, during periods of remission following antibody therapy is also frequently done. Lastly, again in parallel with the OKT3 therapeutic monitoring model, flow cytometric immunophenotyping can be useful in monitoring regeneration of the B cell compartment following cessation of therapy, as interestingly, return of normal B cell levels in the peripheral blood can take many months. [9,25,26]

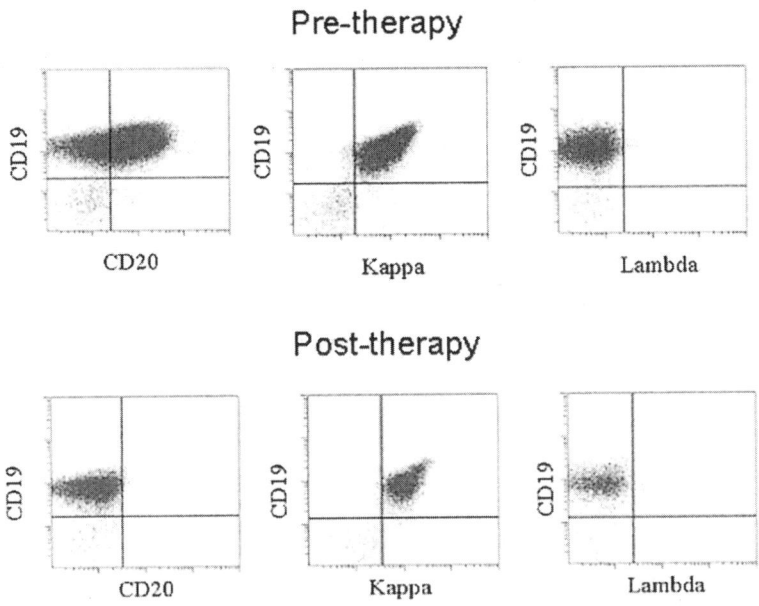

Figure 10-1. Analysis of CD19, CD20, kappa immunoglobulin light chain, and lambda immunoglobulin light chain staining in a B cell lymphoma patient pre- and post-rituximab therapy. Comparing the left histograms in the top and bottom rows shows the blocking of fluorescently labeled anti-CD20 antibody, however, the positive CD19 staining shows that the B cells were not eliminated in this patient. The two sets of histograms to the right demonstrate that these B cells represent the same kappa restricted B cell clonal population.

Of note are reports of differential cell killing in different tissue compartments following anti-CD52 therapy (Campath).[28-30] In B cell non-Hodgkin's lymphoma, poor responses have been reported in lymph nodes as compared to peripheral blood and bone marrow.[29,30] Also, a case report of a patient with a t(14;18)+ lymphoma in which the peripheral blood and bone marrow remained PCR positive following chemotherapy showed eradication of the B cell clone in the peripheral blood at the PCR level but not in the bone marrow with Campath treatment.[28] It is important to note in the latter case that the bone marrow remained positive for lymphoma by morphology and immunohistochemistry following Campath as well. This differential response in different tissues to therapy has lead to clinical trials assessing the combination of rituximab and Campath in treatment of B cell malignancies.[31] Although significant clinical responses were seen, in initial trials of rituximab addition to Campath treatment of B-CLL patients, eradication of the clonal B cells was still not seen in the bone marrows of these patients.[32] Thus, in the immunophenotypic monitoring of patients treated with Campath, and likely other antibody mediated treatments, examination of not only peripheral blood, but in many patients, simultaneous examination of bone marrow and tissue samples may be equally as important.

Not unexpectedly, a similar testing scenario as that described above for anti-CD20 therapy is being seen in the monitoring of other antigen directed therapies. There is every reason to believe that the numbers of antigen and/or ligand targeted therapies for the treatment of hematopoietic malignancies is only going to grow over the next several years.[10,33] In addition, an increasing utilization of these therapeutic strategies is being seen in a variety of other diseases and treatment settings.[34-44] Thus, an increasing demand for assessment of a large number of therapy related markers can be anticipated in most clinical flow cytometry laboratories. These assays will probably become more complex involving minimally four color analyses, and in many cases more than four colors. This will allow more efficient analysis of the large number of antigens and ligands that will be of interest to the clinician. However, there are more important, and fundamental, reasons for an extension to greater than three or four color techniques. In many instances, assessment of two, three, or even four antigens is necessary to simply specifically identify the aberrant cell in a sample. This may leave only one, or in some cases no, fluorescence color to assess the presence or expression of a potential therapeutic target on the malignant cells or to assess the effect of the therapeutic on those same malignant cells. Thus, effective assessment of therapeutic binding and effects is going to require an extension into more complex analyses. Specifically assessing the effect of the drug on apoptotic and proliferation regulatory pathways will lead to new understanding of the mechanisms of drug action,[45] and as importantly, perhaps mechanisms of resistance. An additional complexity may arise from the need to quantify antigen, or therapeutic target, levels. Golay et al,[46] have shown that at least in vitro the cytotoxic killing of B cells by rituximab correlates with CD20 staining intensity and, although not yet proven, it has been suggested that this may be the case in vivo as well.[47] Further, flow cytometric monitoring may play an important role in assessing cytokine or other treatments designed to modulate the expression level of a therapeutic target, potentially increasing the effectiveness of a directed therapy.[48,49] Thus, the need to quantitatively measure target molecule levels is almost certainly going to be important.

4. FUTURE POTENTIAL ROLES

Perhaps even more exciting is the potential role that cytometric analyses may play in assessing and monitoring of the new generation of therapies such as imatinib mesylate (STI571, Gleevec)[50,51] that more specifically target abnormal or dysregulated proteins in the malignant or abnormal cells in a patient. Driven by the Human Genome and Proteomics initiatives, the pace at which genes and molecules associated with specific diseases are being identified has greatly accelerated as has the understanding of these abnormalities in the context of cell regulation and the biology of disease. This knowledge will foster increasingly rapid development of new therapeutics that, like imatinib mesylate, more specifically target abnormalities or dysregulated functions in the malignant or abnormal cells. Clearly, in treatment of human malignancies, it is believed that development of rational therapies targeted at known abnormalities in tumor cells versus normal cells will produce significant reductions in therapy-induced toxicity compared to conventional chemotherapy. This hope was realized in the treatment of chronic myelogenous leukemia patients with imatinib mesylate, where extremely low toxicity was seen. With this in mind, especially for cancer modalities, previously reliable laboratory endpoints often may not provide adequate information about the effects of treatment during therapy.[52] Not surprisingly, many of the new rationally designed, directed therapies target molecules involved in signal transduction pathways that regulate cell proliferation, apoptosis, differentiation, or angiogenesis.[52-54] The development of new, and novel, flow cytometry cell based assays to measure the impact of therapy on these regulatory pathways, both in the malignant, or abnormal, cells as well as in normal cells, will play a vital role in the monitoring of these therapies as well as development of new therapies. Most regulatory pathways controlling cellular proliferation and apoptosis involve a series, or cascade, of alterations of the state (such as phosphorylation) of a number of molecules, ultimately changing the expression of key proteins such as cyclins, cyclin dependent kinases (CDKs), or apoptosis regulatory proteins that regulate cell growth and cell death. Sophisticated multi-parametric analyses assessing in specific cell sub-populations the targeted protein(s) and the therapeutic as well as the levels and molecular states, such as phosphorylation, of key intermediate molecules in these pathways that are regulated by, and downstream of, the targeted proteins will be required. Further, since multiple regulatory pathways control growth and death, cellular response to drug and emergence of resistance may not be restricted to a single pathway. Thus, the cellular proliferative and apoptotic responses regulated by these disrupted pathways along with the key endpoint regulatory molecules such as cyclins or CDKs will also need to be monitored in the same cell sub-populations as part of these analyses.

Imatinib mesylate therapy[50,51] for chronic myelogenous leukemia (CML) patients represents one of the first successful examples of a paradigm in which a genetic abnormality associated with a disease is identified followed by identification of the gene(s) involved, the characterization of the protein, and development of a new drug specifically targeting this aberrant protein as a therapy. As such it may serve as a model in many respects for the development of not only new drug therapies but for the tools that will be needed to monitor these types of therapies. CML is a chronic leukemia characterized by the accumulation of abnormal myeloid cells harboring the Philadelphia chromosome.[55,56] The Philadelphia chromosome represents a translocation between chromosomes 9 and 22 leading to a fusion between the *BCR* and *c-ABL* genes. This leads to the production of a fusion protein, BCR-ABL kinase, having abnormal kinase activity, which plays a key role in the development and progression of the disease.[55-57] Imatinib mesylate represents a kinase inhibitor developed as a therapeutic for the treatment of CML.[50,51] It has high specificity for inhibition of the BCR-ABL kinase, although at higher concentrations it does show inhibition of other kinases such as c-kit and PDGF receptor. Initial response to imatinib mesylate has been spectacular with most patients rapidly achieving a complete clinical remission.[50,51] However, a very high percentage of these patients relapse, or develop resistance to imatinib therapy.[50,51,58]

Several roles for cytometric (cell based) monitoring of these patients, and as a model other kinase inhibitor treated patients as well, may arise. Interestingly, during escalation of dose in imatinib mesylate clinical trials, only limited toxicity was seen. Thus, the paradigm of determining toxic drug levels during clinical trials and to use that information in assessing relevant treatment dose is less applicable with imatinib mesylate. As mentioned above, this may be a common theme as more rational targeted therapies become available. An alternative that may provide an adjunct to determining effective doses in vivo will be monitoring the phosphorylation of key molecules that are regulated through phosphorylation by kinases targeted by the drug used,[59] in the case of imatinib, the BCR-ABL kinase. The development of antibody reagents highly specific for phosphorylated epitopes on signal transduction protein intermediates will permit one, in single cell measurements, to functionally assess whether a kinase upstream of the protein intermediate being measured is active or not. Immediate downstream phosphorylation targets of the BCR-ABL kinase which may be suitable monitors of BCR-ABL kinase activity include Crkl as well as members of the Jak-Stat pathway,[60-65] specifically Stat1 and Stat5-- targets which BCR-ABL kinase is able to directly phosphorylate independent of Jak activation.[60,64] Additionally, the autophosphorylation site on BCR-ABL could also be included. An example of the cytometric application of these reagents in a model system highlighting their specificity for detection of phosphorylated Stat5 (p-Stat5) is shown in Figure 10-2. These data supporting the specificity of these reagents comes from stimulation of peripheral T cells[66] with the cytokines, IL-2 and IL-4. IL-2 activates the Jak-Stat pathway leading to phosphorylation of a number of Stat molecules including Stat5,[67] and T cells stimulated with IL-2 show significant increased staining for p-Stat5[66] as opposed to unstimulated controls or cells stimulated with the cytokine IL-4, which also stimulates the Jak-Stat pathway but primarily other stat molecules and not Stat5.[67,68] In the specific case of monitoring BCR-ABL kinase activity, we, in collaboration with several other laboratories (Clinical Cytometry Consortium; Drs. Hedley, Jacobberger, and Shankey), have developed multi-parametric assays to measure p-Stat5 in clinical specimens. As a model for this application, K562 cells, a CML cell line constitutively expressing BCR-ABL kinase and having high level of expression of p-Stat5,[60] were spiked into normal peripheral blood mononuclear cells.

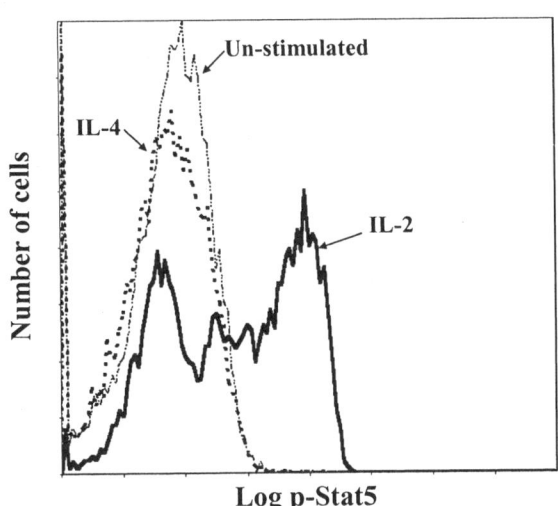

Figure 10-2. Distribution of the number of cells versus log p-Stat5 staining intensity. Peripheral blood mononuclear cells isolated by ficoll-hypaque separation were either stimulated with IL-2, IL-4, or not stimulated as shown.

Figure 10-3 illustrates the ability to detect the high levels of p-Stat5 in the spiked K562 cells based on their expression of CD15 and high level p-Stat5, and to modulate that expression in vitro with imatinib mesylate treatment. In general, coupling the measurement of P-Stat5 with immunophenotypic markers to identify or enrich for the abnormal malignant cells allows rapid determination in vivo of whether imatinib treatment has inhibited BCR-ABL kinase activity specifically in the malignant cells through assessment of p-Stat5 levels. The potential for this approach looks extremely promising and this assay is currently being implemented in several imatinib mesylate clinical trial centers. Recent articles by Hedley et al[59] and Nolan et al[69] demonstrates the applicability of these types of assays in other signaling pathways as well. Specifically, in the work of Hedley et al, monitoring of p-Mek and p-Erk, signaling intermediates in the MAP kinase pathway, in the presence or absence of a raf kinase inhibitor, points to the potential for the application of similar approaches in monitoring of patients during clinical trials of this inhibitor as well.

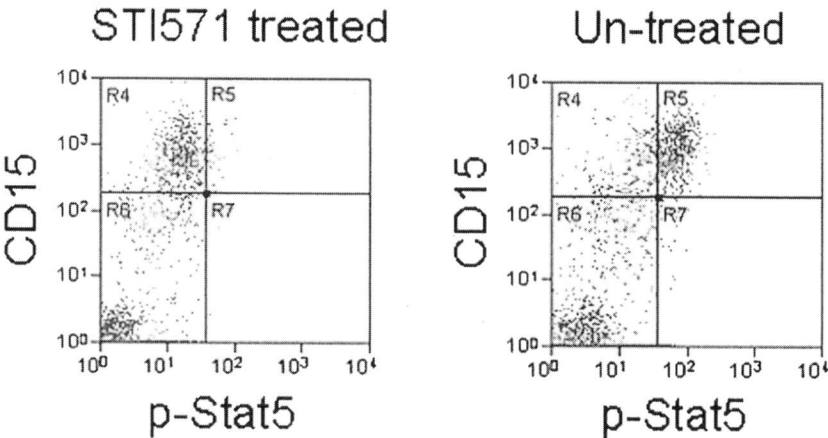

Figure 10-3. Histogram of anti-CD15 and anti-phospho-Stat5 staining in a peripheral blood mononuclear cell sample spiked with K562 cells, a BCR-ABL positive cell line that shows constitutive activation of Stat5. These results show detection of the constitutive high expression p-Stat5 in the CD15+ K562 cells and the ability to modulate that expression with imatinib mesylate (STI571) treatment.

The importance of single cell measurements, as opposed to bulk measurements on cell lysates, in assessing phosphorylation, or activity, of key molecules in signaling cascades was also noted. It was clear that in this experimental setting the MAPK pathway was either on or off,[59] a determination that would have been difficult using methods that assess whole cell lysates to measure the same endpoints. Whether this on/off signaling at the single cell level is also true in more physiological settings will be of great interest and these techniques provide the tools to directly address that question. Thus, single cell measurements of signaling mechanisms critical to clinical monitoring of patients (as discussed in more detail below) may also be crucial to understanding the more basic biology of signaling processes as well.

Although potentially important to understanding the biology of signaling processes and the effects of the kinase inhibitors used, how important is the determination of these phosphorylation events on a single cell basis versus more traditional assays employing cell lysates in a clinical setting? Some argument can be made that during overt disease, when the malignant population is the predominant population present, bulk methods employing lysis of all cells and measurement of phosphorylated targets such as p-Stat5 in Western analyses or other techniques may be adequate. However, as patients respond, and the malignant population decreases, utilization of bulk assessment techniques will less reflect the therapeutic impact on the malignant cells and more reflect the impact on the normal cells in the patient. In fact, when morphologic and clinical remission is reached, bulk methods will predominantly be a reflection of only the normal cell response. Bulk methods will rarely be effective in identification of rare malignant cells that are resistant to drug therapy or in the sensitive, early detection of resistant cells before overt relapse occurs. These are two arenas in which flow cytometry based single cell measurements will be exquisitely sensitive in assessing phosphorylation, or activation state, of multiple proteins in rare cells. These measurements could also play a key role in selection of the most appropriate co-therapy when resistance to an initial kinase inhibitor drug arises.

Further, single cell measurement techniques will almost certainly be important in understanding the mechanisms of drug resistance in individual patients. These techniques afford a sensitive assessment of re-activation of a signaling pathway despite presence of drug. For example, in development of resistance to imatinib mesylate therapy, in general, one sees continued, or recurrent, high level expression of p-Stat5 in the presence of imatinib mesylate[58] due to either amplification of *BCR-ABL* or mutation of that locus. During remission, flow cytometry techniques to measure rare, resistant cells emerging early in development of resistance will almost certainly be a more sensitive technique for monitoring development of imatinib resistance. However, whether this will be useful in management decisions of CML patients where all patients develop resistance and combination therapies are becoming commonplace remains to be seen. Nonetheless, this paradigm applies more generally and undoubtedly will play a role in this arena at some level in not only imatinib but other targeted therapies as well.

With appropriate reagents, single cell measurements may be a useful adjunct in acquiring an understanding of the development of resistance to targeted therapies. Was resistance due to inhibition of drug uptake, or alternatively, to other mechanisms of drug inhibition? Development of resistance may in some instances be more complex than simply altering drug uptake or development of mechanisms to inhibit drug action with subsequent re-activation of the relevant pathway. Regulation of cell proliferation and apoptosis occurs through a number of alternative, and in some cases redundant, pathways. Thus, in some instances, development of resistance will arise through cells utilizing alternative signaling pathways to the one which is blocked. Multi-parametric approaches coupling measurement of specific inhibition of one pathway as described above along with measurement of other relevant regulatory pathways and functional endpoint measurements of cell proliferation, cell regulatory molecules (cyclins, cyclin dependant kinase, etc), apoptosis, or apoptosis regulatory molecules may be useful in identifying emergence of resistance even when the therapeutic drug is still effectively blocking its target molecule. The ability to utilize these techniques to simultaneously measure multiple pathways has clearly been demonstrated.[69] In addition, knowing what these responses are and expression of which molecules have been altered may point to the mechanism of resistance, to what other pathways may need to be monitored, and to potentially appropriate additional therapies.

In addition, particularly when one moves outside of the realm of hematopoietic malignancies, only rarely are single kinase abnormalities going to be the primary, or only, abnormality responsible for disease.[52] Even in the setting of CML, these techniques may be key in assessing the effects of combination therapies used with imatinib mesylate and helping to determine on a patient specific basis what the most effective combination of treatments may be. Although most CML patients in chronic phase respond to imatinib, response in accelerated and blast crisis phase is more heterogeneous. Before initiation of therapy, assessment of in vitro response to imatinib may be useful in determining which of these patients are likely to respond to imatinib in vivo.

Another exciting arena over the last several years has been development of gene therapy options.[70-73] Insertion and expression of specific genes into abnormal cells designed to functionally correct the defect in these cells is an exciting prospect. Initial forays into this arena have meet with some well publicized problems, nonetheless, this approach remains promising and is rapidly evolving. The potential heterogeneity in expression of an inserted foreign gene into the abnormal cells and its effectiveness in restoring normal function or overcoming the effects of an abnormal protein lends itself to cytometric techniques facilitating evaluation of transfected gene expression and its effects on specific regulatory pathways and in specific cell sub-populations that would be difficult by other technologies. Flow cytometric approaches will play a role in the process of generation of transfected cells for these therapeutic approaches. For some time, flow cytometry approaches have been employed to measure the expression level of a transfected or transduced gene into a cell.[74-80] Sorting of cells can also be used in lieu of drug selection to establish stable transfected cell lines as well as for selection of cells having a specific expression level of a transfected gene (protein) from the heterogeneous expression typically seen to generate cell lines having homogeneous, typically high, expression levels.[81]

Far more exciting, however, is an elegant example of the use of flow cytometry to monitor the effectiveness in correcting a regulatory defect by induction of a normal transfected gene, in this case wild-type p53, into a background with abnormal expression using an adenovirus delivery system recently shown by Jaccobberger et al.[82] Not only did these approaches prove to be a sensitive way of confirming successful, high expression of the wild-type p53, but more importantly, the sophisticated multi-parametric approaches were able to clearly show that this protein was functionally interacting with other cellular proteins to restore normal p53 function in these cells. It is likely that cytometric approaches will play a significant role not only in the laboratory aspects of generation and characterization of these therapeutic agents but also in the monitoring of successful function and maintenance of these cells in the patient.

5.   SUMMATION

Over the last twenty years, cytometric evaluation of hematopoietic malignancies has evolved from an adjunctive test which was secondary in the diagnostic work-up, typically following by several days the primary diagnostic work-up, to one which although still adjunctive to morphology is now a key aspect of the primary diagnostic package. The maturing of the technology in this setting is satisfying; however, more exciting are the glimpses of the next evolution of this technology in a clinical setting, perhaps first to be seen in the realm of hematopoietic malignancies. Rapid movement of cytometric approaches into the arena of therapeutic management and monitoring of patients is being seen. This movement involves more complex multi-parametric approaches than previously have been employed in most clinical cytometry laboratories with five, six, seven, or even more color analyses finding their way into the clinical setting. These developments and needs are going to require cytometry technologists with extensive experience and training along with laboratory directors, pathologists, and clinicians who are knowledgeable about the analyses along with interpretation and application of the results. Interpretation of these experimental results will require sophisticated cytometry skills as well as a detailed knowledge of the signaling and regulatory pathways in which the measured molecules function. This is a very exciting time in clinical cytometry, perhaps the most exciting time yet, but a challenge remains in providing the appropriate training mechanisms and tools to ensure that these analyses can be adequately performed in a wide range of clinical laboratories.

REFERENCES

1. Jennings CD, Foon KA. Recent advances in flow cytometry: Application to the diagnosis of hematologic malignancy. Blood 1997; 90:2863-2892.
2. Peterson LC, Goolsby C. Flow cytometric immunophenotyping of hematological malignancies involving the blood and bone marrow. A Review. Curr Diag Path 1997;4:187-195.
3. Liu Z. Hultin LE. Cumberland WG. Hultin P. Schmid I. Matud JL. Detels R. Giorgi JV. Elevated relative fluorescence intensity of CD38 antigen expression on CD8+ T cells is a marker of poor prognosis in HIV infection: results of 6 years of follow-up. Cytometry. 1996;26:1-7.
4. Del Poeta G, Maurillo L, Venditti A, Buccisano F, Epiceno AM, Capelli G, Tamburini A, Suppo G, Battaglia A, Del Principe MI, Del Moro B, Masi M, Amadori S. Clinical significance of CD38 expression in chronic lymphocytic leukemia. Blood 2001;98:2633-2639.
5. Damle RN, Wasil T, Fais F, Ghiotto F, Valetto A, Allen SL, Buchbinder A, Budman D, Dittmar K, Kolitz J, Lichtman SM, Schulman P, Vinciguerra VP, Rai KR, Ferrarini M, Chiorazzi N. Ig V gene mutation status and CD38 expression as novel prognostic indicators in chronic lymphocytic leukemia. Blood 1999;94:1840-1847.
6. Hamblin TJ, Davis Z, Gardiner A, Oscier DG, Stevenson FK. Unmutated Ig V_h genes are associated with a more aggressive form of chronic lymphocytic leukemia. Blood 1999;94:1848.
7. Crespo M, Bosch F, Villamor N, Bellosillo B, Colomer D, Rozman M, Marce S, Lopez-Guillermo A, Campo E, Montserrat E. ZAP-70 expression as a surrogate for immunoglobulin-variable-region mutations in chronic lymphocytic leukemia. N Eng J Med 2003;348:1764-1775.
8. Nolan GP. Multiparameter Kinase Profiling in Primary and Cancer Cells. Presented at the AACR-NCI-EORTC International Conference On Molecular Targets and Cancer Therapeutics. Discovery, Biology and Clinical Applications. Boston, MA November, 2003.

9. Douglas VK, Gordon LI, Goolsby CL, White CA, Peterson LC. Lymphoid aggregates in bone marrow mimic residual lymphoma after Rituximab therapy for non-Hodgkin lymphoma. Am J Clin Pathol 1999;112:844-853.

10. Illidge TM, Bayne MC. Antibody therapy of lymphoma. Exp Opin Pharmacother 2001;2:953-961.

11. Syrigos KN, Pliarchopoulou K, Harrington KJ. The development of monoclonal antibody therapy in leukemias. Hybridoma 2001;20:145-148.

12. White CA, Weaver RL, Grillo-Lopez AJ. Antibody-targeted immunotherapy for treatment of malignancy. Annu Rev Med 2001;52:125-145.

13. Siegel AB, Goldenberg DM, Cesano A, Coleman M, Leonard JP. CD22-directed monoclonal antibody therapy for lymphoma. Sem in Oncology 2003;30:457-64.

14. Flynn JM, Byrd JC. Campath-1H monoclonal antibody therapy. Curr Opin Oncol 2000;12:574-581.

15. Koon HB, Junghans RP. Anti-CD30 antibody-based therapy. Curr Opin Oncol 2000;12:588-593.

16. Radich J, Sievers E. New developments in the treatment of acute myeloid leukemia. Oncology 2000;14:125-131.

17. Ruffner KL, Matthews DC. Current uses of monoclonal antibodies in the treatment of acute leukemia. Sem Oncol 2000;27:531-539.

18. Sievers EL. Targeted therapy of acute myeloid leukemia with monoclonal antibodies and immunoconjugates. Can Chemotherapy & Pharmacology 2000;46:S18-22.

19. Foss FM. Interleukin-2 fusion toxin: Targeted therapy for cutaneous T cell lymphoma. Ann New York Acad Sci 2001;941:166-176.

20. Cinti P, Cociolo P, Evangelista B, Orlandini AM, Bruzzone P, Renna Molajoni E, Cortesini R. OKT3 prophylaxis in kidney transplant recipients: Drug monitoring by flow cytometry. Transplantation Proc 1996;28:3214-3216.

21. Hammond EA, Yowell RL, Greenwood J, Hartung L, Renlund D, Wittwer C. Prevention of adverse clinical outcome by monitoring of cardiac transplant patients for murine monoclonal CD3 antibody (OKT3) sensitization. Transplantation 1993;55:1061-1063.

22. Harford AM, Shopp GM, Ashmore LM, Seppelt JE, Mosdell DM, Gibel LJ, Sterling WA. OKT3-treated kidney transplant patients: Monitoring of effects on peripheral blood mononuclear cells by using two-color flow cytometry. Transplantation Proc 1988;20:245-248.

23. Lim VL, Gumbert M, Garovoy MR. A flow cytometric method for the detection of the development of antibody to Orthoclone OKT3. J Immunol Meth 1989;121:197-201.

24. McIntyre JA, Kincade M, Higgins NG. Detection of IGA anti-OKT3 antibodies in OKT3-treated transplant recipients. Transplantation 1996;61:1465-1469.

25. McLaughlin P, Grillo-Lopez AJ, Link BK, Levy R, Czuczman MS, Williams ME, Heyman MR, Bence-Bruckler I, White CA, Cabanillas F, Jain V, Ho AD, Lister J, Wey K, Shen D, Dallaire BK. Rituximab chimeric anti-CD20 monoclonal antibody therapy for relapsed indolent lymphoma: Half of patients respond to a four-dose treatment program. J Clin Oncol 1998;16:2825-2833.

26. Reff ME, Carner K, Chambers KS, Chinn PC, Leonard JE, Raab R, Newman RA, Hanna N, Anderson DR. Depletion of B-cells in vivo by a chimeric mouse human monoclonal antibody to CD20. Blood 1994;83:435-445.

27. Rawstron AC, Kennedy B, Evans PA, Davies FE, Richards SJ, Haynes AP, Russell NH, Hale G, Morgan GJ, Jack AS, Hillmen P. Quantitation of minimal disease levels in chronic lymphocytic leukemia using a sensitive flow cytometric assay improves the prediction of outcome and can be used to optimize therapy. Blood 2001;98:29-35.

28. DelleKarth G, Laczika K, Scholten C, Lechner K, Jaeger U. Clearance of PCR-detectable lymphoma cells from the peripheral blood, but no bone marrow after therapy with Campath-1H. Am J Hematol 1995;50:146-152.

29. Lim SH, Davey G, Marcus R. Differential response in a patient treated with Campath-1H monoclonal antibody for refractory non-Hodgkin lymphoma. Lancet 1993;341:432-433.

30. Poynton CH, Mort D, Maughan TS. Adverse reactions to Campath-1H monoclonal antibody. Lancet 1993;341:1037.

31. Nabhan C, Tallman MS, Riley MB, Fitzpatrick J, Gordon LI, Gartenhaus R, Kuzel T, Siegel R, Rosen ST. Phase I study of Rituximab and Campath-1H in patients with relapsed or refractory chronic lymphocytic leukemia. Abst. Blood 2001;98:365a.

32. Lal A, Nabhan C, Rosen S, Goolsby C, Peterson L. Peripheral blood (PB), bone marrow (BM) and flow cytometric (FC) changes in patients with chronic lymphocytic leukemia (CLL) treated with Campath-1H and Rituximab. Presented at USCAP meeting, Chicago, February 2002.

33. Davis AT. Monoclonal antibody-based therapy of lymphoid neoplasms: What's on the horizon? Sem Hematol 2000;37:34-42.

34. Bukowski RM. Cytokine therapy for metastatic renal cell carcinoma. Sem Urol Oncol 2001;19:148-154.

35. Graca L, Honey K, Adams E, Cobbold SP, Waldmann H. Cutting edge: Anti-CD154 therapeutic antibodies induce infectious transplantation tolerance. J Immunol 2000;165:4783-4786.

36. Hale G, Jacobs P, Wood L, Fibbe WE, Barge R, Novitzky N, Toit C, Abrahams L, Thomas V, Bunjes D, Duncker C, Wiesneth M, Selleslag D, Hidajat M, Starobinski M, Bird P, Waldmann H. CD52 antibodies for prevention of graft-versus-host disease and graft rejection following transplantation of allogeneic peripheral blood stem cells. Bone Marrow Transplantion 2000;26(1):69-76.

37. Issacs JD, Greer S, Sharma S, Symmons D, Smith M, Johnston J, Waldmann H, Hale G, Hazleman BL. Morbidity and mortality in rheumatoid arthritis patients with prolonged and profound therapy-induced lymphopenia. Arth Rheum 2001;44:1998-2008.

38. Kottaridis PD, Milligan DW, Chopra R, Chakraverty RK, Chakrabarti S, Robinson S, Peggs K, Verfuerth S, Pettengell R, Marsh JC, Schey S, Mahendra P, Morgan GJ, Hale G, Waldmann H, de Elvira MC, Williams CD, Devereux S, Linch DC, Goldstone AH, Mackinnon S. In vivo Campath-1H prevents graft-versus-host disease following non-myeloablative stem cell transplantation. Blood 2000;96:2419-2425.

39. Mitsuyasu RT. The potential role of interleukin-2 in HIV. AIDS 2001;15:S22-27.

40. Philip PA, Flaherty LE. Biochemotherapy for melanoma. Curr Oncol Rep 2000;2:314-321.

41. Ratanatharathorn V, Ayash L, Lazarus HM, Fu J, Uberti JP. Chronic graft-versus-host disease: clinical manifestation and therapy. Bone Marrow Trans 2001;28:121-129.

42. Simpson D. New developments in the prophylaxis and treatment of graft versus host disease. Exp Opin Pharmacother 2001;2:1109-1117.

43. Smith KA. Low-dose daily interleukin-2 immunotherapy: Accelerating immune restoration and expanding HIV-specific T-cell immunity without toxicity. AIDS 2001;15:S28-35.

44. Zecca M, DeStefano P, Nobili B, Locatelli F. Anti-CD20 monoclonal antibody for the treatment of severe, immune-mediated, pure red cell aplasia and hemolytic anemia. Blood 2001;97:3995-3997.

45. Mathas S, Rickers A, Bommert K, Dorken B, Mapara MY. Anti-CD20- and B-cell receptor-mediated apoptosis: Evidence for shared intracellular signaling pathways. Cancer Res 2000;60:7170-7176.

46. Golay J, Lazzari M, Facchinetti V, Bernasconi S, Borleri G, Barbui T, Rambaldi A, Introna M. CD20 levels determine the in vitro susceptibility to rituximab and complement of B-cell chronic lymphocytic leukemia: further regulation by CD55 and CD59. Blood 2001;98:3383-3389.

47. Huh YO, Keating MJ, Saffer HL, Jilani I, Lerner S, Albitar M. Higher levels of surface CD20 expression on circulating lymphocytes compared with bone marrow and lymph nodes in B-cell chronic lymphocytic leukemia. Amer J Clin Path 2001;116:437-43.

48. Treon SP, Shima Y, Preffer FI, Doss DS, Ellman L, Schlossman RL, Grossbard ML, Belch AR, Pilarski LM, Anderson KC. Treatment of plasma cell dyscrasias by antibody-mediated immunotherapy. Sem Oncol 1999;26:97-106.

49. Venugopal P, Sivaraman S, Huang XK, Nayini J, Gregory SA, Preisler HD. Effects of cytokines on CD20 antigen expression on tumor cells from patients with chronic lymphocytic leukemia. Leuk Res 2001;25:99-100.

50. Brunstein CG, McGlave PB. The biology and treatment of chronic myelogenous leukemia. Oncology 2001;15:23-31.

51. Maslak P, Scheinberg D. Targeted therapies for the myeloid leukaemias. Exp Opin Invest Drugs 2000;9:1197-1205.

52. Druker BJ, Lydon NB. Lessons learned from the development of an Abl tyrosine kinase inhibitor for chronic myelogenous leukemia. J Clin Invest 2000;105:3-7.

53. Al-Obeidi FA, Lam KS. Development of inhibitors for protein tyrosine kinases. Oncogene 2000;19:5690-5701.

54. Seidel HM, Lamb P, Rosen J. Pharmaceutical intervention in the JAK/STAT signaling pathway. Oncogene 2000;19:2645-2656.

55. Blennerhasset GT, Furth M, Anderson A, Burns JP, Chaganti RS, Blick M, Talpaz M, Dev VG, Chan LC, Wiedemann LM. Clinical evaluation of a DNA probe assay for the Philadelphia (Ph1) translocation in chronic myelogenous leukemia. Leukemia 1988;2:648-657.

56. Sawyers CL. The bcr-abl gene in chronic myelogenous leukaemia. In: Cancer Surveys, Vol 15, Oncogenes in the Development of Leukaemia, Imperial Cancer Research Fund, pp 37-51, 1992.

57. Van Etten RA. Malignant transformation by abl and bcr/abl. In: Oncogenes and tumor suppressor genes in human malignancies, pp 167-192, 1993.

58. Gorre ME, Mohammed M, Ellwood K, Hsu N, Paquette R, Rao PN, Sawyers CL. Clinical resistance to STI-571 cancer therapy caused by BCR-ABL gene mutation or amplification. Science 2001;293:876-880.

59. Chow S, Patel H, Hedley DW. Measurement of MAP kinase activation by flow cytometry using phospho-specific antibodies to MEK and ERK: Potential for pharmacodynamic monitoring of signal transduction inhibitors. Comm Clin Cytometry 2001;46:72-78.

60. Carlesso N, Frank DA, Griffin JD. Tyrosyl phosphorylation and DNA binding activity of signal transducers and activators of transcript (STAT) proteins in hematopoietic cell lines transformed by Bcr/Abl. J Exper Med 1996;183:811-820.

61. Chai SK, Nichols GL, Rothman P. Constitutive activation of JAKs and STATs in BCR-Abl-expressing cell lines and peripheral blood cells derived from leukemic patients. J Immunol 1997;159:4720-4728.

62. Coffer PJ, Koenderman L, de Groot RP. The role of STATs in myeloid differentiation and leukemia. Oncogene 2000;19:2511-2522.

63. Frank DA. STAT signaling in the pathogenesis and treatment of cancer. Molec Med 1999;5;432-456.

64. Ilaria RL Jr, Van Etten RA. P210 and P190$^{BCR/ABL}$ induce the tyrosine phosphorylation and DNA binding activity of multiple specific STAT family members. J Biol Chem 1996;271:31704-31710.

65. Nieborowska-Skorska M, Wasik MA, Slupianek A, Salomoni P, Kitamura T, Calabretta B, Skorski T. Signal transducer and activator of transcription (STAT)5 activation by BCR/ABL is dependent on intact Src homology (SH)3 and SH2 domains of BCR/ABL and is required for leukemogenesis. J Exp Med 1999;189:1229-1242.

66. Jacobberger J, Sramkowski R, Feisa P, Ye P, Gottlieb M, Hedley D, Shankey T, Smith B, Paniagua M, Goolsby C. Immunoreactivity of stat5 phosphorylated on tyrosine 694 as a cell-based measure of Bcr/Abl kinase activity. Cytometry 54A, 75-88 2003.

67. Lin J-X, Migone T-S, Tsang M, Friedmann M, Weatherbee JA, Zhou L, Yamauchi A, Bloom ET, Mietz J, John S, Leonard WJ. The role of shared receptor motifs and common stat proteins in the generation of cytokine pleiotropy and redundancy by IL-2, IL-4, IL-7, IL-13 and IL-15. Immunity 1995;2:331-339.

68. Jiang H, Marris MB, Rothman P. IL-4/IL-13 signaling beyond JAK/STAT. J All Clin Immunol 2000;105:1063-1070.

69. Perez OD, Nolan GP. Simultaneous measurement of multiple active kinase states using polychromatic flow cytometry. Nature Biotechnology 2002;20:155-62.

70. Brenner MK. Gene transfer and the treatment of haematological malignancy. J Int Med 2001;249:345-358.

71. Cusack JC Jr, Tanabe KK. Cancer gene therapy. Surg Oncol Clin North Am 1998;7:421-469.

72. Pandha HS, Martin LA, Rigg AS, Ross P, Dalgleish AG. Oncological applications of gene therapy. Curr Opin Invest Drugs 2000;1:122-134.

73. Roskrow MA, Gansbacher B. Recent developments in gene therapy for oncology and hematology. Crit Rev Oncol-Hematol 1998;28:139-151.

74. Fiering SN, Roederer M, Nolan GP, Micklem DR, Parks DR, Herzenberg LA. Improved FACS-Gal: Flow cytometric analysis and sorting of viable eukaryotic cells expressing reporter gene constructs. Cytometry 1991;12:291-301.

75. Jasin M, Zalamea P. Analysis of Escherichia coli beta-galactosidase expression in transgenic mice by flow cytometry of sperm. Proc Natl Acad Sci USA 1992;89:10681-10685.

76. Klein D, Indraccolo S, von Rombs K, Amadori A, Salmons B, Gunzburg WH. Rapid identification of viable retrovirus-transduced cells using the green fluorescent protein as a marker. Gene Ther 1997;4:1256-1260.

77. Mazurier F, Moreau-Gaudry F, Maguer-Satta V, Salesse S, Pigeonnier-Lagarde V, Ged C, Belloc F, Lacombe F, Mahon FX, Reiffers J, de Verneuil H. Rapid analysis and efficient selection of human transduced primitive hematopoietic cells using the humanized S65T green fluorescent protein. Gene Ther 1998;5:556-562.

78. Puchalski RB, Manoharan TH, Lathrop AL, Fahl WE. Recombinant glutathione S-transferase (GST) expressing cells purified by flow cytometry on the basis of a GST-catalyzed intracellular conjugation of glutathione to monochlorobimane. Cytometry 1991;12:651-665.

79. Wiechen K, Zimmer C, Dietel M. Selection of a high activity c-erbB-2 ribozyme using a fusion gene of c-erbB-2 and the enhanced green fluorescent protein. Cancer Gene Ther 1998;5:45-51.

80. Wittrup KD, Bailey JE.   A single-cell assay of beta-galactosidase activity in Saccharomyces cerevisiae. Cytometry 1988;9:394-404.

81. Van Tendeloo VF, Ponsaerts P, Van Broeckhoven C, Berneman ZN, Van Bockstaele DR. Efficient generation of stably electrotransfected human hematopoietic cell lines without drug selection by consecutive FAC sorting. Cytometry 2000;41:31-35.

82. Jacobberger JW, Sramkoski RM, Zhang D, Zumstein LA, Doerksen LD, Merritt JA, Wright SA, Shults KE. Bivariate analysis of the p53 pathway to evaluate Ad-p53 gene therapy efficacy. Comm Clin Cytometry 1999;38:201-213.

Chapter 11

HODGKIN LYMPHOMA
Clinical, Morphologic, Immunophenotypic, and Molecular Characteristics

Bertram Schnitzer and Riccardo Valdez
University of Michigan Medical School, Ann Arbor, Michigan

1.   INTRODUCTION

The most controversial and baffling of the lymphomas, and the one that continues to fascinate both clinicians and pathologists, is Hodgkin lymphoma, formerly known as Hodgkin's disease.[1] The nature of this disorder – that is whether it is an infectious or an inflammatory process, an unusual immunologic reaction, or a true malignancy – has been debated for more than a century. In the past three decades, however, the application of new technologies including monoclonal antibody production, immunohistochemical techniques, and such molecular innovations as immunoglobulin and T-cell receptor gene rearrangements, as well as PCR to detect clonality, and isolation of single neoplastic cells from tissue sections, have all played a crucial role in advancing our understanding of this disease. In this chapter, we review the evolution of the classification schemes of Hodgkin lymphoma, emphasizing the recently described histologic subtypes, and we discuss the application of immunohistochemical and molecular analysis in determining the nature of the elusive Reed-Sternberg cell.

2.   CLINICAL, MORPHOLOGIC, AND
        IMMUNOPHENOTYPIC CHARACTERISTICS
        OF HODGKIN LYMPHOMA

2.1   Historical Perspective

In 1832, Thomas Hodgkin[2] reported seven autopsy cases of a disorder that Sir Samuel Wilks in his 1865 publication termed "Hodgkin's disease".[3] Langhans in 1872[4] and Greenfield in 1878[5] both described the histologic features of this disorder, but it was Carl Sternberg in Germany in 1898[6] and Dorothy Reed at Johns Hopkins in 1902[7] who first described the cytologic characteristics of the giant cells that must be present for a diagnosis of Hodgkin's disease to be established. The latter two pathologists are also credited with the first definitive microscopic description of the disorder. The large cells, which are now known to be the malignant cells in Hodgkin's disease, are called Reed-Sternberg (RS) cells or, alternately, Sternberg-Reed cells, and Hodgkin (H) cells.

Hodgkin's disease, or Hodgkin lymphoma (now the official WHO designation) is an unusual malignancy, both in its clinical presentation and in its histologic findings. It may in some cases present more like an infectious process rather than a malignant disorder, in that the patient not infrequently exhibits symptoms of fever and drenching night sweats. In fact, both Sternberg and Reed did not consider Hodgkin's disease (HL) to be a malignancy. Sternberg believed that it was a type of tuberculosis, because tuberculosis was often seen in conjunction with HL, whereas Reed considered HL to be an inflammatory process distinct from tuberculosis.[8] Whether or not HL was an infectious or malignant process was a question debated for many years, during which the search to identify a causative agent resulted in failure. Finally, in 1962, cytogenetic studies conclusively showed that RS cells were neoplastic, because they were both aneuploid and of clonal derivation.[9]

2.2   Clinical Features

HL accounts for approximately 30% of all lymphomas. In industrialized nations, HL has a bimodal age distribution with the first peak occurring between the ages of 15 and 35 years and the second peak seen in the sixth decade.[10] Nodular sclerosis HL is responsible for the first peak, whereas the MC type occurs more often in the older age group.

Most patients present with localized lymphadenopathy limited to one or two lymph nodes, often in the cervical region. Mediastinal involvement may be present with or without peripheral adenopathy. Mediastinal disease may be detected in an asymptomatic patient by routine chest x-ray, or else the patient may complain of symptoms which are secondary to enlarged mediastinal lymph nodes or a mediastinal mass. In rare instances, a paraneoplastic symptom specific for HL, pain in lymph nodes involved by HL, occurs when the patient drinks alcoholic beverages.[11] Occasionally, patients present with cyclic bouts of a fever called "Pel-Ebstein" fever, named after the two physicians who first described it.[12]

The histologic features of Hodgkin lymphoma are also unusual for a malignancy, whether it be non-Hodgkin's lymphoma, carcinoma, or sarcoma. In malignant neoplasms other than Hodgkin's disease, the tumor is composed predominantly of malignant cells, and the neoplasm is named and classified according to the cell of origin. In contrast, the enlarged lymph nodes in Hodgkin's disease consist predominantly of benign reactive inflammatory cells, whereas malignant cells are in the vast minority and may be very difficult to find. The paucity of RS cells in most cases of Hodgkin's disease has until recently (vide infra) hindered attempts to identify their cellular origin and lineage. Furthermore, the classification of Hodgkin's disease is based primarily not on the malignant cell but on the benign inflammatory infiltrate as well as on the immunomorphologic features of the RS cells.

2.3   Classifications of Hodgkin's disease

In contrast to non-Hodgkin's lymphomas (NHL), which have undergone many changes in classification, the organizational scheme for Hodgkin's disease has remained remarkably stable for almost 40 years.

The first useful classification of Hodgkin's disease was published in 1947 by Jackson and Parker in their book "Hodgkin's Disease and Allied Disorders".[13] HL was divided into three histologic types: paragranuloma, granuloma, and sarcoma (Table 11-1). However, this division was not helpful in predicting the outcome of the disease, since approximately 90% of cases fell into the morphologically and prognostically heterogeneous granuloma type. It was not until 1966, when Lukes and Lukes and Butler published their morphologic classification, that the heterogeneous granuloma type of HL was divided into the nodular sclerosis type[14, 15] (which was first described as "nodular granuloma" by Smetana and Cohen in 1956[16]) and the mixed cellularity type. The name of the paragranuloma subtype was changed to the morphologically descriptive lymphocytic and/or histiocytic (L&H) type with either a diffuse or nodular pattern. The sarcoma group was divided into the reticular and the less common diffuse fibrosis types. The six subtypes of the Lukes/Butler classification were found to be too cumbersome for clinical use, and consequently, at a meeting in Rye, NY, the six subtypes were modified and condensed into four types (hence, came the name for the Rye classification). The revision still retained the prognostic relevance of the Lukes/Butler scheme.[17] The four histologic types of the Rye classification included: 1) lymphocyte predominance, in which there was a preponderance of small lymphocytes and few RS cells and which was associated with a prolonged outcome, a finding first noted many years earlier by Rosenthal,[18] 2) nodular sclerosis, a disorder with frequent mediastinal involvement, which is found in equal distribution in young women and men, 3) mixed cellularity, characterized by a mixture of inflammatory cells, which include lymphocytes, eosinophils, plasma cells, and histiocytes, and 4) lymphocyte depletion, a term that replaced the designation reticular and diffuse fibrosis types of HL, which is characterized by few lymphocytes and many RS cells (Table 11-1). In the Lukes-Butler/Rye classifications, lymphocyte predominance HL was associated with an indolent course and a favorable prognosis, whereas the lymphocyte depletion type was associated with an aggressive course and a poor prognosis. The prognostic significance of such classifications, however, has become less relevant since the advent of modern therapy, and survival is now considered to be dependent on the extent of involvement of the disease (i.e. stage).

Table 11-1. Classifications of Hodgkin Lymphoma (HL)

Jackson and Parker (1947)	Lukes and Butler (1966)	Rye (1966)	REAL/WHO (1994/2001)
Paragranuloma	Lymphocytic and/or histiocytic, **nodular**	Lymphocytic predominance	Nodular lymphocyte predominanat
	Lymphocytic and/or histiocytic, **diffuse**	Lymphocytic predominance	Lymphocyte-rich classical HL*
Granuloma	Nodular Sclerosis	Nodular Sclerosis	Nodular Sclerosis
	Mixed Cellularity	Mixed Cellularity	Mixed Cellularity
Sarcoma	Diffuse fibrosis	Lymphocyte depletion	Lymphocyte depletion
	Reticular		

*Lymphocyte rich classical was a provisional entity in the REAL classification

The Lukes-Butler/Rye classifications remained unchanged until publication of the REAL (Revised European American Lymphoma) classification in 1994.[19] In the latter classification scheme (Table 11-1), the sole change with respect to HL was the addition of a new subtype of HL as a provisional entity: lymphocyte-rich classical Hodgkin's disease (LRC HL). In the WHO classification (Table 11-1), an updated version of the REAL scheme published in 2001,[1] the LRC HL subtype was accepted as a distinct separate and entity and four additional changes were made: 1) Hodgkin lymphoma (HL) is now the designation preferred to Hodgkin's disease, because recent clinical and biological studies have shown that HL is truly a lymphoma, since its neoplastic cells are of lymphoid origin. 2) HL is divided into two distinct clinical and biological entities: nodular lymphocyte predominance HL and classical HL (Table 11-1). The two types of HL differ from each other in their natural history, clinical features, epidemiology, immunophenotypes, genetics, and association with the Epstein-Barr virus. Despite the fact that these two types of HL are clinically and biologically different, they share certain features, namely, a paucity of neoplastic cells (Hodgkin and Reed-Sternberg cells) against a background of benign inflammatory cells. The two types of HL also resemble one another in that both exhibit frequent involvement of cervical lymph nodes and localized disease at the time of presentation, and both occur frequently in young adults. In addition, recent studies have demonstrated that in the vast majority of cases, the RS cells in both types of HL are of germinal center B-cell origin (vide infra).[20, 21] 3) Diffuse LP HL is not recognized as a separate subtype but may be seen rarely in conjunction with NLP type (NLP HL with diffuse areas). 4) Nodular sclerosis has been divided into two histologic grades based on the number of RS cells within the nodules.

Classical HL is subdivided into categories that previously had been part of the Lukes/Butler and Rye classifications and include: nodular sclerosis, mixed cellularity, the rare lymphocyte depletion, and the newly added LRC type (Table 11-1).

2.4   Reed-Sternberg Cell

The classic Reed-Sternberg (RS) cell or a variant RS cell (L&H cell, lacunar cell) must be present for a diagnosis of HL to be made. Not only must this cell be present, but it must be found in a cellular milieu of one of the five histologic subtypes of HL, because cells morphologically indistinguishable from RS cells may also be found in benign lymphoid proliferations as well as in non-Hodgkin's lymphomas. There are three types of RS cells: 1) classic, 2) lacunar cell, and 3) lymphocytic and/or histiocytic (L&H) cell (from Lukes/Butler classification).[14, 15] The classic and lacunar types are seen in classical HL but not in NLP, whereas the L&H cell is characteristic of the NLP type of HL. The classic binucleate or "owl eye" cell is found in all subtypes of classical HL but is most abundant in the MC type (Figure 11-1). The lacunar variant of the RS cell is present in NS HL, although it may also be seen in NLRC HL and in small numbers in MC HL. Because of its resemblance to exploded kernels of corn, the L&H cell is also called "popcorn" cell, a variant that is present in the NLP type.[22] The RS cells found in the very rare lymphocyte depletion type have been referred to as pleomorphic, anaplastic, or sarcomatoid.[14, 17] Mononuclear cells with cytologic features of classic RS cells have been called Hodgkin (H) cells

(Figure 11-1). The RS/H cells are the malignant cells within the benign inflammatory infiltrate of HL.

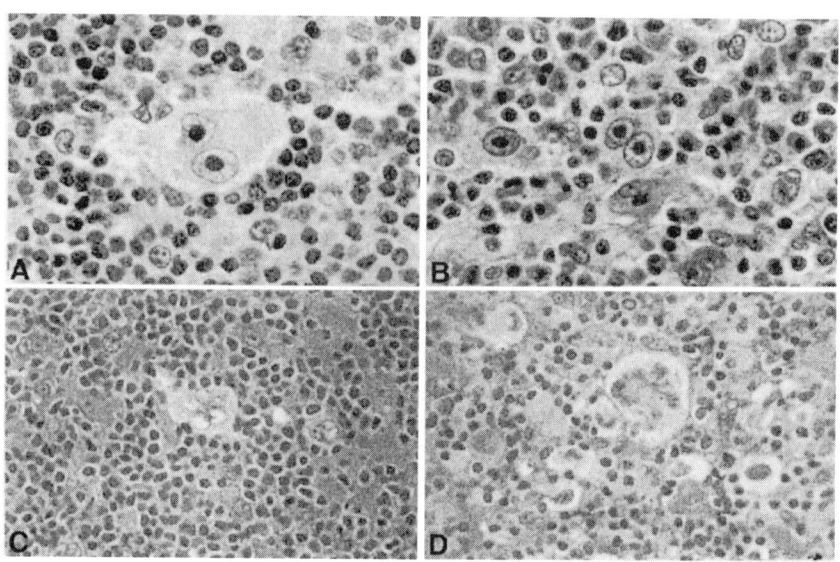

Figure 11-1. Reed-Sternberg cells and variants. A) Classic binucleated "owl eye" Reed-Sternberg cell containing two nuclei with prominent, inclusion-like nucleoli. B) Classic Reed-Sternberg cell and a Hodgkin cell. C) L&H variant ("popcorn" cell) showing lobulated nucleus. D) Lacunar variant of Reed-Sternberg cell showing multilobated nucleus.

The classic RS cells are binucleated, lobulated, or multinucleated giant cells with prominent eosinophilic, inclusion-like nucleoli surrounded by a clear halo in each nucleus or lobe. The cells have abundant amphophilic or eosinophilic cytoplasm. Apoptotic classic RS cells, referred to as "mummified" or "zombie" cells and characterized by pyknotic chromatin, barely recognizable nucleoli, and eosinophilic (and occasionally retracted) cytoplasm, are found in all types of classical HL. Lacunar cells are so named because they are found in clear spaces (lacunae), which are artifacts of formalin fixation. The cytoplasm is retracted around the nucleus, thus leaving a space around the cells. This diagnostically useful artifact is not seen in tissue processed in mercury-containing fixatives (e.g. B5) in which lacunar cells have ample pale-staining cytoplasm. However, lacunar cells are still recognized by such characteristic cytologic features as their hyperlobated nuclei and their small but conspicuous eosinophilic nucleoli (Figure 11-1). Bizarre-appearing, pleomorphic lacunar-type cells may be present, particularly in cases of the syncytial variant of NS HL (vide infra). L&H variants are large cells with complex lobulations of their nuclei containing nucleoli that are smaller than those in classic RS cells, and these variants have only a small amount of cytoplasm (Figure 11-1). Although these are the predominant types of RS cells in NLP HL, some L&H cells may contain prominent nucleoli, thus resembling classical HL.

2.5 Immunophenotype

Immunophenotyping in paraffin sections is exceedingly useful in the diagnosis and subclassification of HL. Because no single marker is highly sensitive nor specific for RS cells, a panel of antibodies must be employed to characterize these cells including: CD15, CD30, CD45, CD20, and CD3. In problematic cases, EMA, bcl-6, fascin, EBV-latent membrane protein (LMP), and additional B- and T-cell antibodies may be added to the panel.[1]

While the immunophenotype of RS cells in all types of classical HL are similar, the presentation, sites of involvement, age of the patients at presentation, and natural history of classical HL vary among the different subtypes. In most cases, classic RS cells express CD15, CD30, and fascin, and they are negative for CD45 (common leukocyte antigen).[1,23] (Table 11-2)

The immunophenotype of classic RS cells may differ from case to case, and not all RS cells in a single case are positive for a specific marker. In a recent study of 1751 cases in which antigen retrieval and an IgM secondary antibody were used, 83% of cases of classical HL had CD15-positive RS cells, whereas in 96% of cases RS cells were CD30-positive, and in 5% of cases RS cells expressed CD20.[24] The low percentage of CD20-positive RS cells in the latter study differs markedly from one previously reported series, in which the percentage of cases of NS and MC HL where RS cells expressed the B-cell markers CD20 and/or CD79a was 60%.[25] Absence of CD15 or CD30 staining (but not both) of RS cells does not exclude a diagnosis of HL. A lack of CD15 staining is usually seen in older, predominantly male patients with advanced stage disease, and by multivariate analysis this absence has been found to be an independent adverse prognostic indicator.[24] Moreover, not all RS cells in a given case of classical HL will express CD15, but only a major or minor subset of RS cells may express this marker in a membrane and/or focal cytoplasmic (Golgi) staining pattern. When RS cells express CD20, only a minor subset of cells are positive, and the intensity of staining with CD20 is usually variable, with a majority of positive cells showing weak expression.[26] CD79a may also stain classic RS cells.[25] Cases in which RS-like cells are negative for both CD15 and CD30 and positive for CD20 are probably not HL, but rather, these cases are most likely examples of T cell/histiocyte-rich B-cell lymphomas (TC/HRBCL).[27] As previously mentioned, none of the antibodies are specific for RS cells.   CD15 also stains myeloid cells, approximately two-thirds of cases of acute myelogenous leukemia, and some adenocarcinomas, especially primary pulmonary types.[28]   CD30 also stains anaplastic large cell lymphomas (ALCL), activated T- and B-cells, and plasma cells as well as embryonal cell carcinoma.[29]   Fascin is expressed by dendritic cells, some cases of ALCL, and some large cell lymphomas.[30, 31]

Table 11-2. Immunophenotype of Reed-Sternberg Cells

Immunophenotypic Marker	"Classic" Reed Sternberg Cells	L & H Cells
CD15	+	-
CD20 (L26), CD79a	-/+	+
CD30	+	-
CD45 (LCA)	-	+
Bcl-6	-	+
CDw75 (LN1)	-	+
EMA	-	+ (50%)
J Chain	-	+
EBV	+ (40-70%)	-
Oct2	-	+
BOB.1	-	+
PU.1	-	+

In contrast to classic RS cells, L&H cells do not express CD15, CD30, or fascin, but they do express B-cell markers CD20, CD79a, and CD75 as well as CD45[32-36].   In addition, L&H cells express BCL-6 (attesting to their germinal center origin), EMA in approximately 50% of cases, and they also synthesize J chains (a feature of B-cells).[1,34-37]   They are also positive for OCT 2, BOB.1, and PU.1, whereas classic RS cells are almost always negative.[38, 39]   Light chain restriction in RS cells has been demonstrated by immunohistochemistry, and clonality of the RS cells can be shown by molecular studies of isolated RS cells (vide infra).[20, 21, 40]   The immunophenotype of the background lymphocytes in NLP HL is also different from that of CHL (with the exception of the NLRC type) in that the former are mostly CD20 and CD79a-positive B-cells, whereas the background small lymphocytes in CHL are T-cells (Table 11-3).   In both NLP and NLRC HL, the RS cells are rosetted by T-lymphocytes.[34, 41, 42]   CD21 outlines a prominent, expanded, concentric meshwork of follicular dendritic cells in NLP HL, whereas in NLRC HL it highlights residual germinal centers as well as the extension of the follicular dendritic network into the expanded mantle zones.[35]   The nodules of NLP HL are composed predominantly of small polyclonal B-cells with a mantle cell phenotype (IgM+, IgD+).

Table 11-3. Immunophenotype of small lymphocytes in Hodgkin lymphoma (HL)

	Classical (except LRC)	NLP HL	NLRC HL
B cells	-	+	+
T cells	+	+, ring RS cells	+, ring RS cells
CD57+ cells	-	+, ring RS cells	-/+, rarely ring RS cells

As stated earlier, RS cells must be found in a proper cellular environment of one of the subtypes of HL. Cells indistinguishable from classic RS cells may be present in benign or other malignant lymphoid proliferations, which usually (with the exception of some peripheral T-cell lymphomas) do not have the inflammatory background of one of the subtypes of HL. Viral disorders, such as infectious mononucleosis, may harbor cells indistinguishable from classic RS cells (RS-like cells), but the background inflammatory population differs from that seen in HL. The RS-like cells in infectious mononucleosis (IM) are immunoblasts that are CD15 negative but, as in classic HL, they express CD30.[43] In contrast to the RS cells in classical HL, the RS-like cells of IM usually express CD45, and like the other immunoblasts that are present, consist of mixtures of B- and T-cells. Non-Hodgkin's lymphomas, especially peripheral T-cell lymphomas (PTCL) and T cell/histiocyte-rich B-cell lymphomas (TC/HRBCL), may contain classic or occasionally L&H-type RS-like cells.[40,43,44] It is of utmost importance to differentiate these NHL from HL because the former are aggressive neoplasms associated with a poor prognosis. PTCL may even have a background polymorphous infiltrate indistinguishable from that of MC HL. However, the impostor RS-like cells in PTCL stain as T-cells, are usually CD15 and CD30 negative, and often express CD45, whereas in TC/HR BCL the RS-like cells express the B-cell markers CD20 and CD79a and are CD15 and usually CD30 negative. In cases in which the RS-like cells resemble L&H variants, the differential diagnosis between these two lymphomas may be difficult; however, a nodular pattern composed of B-cells is characteristic of NLP HL, whereas a diffuse proliferation of T-cells (>90%) tends to be diagnostic of TC/HRLCL.[40,44] The expanded follicular dendritic cell (FDRC) meshwork that is present within the nodules of NLP HL is absent in TC/HR BCL. The number of small B-cells in NLP HL is generally much greater than in TC/HRLCL, where small B-lymphocytes are rare. In addition, double staining has shown rosetting Bcl-6 + /CD57+ lymphocytes around CD20+/Bcl-6+ RS variants in NLP HL. The presence of these lymphocytes is useful in the differential diagnosis of NLP HL from LRC HL and TC/HRBCL, which do not contain Bcl-6+/CD57+ cells.[45]

2.6   Nodular Lymphocyte Predominant Hodgkin Lymphoma

In the Lukes/Butler classification, NLP HL was divided into two morphologic subtypes: nodular and diffuse.[14,15] In the Rye scheme, it was simply called NLP HL.

In the REAL/WHO classification, NLP HL is defined as having at least a partially nodular growth pattern, although diffuse areas may be present in a minority of cases.[1,19] (Table 11-1) Although there is still controversy about whether a purely diffuse LP HL exists, this entity is not recognized as a distinct category in the WHO scheme. The studies by the German Hodgkin Study Groups[34,46] showed that immunophenotyping is essential for a diagnosis of NLP HL.

2.6.1   Clinical Features

The clinical features of the NLP type of HL are well known and are distinct from those of CHL with the exception of the LRC type.[1,47,48] The disorder is uncommon, comprising only about three to eight percent of HL and affects predominantly males (male to female ratio 3:1) in their fourth decade, although this entity may also be seen in children and older adults.[47] Peripheral lymph nodes are involved, but mediastinal disease is distinctly uncommon. The vast majority of patients present with stage I/II disease, and most patients achieve complete remission after standard therapy for CHL, with approximately 80 to 90% being alive after 10 years.[48] Advanced stage and older age are likely to be associated with shorter overall survival. There tends to be a greater number of relapses compared to patients with CHL, but these recurrences are not associated with a poor survival.[49-52] Late relapses (after 10 to 13 years) are characteristic of NLP HL, whereas they are distinctly unusual in CHL, including the NLRC type.[34,47,48] Therefore, continued surveillance for late relapse is indicated in these patients. However, these patients usually do not die of their HL but rather succumb to cardiovascular disease, various complications of therapy, or other neoplasms.[50,52] Although NLP HL is a B-cell lymphoma with a prolonged clinical course characterized by multiple relapses akin to low-grade, especially follicular non-Hodgkin's lymphomas, the suggestion that NLP HL be classified as a type of NHL is unwarranted for several reasons.[35,50] Unlike low-grade NHLs, NLP HL presents with localized rather than widespread disease, and the paucity of neoplastic cells among the majority of benign inflammatory cells seems more consistent with HL than with NHL. In addition, patients with NLP HL are younger than those with low-grade NHL, and NLP HL responds well to localized therapy, whereas low-grade NHLs generally do not.

2.6.2   Histologic Features

The nodal architecture is generally completely effaced by a nodular (or rarely by a nodular and diffuse) infiltrate of small B-lymphocytes and varying numbers of epithelioid histiocytes, within or occasionally ringing nodules, as well as scattered lymphocytic and/or histiocytic (L&H) variants of RS cells (Figure 11-2).[35,46] If uninvolved nodal tissue remains, it is usually found as a compressed rim of tissue at the periphery of the lymph node. The RS cells may be difficult to find, or, less often, they may be readily detected within the nodules in H&E-stained sections. They are usually highlighted by CD20, which is expressed with greater intensity on RS cells than in the population of small lymphocytes within the nodules. Not only are these RS variants morphologically different from classic and lacunar types of RS cells, but they are also immunophenotypically different (Table 11-2). They express B-cell markers CD20, CD79a, CD45 (LCA), BCL-6, EMA (approximately 50% of cases), OCT2, BOB.1, PU.1 and they produce J chains.[34,36,38,39,41] They do not express antigens present on classic RS cells such as CD15, CD30, or fascin. As such, they have features of B-cells. Molecular analysis of isolated RS cells has provided additional evidence that the RS cells in NLP HL are clonal B-cells that are derived from germinal center cells (vide infra).[20,21,37]

2.7   Lymphocyte-rich Classical Hodgkin Lymphoma

2.7.1   Clinical features

LRC HL shares many of the clinical features of NLP HL that are distinct from other forms of CHL. It comprises about five percent of all HL.[34,41] There is a male predominance (approximately 70%), and the median age at diagnosis is greater than that of other types of classical HL as well as that of NLP HL. Like patients with NLP HL, patients with NLRC HL present with low stage disease (stages I/II) and usually lack B symptoms, bulky disease, and mediastinal involvement. In contrast to NLP HL, this type of HL is less often associated with multiple relapses, and the overall survival is favorable, although it is not as good as that of patients with NLP HL.[34,41] The prognosis is less favorable for patients who have relapses than it is for those patients with relapsed NLP HL.[34,47,48]

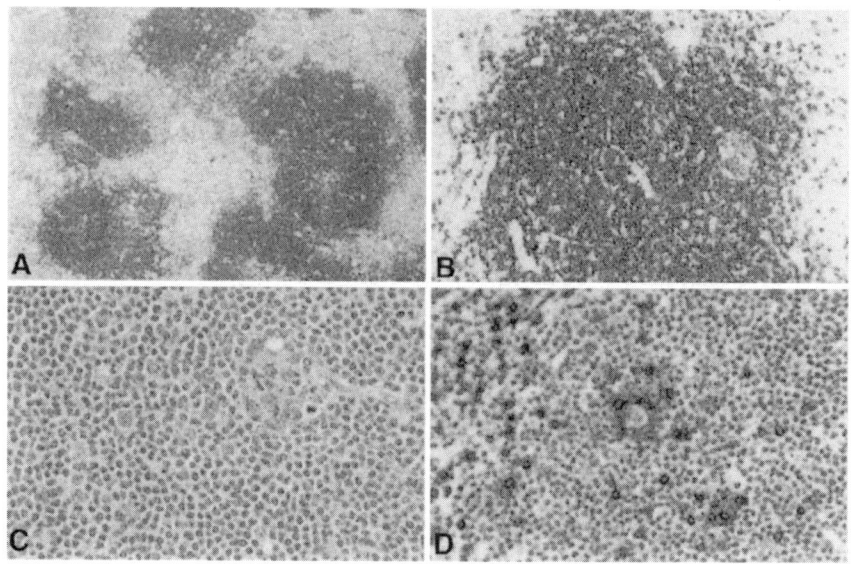

Figure 11-2. Nodular lymphocyte-rich classical Hodgkin lymphoma. A) CD20 positive nodules composed of expanded mantle zones. B) Higher magnification of CD20 positive expanded mantle zone containing an atrophic, eccentrically-placed germinal center. C) H&E section of an atrophic germinal center within the mantle zone. D) CD3 positive lymphocytes ring a Reed-Sternberg cell.

2.7.2   Histologic features

As the name LRCHL implies, the histologic features of this type of HL are characterized by a predominance of small lymphocytes and few, if any, other inflammatory cells.   LRC HL is further divided into two subtypes: nodular and diffuse.   NLRC HL, first described in 1992 and called "follicular HL"[53,55] is much more common than the diffuse type.[1,19,34,47] The nodular pattern, which may simulate the nodularity of NLP HL, is formed by expanded mantle zone B-lymphocytes that may or may not contain eccentrically-placed, residual atrophic or occasionally even hyperplastic germinal centers (Figure 11-3).[53]   Classic types of RS cells and/or lacunar cell variants of RS cells are present in varying numbers within the expanded mantle zones, and it is the presence of these classic RS cells that aids in the diagnosis.   Occasionally cells resembling L&H variants of RS cells may also be present.   Most of the RS cells are seen within the mantle zone or at its junction with internodular areas, whereas occasionally RS cells may be present in the internodular areas composed of residual paracortical T-cells. If, in the future, the indolent, NLP HL stage I disease is handled with a watch-and-wait approach, or if treatment intensity is reduced, or if the disorder is treated with such chemotherapeutic agents as rituximab (anti-CD20 antibody), it will be of the utmost importance to differentiate the two subtypes of HL.[54]

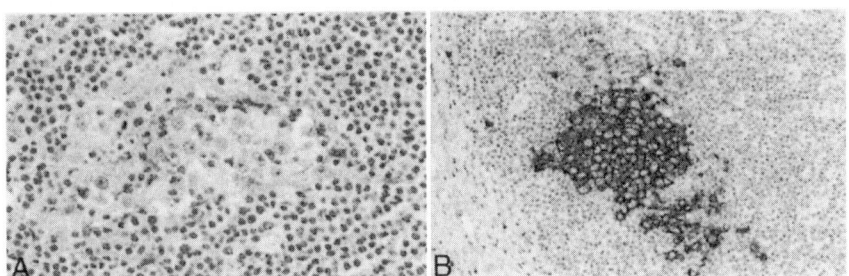

Figure 11-3. Syncytial variant of nocular sclerosis Hodgkin lymphoma. A) Nodule composed of large cells. B) CD15 positivity identifies the large cells as lacunar cell variants.

2.7.3 Differential Diagnosis

NLRC HL has in the past been frequently misinterpreted as NLP HL, which is still the major differential diagnostic consideration. The difficulty in differentiating NLP HL from NLRC HL is confirmed by a study of a large number of cases in which approximately 30% of cases originally diagnosed as NLP HL were found instead to be NLRC HL and in which the immunophenotype of the RS cells was essential in eventually establishing the correct diagnosis.[34] Histologically, both NLP and LRC HL have a nodular pattern, and the nodules in both are composed predominantly of small B- lymphocytes. In contrast to NLRC HL, the B-cell nodules in NLP HL are, in most instances, larger than those in NLRC HL, and they do not contain germinal centers. In addition, the RS cells in NLP HL cells are not of the classic type and are immunologically different as well (CD20+, CD79a+, CD45R+, BCL-6+, EMA+/-, CD15-, CD30-, fascin-). In both subtypes, the T-cells that rosette around RS cells are readily recognized even under low magnification, because they are surrounded by negative-staining B-cells. In addition, CD21 and CD35 outline a prominent, expanded, concentric meshwork of follicular dendritic cells in NLP HL (which in NLRC HL is less extensive). In addition, these markers highlight a densely staining meshwork of residual germinal centers when present as well as FDC network extension into the expanded mantle zone.[1,34] CD57-positive cells are scattered throughout the nodules of NLP HL, sometimes encircling L&H cells, whereas in NLRC HL, they are largely confined to residual germinal centers with occasional CD57-positive cells within mantle zones, rarely encircling RS cells.[1,34,53]

The less common diffuse (D) type of LRC HL is characterized histologically by a diffuse proliferation of small T-lymphocytes with occasional interspersed RS cells of the classic or lacunar cell type.[1] Eosinophils and plasma cells are rare or absent, and necrosis is not seen. Histiocytes may be interspersed among the small lymphocytes. In the past, prior to the availability of immunophenotyping, most cases with the histologic features of DLRC HL were interpreted as either diffuse lymphocyte predominance (DLP) HL, a condition that probably does not exist in the pure form but one that may be associated with NLP HL/NLP with diffuse areas or occasionally as NLP HL, or else categorized as the mixed cellularity (MC) type. On purely morphologic grounds, DLRC HL may also resemble T cell/histiocyte-rich B-cell lymphoma; however, these two lymphomas are immunophenotypically distinct.[40,57] CD15, CD30, CD45, and CD20 are helpful in the differential diagnosis of these lymphomas. In DLRC HL, RS cells are CD15-positive, CD30-positive, and CD45-negative, and the background lymphocytes are mostly T-cells, whereas in NLP HL, RS cells are CD20-positive, CD45-negative, CD15-negative, CD30-negative, and the background lymphocytes are largely B-cells. In TC/HRBCL the large cells are CD15-negative, CD30-negative, CD45-positive, CD20-positive, and the background lymphocytes are predominantly T-cells.[44]

2.8   Nodular Sclerosis HL

2.8.1   Clinical Features

NS HL is the most common subtype of classical HL in developed nations, accounting for 60-80% of cases.[1] It is also the most common type of HL found in adolescents and young adults, and the median age at diagnosis is 28 years. It is the only subtype in which there is no male predominance, with an almost equal male to female ratio.[14, 15] A high percentage of patients present with mediastinal involvement (80%), and massive mediastinal disease is an adverse risk factor.[56]

2.8.2   Morphologic Features

The characteristic histologic features include a thickened nodal capsule from which collagen bands emanate to form multiple nodules containing inflammatory cells as well as varying numbers of lacunar variants of RS cells.[14,15] There is a variable inflammatory component, ranging from that seen in LP to LD HL. The only newly described morphologic entity since the Lukes/Butler classification is the syncytial variant of NS HL.[58,59] This variant is characterized by prominent aggregates of large and often pleomorphic cells, some with the appearance of lacunar cells (Figure 11-3). A grading scheme for NS HL is also included in the REAL/WHO classifications, although it is not required for routine clinical purposes at present.[1] Two histologic grades are identified: grades 1 and 2. The vast majority of cases (75-85%) are grade 1 with 15-25% classified as grade 2. Grade 1 NS HL is characterized by 75% or more of the nodules containing scattered RS cells in a background of lymphocyte predominance or a mixed inflammatory infiltrate. In grade 2, increased numbers or sheets of RS cells (filling a 40x hpf) in at least 25% of nodules must be present. Grade 2 NS HL[1,60,61] appears to be similar or identical to the syncytial variant and has also been referred to as the lymphocyte depletion variant of NS HL.[62] The worse prognosis initially reported to be associated with grade 2 NS HL has not been substantiated in more recent studies.[63-66] The prognosis of NS HL is slightly better than the prognoses of MC and LD HL, probably due partly to presentation with low stage disease. Differential diagnosis of the syncytial variant of NS includes both NHL as well as necrotizing granulomas. Some of the large cells may be morphologically indistinguishable from cells of anaplastic large cell lymphoma or cells of large cell non-Hodgkin's lymphoma. Moreover, because of the clustering of the RS cells, the syncytial variant may even resemble a carcinoma, especially in poorly cut sections. Therefore, the differential diagnosis, especially in a small biopsy in which the characteristic features of NS HL are absent, includes large cell lymphoma, anaplastic large cell lymphoma, and non-hematopoietic neoplasms.[67] Appropriate immunohistochemical stains are helpful in differentiating between these neoplasms (e,g large cell lymphomas of B- or T-cell type stain with either B- or T-cell markers and often CD45; anaplastic large cell lymphoma is CD45-positive/negative, CD30-positive, CD15-negative, T-cell antibody positive/negative, B-cell antibody negative, EMA-positive/negative, and ALK-positive/negative; and non-hematopoietic tumors often express cytokeratin markers). Areas of coagulative or suppurative necrosis, simulating necrotizing granulomas, are often present within the syncytia of RS cells. The suppurative foci must be differentiated from those seen in cat scratch disease; however, atypical RS-like cells are never present in infectious granulomas.

2.9   Mixed Cellularity HL

Approximately 20-25% of cases of HL are of the MC type.[1] In the Lukes/Butler and Rye schemes, MC HL included not only cases conforming to the classical description of this entity (classic RS cells in a diffuse or vaguely nodular mixed inflammatory background in the absence of a nodular sclerosing fibrosis), but it also served as a "wastebasket" for cases that did not readily fit into any of the other subtypes. Cases that cannot be subclassified in the REAL/WHO scheme are should be diagnosed as "unclassifiable".[1,19]

2.9.1   Clinical Features

The median age at presentation is 37 years and almost 70% are male. The bimodal age distribution seen in the NS type is not present. Both MC and LD subtypes are seen primarily in non-industrialized nations and in HIV+ patients. Patients often present with high stage disease (III/IV) and B symptoms. Abdominal involvement and splenic disease are more common than in NS.[1]

2.9.2   Histologic Features

As the name implies, classic RS/H and rare lacunar cells are readily found in a mixed cellular inflammatory background that includes lymphocytes, plasma cells, eosinophils, neutrophils, and histiocytes. EBV encoded LMP-1 is expressed by RS/H cells in approximately 75% of cases, which is much more frequent than in NS and LRC HL.[68] Both MC as well as NS HL may involve interfollicular areas of lymph nodes with prominent follicular hyperplasia possibly masking the HL. Such cases are also referred to as "interfollicular" HL.[69]   The differential diagnosis of MC HL includes peripheral T-cell lymphoma (PTCL). Immunophenotyping must always be carried out in cases resembling MC HL in order to differentiate this subtype of HL from peripheral T-cell lymphoma, because the two may be indistinguishable on morphologic grounds alone.[70] The mixed inflammatory infiltrate may closely resemble that found in MC HL, and RS-like cells may be present in some cases of PTCL. The large cells resembling RS/H cells are most often CD15-negative, stain with one or more T-cell markers, and are usually CD45-positive. In difficult cases, T-cell receptor gene rearrangement studies are required to determine whether or not a clonal T-cell population can be demonstrated to indicate a PTCL.

2.10   Lymphocyte depletion HL

The number of cases diagnosed as LD HL has decreased since immunophenotyping became available. LD HL is the most rare subtype (< 1%)[71] and cases classified as LD in the past are now considered to be mostly non-Hodgkin's lymphoma (especially large cell lymphomas, anaplastic large cell lymphoma), other subtypes of HL (e.g syncytial variant of NS), or occasionally non-hematopoietic neoplasms.[1,71,72]

2.10.1 Clinical Features

The lymphocyte depletion subtype is associated with advanced stage and B symptoms in the majority of cases.[1,71,72] Today, it is seen most often in HIV-infected patients and in individuals in developing countries.[73] Most cases occurring in HIV-positive patients contain EBV-infected RS cells that stain positively with LMP.[68]

2.10.2 Histological Features

In the past, most cases were reported in older individuals with abdominal lymphadenopathy, absence of peripheral lymph node involvement, and advanced stage disease (splenic, liver, and bone marrow involvement). Response to modern chemotherapy is similar to that of other types of classical HL.[72] Histologically, the lymph node is hypocellular due to fibrosis and/or necrosis. There is a paucity of lymphocytes and other inflammatory cells, whereas there is an abundance of anaplastic or "sarcomatous"-appearing RS cells that may be found in confluent sheets. Immunophenotyping is required before a diagnosis of LD HL can be made. The cells with features of RS cells are CD15-positive, CD30-positive, CD45-negative. In addition, they are negative for B- and T-cell markers. Although LD HL in the past behaved more aggressively than other types, with the advent of modern therapy its course is similar to that of other types of classical HL.[71]

3. MOLECULAR AND CELLULAR BIOLOGY OF HODGKIN LYMPHOMA

3.1 Introduction

Since the time of its original description by Sir Thomas Hodgkin in 1832, the pathogenesis of what we now know as Hodgkin lymphoma has been the focus of extensive study. Despite decades of great strides, however, significant advances leading to an improved understanding of the molecular alterations present in Hodgkin lymphoma have only recently been realized, largely through ongoing improvements in molecular biologic techniques.

The ability to isolate single malignant cells through microdissection methods combined with the capacity to apply the polymerase chain reaction (PCR) technique to fresh, frozen, and paraffin-embedded tissues has significantly impacted the study of Hodgkin lymphoma over the past few years. Today even more sophisticated technologic advances, such as novel gene array platforms capable of evaluating the expression patterns of thousands of genes, are producing valuable data that will undoubtedly further expand our knowledge of the biology and pathogenesis of Hodgkin lymphoma. The following is a brief synopsis of the current understanding of the molecular basis of classical Hodgkin lymphoma and nodular lymphocyte predominant Hodgkin lymphoma.

3.2   Classical Hodgkin lymphoma

3.2.1   Clonality and Cell of Origin Studies

It is generally accepted that the malignant cells of Hodgkin lymphoma are the Hodgkin/Reed-Sternberg (HRS) cells. In most cases, the HRS cells comprise less than 1% of all cells in involved tissues, and they are characteristically surrounded by an inflammatory milieu consisting of granulocytes, plasma cells, and a mixture of B- and T-lymphocytes. As discussed earlier in this chapter, the HRS cells are further unique in that they are known to express a variety of leukocyte markers including myeloid markers (e.g., CD15), B-cell markers (e.g. CD19, CD20, CD79a), T-cell markers (CD2, CD4, granzyme B), and characteristically, the lymphocyte activation marker, CD30. Because of these unusual features, particularly the relatively low number of malignant cells present in involved tissues, molecular investigations of Hodgkin lymphoma could not be performed as readily nor with the same reproducibility as they could in other malignant tumors, including the non-Hodgkin lymphomas. As such, the normal cellular counterpart of the HRS cell remained a mystery for a long time. The advent and perfection of single cell microdissection (first by hand-driven pipette methods and then more recently by laser capture techniques), which allowed for the precise isolation of homogeneous, morphologically recognizable cell populations, was pivotal in addressing these problems, and ultimately led the way to an improved understanding of Hodgkin lymphoma. Combined with the highly sensitive technique of PCR, microdissection of individual neoplastic cells enabled detailed characterization of specific HRS cell populations.

The first series of single cell experiments on HRS cells produced heterogeneous results, ranging from non-detection of immunoglobulin gene rearrangement to detection of rearranged immunoglobulin genes in some or in all cases studied.[74-80] The pattern of immunoglobulin gene rearrangement observed in Hodgkin lymphoma cases also differed in the various initial studies. Whereas Kanzler et al[78] and Kuppers et al[79] found a predominance of identical immunoglobulin gene rearrangements in the HRS cell population of 12 of 13 cases, Delabie et al[75] reported the mere finding of non-identical rearrangements indicative of a polyclonal proliferation of HRS cells. Other groups found a mixture of monoclonal and polyclonal HRS cell populations as well as individual HRS cells with both monoclonal and polyclonal rearrangements in similar numbers of cases studied.[77, 78]

Further refinement and optimization of HRS cell isolation techniques and the PCR procedure, however, eventually led to more consistent and reproducible results. Marafioti et al[20] examined a large number of HRS cells isolated from 25 cases of Hodgkin lymphoma and found two hundred and ninety-one identical and only three non-identical rearrangements among 24 analyzable cases. The three non-identical rearrangements lacked evidence of somatic mutation, which was in contrast to the identically rearranged immunoglobulin genes that contained somatic mutations in all cases and suggested that the three non-identical rearrangements were contaminations and technical artifacts.

Although the initial studies produced contradictory results, the subsequent work of multiple separate investigative groups has unequivocally demonstrated that HRS cells are monoclonal cells, and furthermore, it is now widely accepted that HRS cells are of B-cell lineage with rearrangements of the V, D, and J (VDJ) segments of the immunoglobulin heavy chain gene.[81] It is also generally acknowledged that the initial studies, which indicated a polyclonal nature of HRS cells, were unfortunately flawed by technical artifacts. From the various series of cases examined to date, it is currently estimated that approximately 98% of classical Hodgkin lymphomas are B-cell derived neoplasms. Phenotypic and genotypic studies of Hodgkin lymphoma-derived cell lines and a few cases of classical Hodgkin lymphoma expressing T-cell associated antigens suggest that at least some of the remaining cases of Hodgkin lymphoma are derived from transformed and clonal T-cells.[82-84]

3.2.2 Germinal Center Derived Cells

Concomitant with the studies that confirmed the clonal nature and B-cell origin of the HRS cells of classical Hodgkin lymphoma and as alluded to in the previous section, nucleotide sequence analysis of the rearranged VDJ regions of HRS cells revealed a high load of somatic mutations, with these mutations frequently resulting non-functional immunoglobulin variable regions.[20,78] In the normal state, naïve B-cells harbor unmutated immunoglobulin variable genes. Following antigen-dependent activation in secondary lymphoid tissues, activated B-cells enter primary follicles and establish germinal centers. It is within these structures that B-cells proliferate and undergo the process of somatic hypermutation, which introduces mutations (mostly point mutations) into rearranged immunoglobulin variable region genes.[85-87] The process of somatic hypermutation occurs strictly in the germinal centers of secondary lymphoid organs, and only cells producing antibody with the appropriate affinity to immunizing antigens are allowed to survive in the germinal center. The presence of somatic mutations in HRS cells, therefore, was evidence that these cells descended from germinal center B-cells as opposed to post-germinal center B-cells. Moreover, these data pointed towards a possible molecular mechanism accounting for the sustained viability of HRS cells in an environment that would normally mark such aberrant cells for death (through apoptosis) without the several rounds of proliferation and mutation required for ultimate positive selection. In a few cases of classical Hodgkin lymphoma, the somatic mutations in HRS cells were associated with the presence of stop codons and deletions that have been termed "crippling" mutations.[81,87] Germinal center B-cells that acquire these types of mutations are efficiently eliminated from the germinal center through apoptosis and are not allowed to leave the germinal center microenvironment. Although only approximately 25% of cases with originally potentially productive variable gene rearrangements carried stop codons, it was speculated that HRS cells in classical Hodgkin lymphoma were derived from crippled, pre-apoptotic germinal center B-cells.[78, 87]

Additional evidence providing support for the germinal center B-cell derivation of HRS cells, as well as furthering the speculation that even the initial transforming event in Hodgkin lymphoma occurred within the germinal center B-cell itself, came from case studies of patients with so-called "composite lymphomas" composed of follicular non-Hodgkin lymphoma (NHL) and classical Hodgkin lymphoma.[21,88] Molecular analysis of the HRS cells and NHL cells from a small series of composite lymphomas demonstrated identical VDJ rearrangements at the immunoglobulin heavy chain gene locus in the two morphologically distinct cell types, indicating derivation of both cell types from the same B-cell precursor. It was further found that all rearrangements in the HRS and NHL cells carried somatic hypermutations; some of these mutations were shared by the HRS and NHL cells, whereas others were found exclusively in one or the other lymphoma cell type. Similar to previous observations in other NHLs, the VDJ rearrangements of the NHL cells in the composite lymphomas showed signs of ongoing mutations, a finding that was not seen in the HRS cells. The presence of shared sequences unequivocally mapped the differentiation stage of the common B-cell precursor as that of a germinal center B-cell and ruled out linear progression of HRS cells to NHL cells. The conclusions drawn from the composite lymphoma studies included: 1) classical Hodgkin lymphomas derive from germinal center B-cells and not from post-germinal center B-cells, 2) the descendants of the common B-cell precursor undergo two separate transforming events, one leading to HRS cells and the other leading to an NHL phenotype, 3) the transforming event(s) producing Hodgkin lymphoma markedly changes the morphology and immunophenotype of the common precursor cell while the transforming event(s) of NHL more or less result in preservation of the features of the precursor B-cell.[89]

3.2.3 Aberrant Immunoglobulin Expression and Transcription Defects

Upon entry of naïve B-cells into the germinal center, the cell death machinery is activated and only those cells receiving positive selection signals are allowed to leave the germinal center to enter the pool of memory B-cells.[87] Cells that do not acquire favorable mutations or that lose the ability to produce antibody are quickly and efficiently eliminated by the process of a programmed cell death (apoptosis). It was known from previous studies that HRS cells lacked B-cell receptor and immunoglobulin mRNA transcripts, and that they were incapable of expressing immunoglobulin or producing functional antibody. Moreover, it was also known that crippling mutations occurred in only 25% of HRS cells.[20] As such, investigators focused on additional cellular abnormalities or mechanisms to account for the inability of HRS cells to express immunoglobulin and to explain how these aberrant cells escaped apoptosis.

Subsequent studies implicated abnormalities in transcription factors resulting in inactivation of the immunoglobulin promoter gene.[38,39,90-92] Expression of rearranged immunoglobulin heavy and light chain genes is critical for B-cell differentiation, and this process is regulated by a complex interaction between regulatory DNA elements and transcription factors.[93] The octamer motif is among the DNA regulatory elements necessary for B-cell-specific transcription. The octamer motif is an important transcriptional regulatory site that is part of promoter and enhancers of ubiquitously expressed genes. The octamer motif is found in all immunoglobulin heavy and light chain promoters as well as in the heavy chain and kappa light chain enhancer elements, and it has been determined to be essential for B-cell specificity and activity of the immunoglobulin promoter and enhancer.[94] The octamer site interacts with transcription factors belonging to the POU family of homeo-domain proteins, binding specifically to the octamer motif via their POU domain.[95]

The transcription factor, OCT.2, whose expression is restricted to B-cells and neuronal cells, in conjunction with its cofactor BOB.1, plays a critical role in immunoglobulin promoter transactivation. In a study by Re et al,[90] which utilized Hodgkin's disease-derived cell lines, it was found that HRS cells lacked expression of OCT.2 and BOB.1. The absence of these transcription factors represented a novel mechanism for immunoglobulin gene deregulation in HRS cells and pointed toward a defect in the transcription factor machinery of HRS cells as the cause of the lack of immunoglobulin gene expression in these cells. This finding was further supported by the work of Stein et al[38] who analyzed 35 cases of nodular lymphocyte predominant Hodgkin lymphoma (NLP HL), 32 cases of classical Hodgkin lymphoma, and 2 Hodgkin's disease cell lines for OCT.2 and BOB.1 expression and demonstrated an absence of OCT.2 and/or BOB.1 in classical Hodgkin lymphoma and a striking over-expression of OCT.2 in NLP HL. Not only did this study yield significant information regarding another mechanism accounting for the lack of antibody production by HRS cells, but it also revealed OCT.2 (as well as BOB.1) as potentially valuable immunohistochemical markers useful in the differentiation of classical Hodgkin lymphoma from NLP HL and other B-cell non-Hodgkin lymphomas.

Following recognition of the importance of transcription factors, such as OCT.2 and BOB.1, in the pathogenesis of Hodgkin lymphoma, researchers using case material from patients with Hodgkin lymphoma and Hodgkin lymphoma-derived cell lines focused on the expression patterns of other transcription factors with known roles in immunoglobulin gene regulation as well as B-cell development. One such significant study, performed by Torlakovic et al,[39] examined the relevance of PU.1 in HRS cells. PU.1 belongs to the Ets-family of transcription factors, and it is necessary for B-cell development.[96,97] Specifically, PU.1 regulates a number of genes important for B-cell differentiation, and among these are the genes for immunoglobulin heavy chain, J chain, and both light chain genes as well as the CD20 gene and the MB-1 gene. PU.1 has been shown to act by cooperating with several other transcription factors such as c-JUN and c-FOS.[98] In their study, Torlakovic et al. examined the expression of PU.1 by Western blotting in four cases of classical Hodgkin lymphoma-derived cell lines and five cases of non-Hodgkin lymphoma-derived cell lines. In addition, they performed immunohistochemistry on 35 cases of classical Hodgkin lymphoma, 15 cases of NLP HL, and 67 cases of non-Hodgkin lymphoma. The findings of this study were significant in that PU.1 expression was strikingly absent in HRS cells of classical Hodgkin lymphoma but uniformly present in all cases of NLP HL. In addition, PU.1 expression was also found in a significant percentage of B-cell non-Hodgkin lymphoma (61 of 67 cases) with the exception of T-cell-rich large B-cell lymphoma. Moreover, PU.1 was not expressed in 17 cases of peripheral T-cell lymphoma nor in 7 cases of anaplastic large cell lymphoma. Lastly, this study was significant in that it also examined the expression of OCT.2 in classical Hodgkin lymphoma and NLP HL, and confirmed the earlier findings of Re et al[90] and Stein et al.[38] Taken together, the studies on the transcription factors OCT.2, BOB.1, and PU.1 yielded important information regarding the pathogenesis of HRS cells, specifically related to the lack of immunoglobulin expression in classical Hodgkin lymphoma. These studies were also relevant in that they provided additional markers in the immunohistochemical arsenal for distinguishing classical Hodgkin lymphoma from NLP HL and other types of B-cell non-Hodgkin lymphoma (summarized in Table 11-2).

3.2.4 Inhibition of Apoptosis

Since B-cells that have lost the capacity to express surface immunoglobulin undergo apoptosis in the normal germinal center reaction, it follows that HRS cells may have some mechanism for escaping the apoptotic pathway. While the complete mechanism has yet to be elucidated, recent studies have implicated nuclear factor kappa B (NFkB) in the protection of HRS cells from programmed cell death.[99,100] NFkB is a ubiquitously expressed transcription factor that regulates several vital cellular functions including apoptosis (specifically preventing it) and cell proliferation and differentiation.[101,102] In addition, NFkB is also known to play a major role in controlling the immune response and inflammation. In most normal cell types, NFkB is only transiently activated, mainly by stress signals and in immune inflammatory signaling events. As a characteristic of HRS cells, a constitutive activation of NFkB has been recognized. Constitutive NFkB accounts for the elevated expression of several genes typically associated with HRS cells, including cell cycle-regulating and anti-apoptotic genes, and contributes to proliferation, apoptosis resistance, and tumorgenicity of HRS cells.[103] The involvement of NFkB in the resistance of HRS cells to apoptosis is supported by in-vitro findings demonstrating that inactivation of NFkB restores the sensitivity of HRS cells to apoptosis. The persistent activation of NFkB is thought to be caused by defects in members of the inhibitors of kappa B (IkB) family, which are natural inhibitors of NFkB, or by the aberrant activation of IkB kinase.[104-106] In a study by Jungnickel et al[106] in which single HRS cells micromanipulated from histologic sections of Hodgkin lymphoma were analyzed, clonal deleterious somatic mutations in the IkB alpha gene were detected, indicating a role for IkB alpha defects in the pathogenesis of Hodgkin lymphoma and moreover suggesting that IkB alpha is a tumor suppressor gene.

3.2.5   Gene Expression Profiling

One reason for the longstanding controversy regarding the cellular origin of HRS cells was their unusual phenotype, which cannot be fully related to any normal cell of the hematopoietic system. Typical B-cell markers such as CD19, CD20, and CD22 in addition to the common leukocyte antigen marker, CD45, are either not expressed or expressed by only a small fraction of the HRS cells of classical Hodgkin lymphoma. These atypical immunophenotypic features, along with recent data showing down-regulation of certain transcription factors with known relevance for proper B-cell function (i.e. OCT.2, BOB.1, and PU.1), suggest that the global B-lineage-specific gene expression program may be altered in the HRS cells of classical Hodgkin lymphoma. In a recent study by Schwering et al.,[107] comprehensive gene expression profiles of Hodgkin lymphoma cell lines and normal B-cell subsets were analyzed with respect to the B-cell phenotype of HRS cells. Not only did this study demonstrate down-regulation of single B-lineage markers in HRS cells, but more importantly, it also revealed a defect in the entire B-lineage gene expression program, with either lacking or greatly reduced RNA expression for nearly all known genes specific for B-cells, lymphocytes, or hematopoietic cells. Based on their results, the authors of this study proposed that the survival of HRS cells without immunoglobulin or B-cell receptor expression could be explained by a loss of their B-cell lineage identity, which may arise from a fundamental defect in their ability to maintain a B-cell differentiation state. In a separate earlier study by Hertel et al.,[108] it was demonstrated that immunoglobulin promoters as well as both intronic and 3' enhancer sequences were transcriptionally inactive in HRS cell lines, and that this inactivity correlated with either reduced levels or a complete lack of B-cell specific transcription factors (including OCT.2, BOB.1, PU.1, and PAX-5) required for their expression. The authors of this study suggested that HRS cells are differentiated B-cells with global down-regulation of B-cell-specific genes.

3.3   Nodular Lymphocyte Predominant Hodgkin Lymphoma

Immunomorphologic investigations have shown that while related, classical Hodgkin lymphoma and NLP HL represent distinct biologic entities. The origin of the tumor cells in NLP HL, which are known as lymphocytic and/or histiocytic (L&H) cells, was clarified in the 1980s by immunophenotyping studies using polyclonal and monoclonal antibodies.[35] The consistent detection of B-cell specific molecules, including J-chain, CD20, and CD79a, in L&H cells provided convincing evidence of their B-cell derivation. Recent single cell molecular studies have formally proven the cellular origin and clonal nature of these cells with the finding of monoclonal immunoglobulin gene rearrangements in the DNA of isolated single L&H cells.[109-111] As in classical Hodgkin lymphoma, the variable region of the immunoglobulin heavy chain gene carries a high load of somatic mutations. Unlike classical Hodgkin lymphoma, however, L&H cells also show evidence of ongoing mutations with intraclonal diversity, and moreover, the rearrangements are usually functional with immunoglobulin mRNA transcripts detectable in the L&H cells of most cases of NLP HL. The ongoing mutations identify mutating germinal center B-cells growing dependent on antigen binding and selection as precursors of the L&H cells in NLP HL. With regard to these genetic characteristics, L&H cells are comparable with follicle center B-cell non-Hodgkin lymphoma cells. Unlike in follicular lymphomas, however, where activation of Bcl-2 is key to the pathogenesis of the lymphoma, the transforming event(s) in L&H cells still remains unknown. Bcl-6, a Kruppel-type zinc finger transcriptional repressor protein normally expressed in the nuclei of germinal center B-cells, was recently shown to be expressed in 75-100% of L&H cells in 19 cases of NLP HL examined; the HRS cells of classical Hodgkin disease on the other hand frequently lack Bcl-6 expression.[37] Taken together, current data indicate that the L&H cells of NLP HL are also derived from germinal center B-cells, but they retain at least part of the germinal center B-cell phenotype, in contrast to HRS cells which appear to lose their B-cell identity in most cases. L&H cells, therefore, are thought to behave like transformed centroblasts, with continued somatic mutation (which may be important for the persistence and expansion of the clonal population) occurring in a germinal center-like environment.[112] The molecular events leading to the transformation of L&H cells remain undefined.

3.4   Further Directions

While the techniques of laser microdissection and PCR have enabled significant successes towards unraveling the mysteries of Hodgkin lymphoma, even newer technologies such as cDNA and tissue microarray analyses show great promise in further divulging the pathogenesis of this intriguing disease through comprehensive gene and protein expression profiling. cDNA arrays are powerful tools useful for the identification of differentially expressed genes in malignant tumors. Similarly, tissue microarrays are powerful for analyzing a large number of molecular variables in a large series of tumors. Both techniques are already being employed to investigate various features of Hodgkin lymphoma, including the expression of B-cell lineage-specific genes and genes associated with B-cell differentiation and maintenance, cell cycle and apoptosis regulatators, and even HRS cell-specific genes. Future advances using these emerging techniques will undoubtedly lead to an enhanced understanding of Hodgkin lymphoma, and they may also eventually yield an improved prognostic classification scheme based on predictable responses to therapy and overall clinical outcome.

REFERENCES

1. Jaffe E, Harris N, Stein H, Vardiman J. World Health Organization Classification of Tumours: Pathology and Genetics of Tumours of Haemopoietic and Lymphoid Tissues; 2001.
2. Hodgkin T. On some morbid appearances of the assorbant glands and spleen. Med Chir Trans 1832(17):69-97.
3. Wilks S. Cases of lardaceous disease and some allied affections with remarks.; 1856.
4. Langhans. Das maligne Lymphoma v kom (Pseudoleukoemic). Virchows Arch Pathol Anat 1872;54:509.
5. Greenfield. Specimens illustrative of the pathology of lymphadenoma and leukocythemic. Trans Pathol Soc 1878:20-272.
6. Sternberg. Ueber eine eigenartige unter dem Bilde der Pseudoleukemic verlaufende Tuberculose des lymphatisshen Apparates. J Heilk 1898;19(21).
7. Reed. On the pathological changes in Hodgkin's disease, with special reference to its relation to tuberculosis. 1902(10):133.
8. Kaplan. Hodgkin's Disease. 2nd edition ed. Cambridge: Harvard University Press; 1980.
9. Spriggs B. Chromosomes of Sternberg-Reed cells. Lancet 1962(2):153.
10. MacMahon B. Epidemiology of Hodgkin's disease. Cancer Res 1966;26(6):1189-201.
11. Atkinson K, Austin DE, McElwain TJ, Peckham MJ. Alcohol pain in Hodgkin's disease. Cancer 1976;37(2):895-9.
12. Gupta RK, Gospodarowicz, Lister TA. Hodgkin's Disease. In: Mauch P, Armitage JO, Diehl V, Hoppe RT, Weiss LM, editors. Philadelphia: Lippincott Williams & Wilkens; 1999.
13. Jackson, Parker. Hodgkin 's Disease and Allied Disorders: New York: Oxford University Press; 1947.
14. Lukes RJ. Relationship of histologic features to clinical stages in Hodgkin's disease. Am J Roentgenol 1963;90:944.
15. Lukes RJ, Butler JJ. The pathology and nomenclature of Hodgkin's disease. Cancer Res 1966;26(6):1063-83.
16. Smetana, Cohen. Mortality in relation to histologic type in Hodgkin's disease. Blood 1956;26:211-224.

17. Lukes RJ, L.F. C, T.C. H, Rappaport H, P. R. Report of the nomenclature committee. Cancer 1966;26:1311-.
18. Rosenthal SR. Significance of tissue lymphocytes in the prognosis of lymphogranulomukosis. Arch Pathol Lab Med 1936(21):628.
19. Harris NL, Jaffe ES, Stein H, Banks PM, Chan JK, Cleary ML, et al. A revised European-American classification of lymphoid neoplasms: a proposal from the International Lymphoma Study Group. Blood 1994;84(5):1361-92.
20. Marafioti T, Hummel M, Foss HD, Laumen H, Korbjuhn P, Anagnostopoulos I, et al. Hodgkin and reed-sternberg cells represent an expansion of a single clone originating from a germinal center B-cell with functional immunoglobulin gene rearrangements but defective immunoglobulin transcription. Blood 2000;95(4):1443-50.
21. Brauninger A, Hansmann ML, Strickler JG, Dummer R, Burg G, Rajewsky K, et al. Identification of common germinal-center B-cell precursors in two patients with both Hodgkin's disease and non-Hodgkin's lymphoma. N Engl J Med 1999;340(16):1239-47.
22. Neiman RS. Current problems in the histopathologic diagnosis and classification of Hodgkin's disease. Pathol Annu 1978;13 Pt 2:289-328.
23. Harris NL. Hodgkin's disease: classification and differential diagnosis. Mod Pathol 1999;12(2):159-75.
24. von Wasielewski R, Mengel M, Fischer R, Hansmann ML, Hubner K, Franklin J, et al. Classical Hodgkin's disease. Clinical impact of the immunophenotype. Am J Pathol 1997;151(4):1123-30.
25. Isaacson PG, Ashton-Key M. Phenotype of Hodgkin and Reed-Sternberg cells. Lancet 1996;347(8999):481.
26. Schmid C, Pan L, Diss T, Isaacson PG. Expression of B-cell antigens by Hodgkin's and Reed-Sternberg cells. Am J Pathol 1991;139(4):701-7.
27. McBride JA, Rodriguez J, Luthra R, Ordonez NG, Cabanillas F, Pugh WC. T-cell-rich B large-cell lymphoma simulating lymphocyte-rich Hodgkin's disease. Am J Surg Pathol 1996;20(2):193-201.
28. Sheibani K, Battifora H, Burke JS, Rappaport H. Leu-M1 antigen in human neoplasms. An immunohistologic study of 400 cases. Am J Surg Pathol 1986;10(4):227-36.
29. Millward, Weidner. CD30 (Ber-H2) expression in nonhematopoietic tumors. Applied Immunohistochemistry 1998;6:164-8.
30. Pinkus GS, Pinkus JL, Langhoff E, Matsumura F, Yamashiro S, Mosialos G, et al. Fascin, a sensitive new marker for Reed-Sternberg cells of hodgkin's disease. Evidence for a dendritic or B cell derivation? Am J Pathol 1997;150(2):543-62.
31. Kempf W, Levi E, Kamarashev J, Kutzner H, Pfeifer W, Petrogiannis-Haliotis T, et al. Fascin expression in CD30-positive cutaneous lymphoproliferative disorders. J Cutan Pathol 2002;29(5):295-300.
32. Pinkus GS, Thomas P, Said JW. Leu-M1--a marker for Reed-Sternberg cells in Hodgkin's disease. An immunoperoxidase study of paraffin-embedded tissues. Am J Pathol 1985;119(2):244-52.
33. Pinkus GS, Said JW. Hodgkin's disease, lymphocyte predominance type, nodular--further evidence for a B cell derivation. L & H variants of Reed-Sternberg cells express L26, a pan B cell marker. Am J Pathol 1988;133(2):211-7.
34. Anagnostopoulos I, Hansmann ML, Franssila K, Harris M, Harris NL, Jaffe ES, et al. European Task Force on Lymphoma project on lymphocyte predominance Hodgkin disease: histologic and immunohistologic analysis of submitted cases reveals 2 types of Hodgkin disease with a nodular growth pattern and abundant lymphocytes. Blood 2000;96(5):1889-99.

35. Mason DY, Banks PM, Chan J, Cleary ML, Delsol G, de Wolf Peeters C, et al. Nodular lymphocyte predominance Hodgkin's disease. A distinct clinicopathological entity. Am J Surg Pathol 1994;18(5):526-30.

36. Stein H, Hansmann ML, Lennert K, Brandtzaeg P, Gatter KC, Mason DY. Reed-Sternberg and Hodgkin cells in lymphocyte-predominant Hodgkin's disease of nodular subtype contain J chain. Am J Clin Pathol 1986;86(3):292-7.

37. Falini B, Bigerna B, Pasqualucci L, Fizzotti M, Martelli MF, Pileri S, et al. Distinctive expression pattern of the BCL-6 protein in nodular lymphocyte predominance Hodgkin's disease. Blood 1996;87(2):465-71.

38. Stein H, Marafioti T, Foss HD, Laumen H, Hummel M, Anagnostopoulos I, et al. Down-regulation of BOB.1/OBF.1 and Oct2 in classical Hodgkin disease but not in lymphocyte predominant Hodgkin disease correlates with immunoglobulin transcription. Blood 2001;97(2):496-501.

39. Torlakovic E, Tierens A, Dang HD, Delabie J. The transcription factor PU.1, necessary for B-cell development is expressed in lymphocyte predominance, but not classical Hodgkin's disease. Am J Pathol 2001;159(5):1807-14.

40. De Wolf-Peeters C, Pittaluga S. T-cell rich B-cell lymphoma: a morphological variant of a variety of non-Hodgkin's lymphomas or a clinicopathological entity? Histopathology 1995;26(4):383-5.

41. Schmid C, Sargent C, Isaacson PG. L and H cells of nodular lymphocyte predominant Hodgkin's disease show immunoglobulin light-chain restriction. Am J Pathol 1991;139(6):1281-9.

42. Poppema S. The nature of the lymphocytes surrounding Reed-Sternberg cells in nodular lymphocyte predominance and in other types of Hodgkin's disease. Am J Pathol 1989;135(2):351-7.

43. Abbondanzo SL, Sato N, Straus SE, Jaffe ES. Acute infectious mononucleosis. CD30 (Ki-1) antigen expression and histologic correlations. Am J Clin Pathol 1990;93(5):698-702.

44. Rudiger T, Ott G, Ott MM, Muller-Deubert SM, Muller-Hermelink HK. Differential diagnosis between classic Hodgkin's lymphoma, T-cell-rich B-cell lymphoma, and paragranuloma by paraffin immunohistochemistry. Am J Surg Pathol 1998;22(10):1184-91.

45. Kraus MD, Haley J. Lymphocyte predominance Hodgkin's disease: the use of bcl-6 and CD57 in diagnosis and differential diagnosis. Am J Surg Pathol 2000;24(8):1068-78.

46. von Wasielewski R, Werner M, Fischer R, Hansmann ML, Hubner K, Hasenclever D, et al. Lymphocyte-predominant Hodgkin's disease. An immunohistochemical analysis of 208 reviewed Hodgkin's disease cases from the German Hodgkin Study Group. Am J Pathol 1997;150(3):793-803.

47. Diehl V, Franklin J, Sextro M, Mauch P. Clinical presentation and tretment of Lymphocyte Predominance Hodgkin's Disease. In: Mauch P, Armitage JO, Diehl V, editors. Hodgkin's Disease. Philadelphia: Lippincott Williams & Wilkins; 1999. p. 563.

48. Diehl V, Sextro M, Franklin J, Hansmann ML, Harris N, Jaffe E, et al. Clinical presentation, course, and prognostic factors in lymphocyte-predominant Hodgkin's disease and lymphocyte-rich classical Hodgkin's disease: report from the European Task Force on Lymphoma Project on Lymphocyte-Predominant Hodgkin's Disease. J Clin Oncol 1999;17(3):776-83.

49. Regula DP, Jr., Hoppe RT, Weiss LM. Nodular and diffuse types of lymphocyte predominance Hodgkin's disease. N Engl J Med 1988;318(4):214-9.

50. Orlandi E, Lazzarino M, Brusamolino E, Paulli M, Astori C, Magrini U, et al. Nodular lymphocyte predominance Hodgkin's disease: long-term observation reveals a continuous pattern of recurrence. Leuk Lymphoma 1997;26(3-4):359-68.

51. Regula DP, Jr., Weiss LM, Warnke RA, Dorfman RF. Lymphocyte predominance Hodgkin's disease: a reappraisal based upon histological and immunophenotypical findings in relapsing cases. Histopathology 1987;11(11):1107-20.

52. Bodis S, Kraus MD, Pinkus G, Silver B, Kadin ME, Canellos GP, et al. Clinical presentation and outcome in lymphocyte-predominant Hodgkin's disease. J Clin Oncol 1997;15(9):3060-6.

53. Kansal R, Singleton TP, Ross CW, Finn WG, Padmore RF, Schnitzer B. Follicular hodgkin lymphoma: a histopathologic study. Am J Clin Pathol 2002;117(1):29-35.

54. Keilholz U, Szelenyi H, Siehl J, Foss HD, Knauf W, Thiel E. Rapid regression of chemotherapy refractory lymphocyte predominant Hodgkin's disease after administration of rituximab (anti CD 20 mono- clonal antibody) and interleukin-2. Leuk Lymphoma 1999;35(5-6):641-2.

55. Ashton-Key M, Thorpe PA, Allen JP, Isaacson PG. Follicular Hodgkin's disease. Am J Surg Pathol 1995;19(11):1294-9.

56. Colby TV, Hoppe RT, Warnke RA. Hodgkin's disease: a clinicopathologic study of 659 cases. Cancer 1982;49(9):1848-58.

57. Achten R, Verhoef G, Vanuytsel L, De Wolf-Peeters C. Histiocyte-rich, T-cell-rich B-cell lymphoma: a distinct diffuse large B-cell lymphoma subtype showing characteristic morphologic and immunophenotypic features. Histopathology 2002;40(1):31-45.

58. Strickler JG, Michie SA, Warnke RA, Dorfman RF. The "syncytial variant" of nodular sclerosing Hodgkin's disease. Am J Surg Pathol 1986;10(7):470-7.

59. Ben-Yehuda-Salz D, Ben-Yehuda A, Polliack A, Ron N, Okon E. Syncytial variant of nodular sclerosing Hodgkin's disease. A new clinicopathologic entity. Cancer 1990;65(5):1167-72.

60. Bennett MH, MacLennan KA, Easterling MJ, Vaughan Hudson B, Jelliffe AM, Vaughan Hudson G. The prognostic significance of cellular subtypes in nodular sclerosing Hodgkin's disease: an analysis of 271 non-laparotomised cases (BNLI report no. 22). Clin Radiol 1983;34(5):497-501.

61. MacLennan KA, Bennett MH, Vaughan Hudson B, Vaughan Hudson G. Diagnosis and grading of nodular sclerosing Hodgkin's disease: a study of 2190 patients. Int Rev Exp Pathol 1992;33:27-51.

62. DeVita VT, Jr., Simon RM, Hubbard SM, Young RC, Berard CW, Moxley JH, 3rd, et al. Curability of advanced Hodgkin's disease with chemotherapy. Long-term follow-up of MOPP-treated patients at the National Cancer Institute. Ann Intern Med 1980;92(5):587-95.

63. d'Amore ES, Lee CK, Aeppli DM, Levitt SH, Frizzera G. Lack of prognostic value of histopathologic parameters in Hodgkin's disease, nodular sclerosis type. A study of 123 patients with limited stage disease who had undergone laparotomy and were treated with radiation therapy. Arch Pathol Lab Med 1992;116(8):856-61.

64. Ferry JA, Linggood RM, Convery KM, Efird JT, Eliseo R, Harris NL. Hodgkin disease, nodular sclerosis type. Implications of histologic subclassification. Cancer 1993;71(2):457-63.

65. Hess JL, Bodis S, Pinkus G, Silver B, Mauch P. Histopathologic grading of nodular sclerosis Hodgkin's disease. Lack of prognostic significance in 254 surgically staged patients. Cancer 1994;74(2):708-14.

66. Harris NL. Hodgkin's lymphomas: classification, diagnosis, and grading. Semin Hematol 1999;36(3):220-32.
67. Bacchi CE, Dorfman RF, Hoppe RT, Chan JK, Warnke RA. Metastatic carcinoma in lymph nodes simulating "syncytial variant" of nodular sclerosing Hodgkin's disease. Am J Clin Pathol 1991;96(5):589-93.
68. Khan G, Norton AJ, Slavin G. Epstein-Barr virus in Hodgkin disease. Relation to age and subtype. Cancer 1993;71(10):3124-9.
69. Doggett RS, Colby TV, Dorfman RF. Interfollicular Hodgkin's disease. Am J Surg Pathol 1983;7(2):145-9.
70. Banks PM. The distinction of Hodgkin's disease from T cell lymphoma. Semin Diagn Pathol 1992;9(4):279-83.
71. Kant JA, Hubbard SM, Longo DL, Simon RM, DeVita VT, Jr., Jaffe ES. The pathologic and clinical heterogeneity of lymphocyte-depleted Hodgkin's disease. J Clin Oncol 1986;4(3):284-94.
72. Greer JP, Kinney MC, Cousar JB, Flexner JM, Dupont WD, Graber SE, et al. Lymphocyte-depleted Hodgkin's disease. Clinicopathologic review of 25 patients. Am J Med 1986;81(2):208-14.
73. Tirelli U, Errante D, Dolcetti R, Gloghini A, Serraino D, Vaccher E, et al. Hodgkin's disease and human immunodeficiency virus infection: clinicopathologic and virologic features of 114 patients from the Italian Cooperative Group on AIDS and Tumors. J Clin Oncol 1995;13(7):1758-67.
74. Trumper LH, Brady G, Bagg A, Gray D, Loke SL, Griesser H, et al. Single-cell analysis of Hodgkin and Reed-Sternberg cells: molecular heterogeneity of gene expression and p53 mutations. Blood 1993;81(11):3097-115.
75. Delabie J, Tierens A, Gavriil T, Wu G, Weisenburger DD, Chan WC. Phenotype, genotype and clonality of Reed-Sternberg cells in nodular sclerosis Hodgkin's disease: results of a single-cell study. Br J Haematol 1996;94(1):198-205.
76. Delabie J, Tierens A, Wu G, Weisenburger DD, Chan WC. Lymphocyte predominance Hodgkin's disease: lineage and clonality determination using a single-cell assay. Blood 1994;84(10):3291-8.
77. Hummel M, Ziemann K, Lammert H, Pileri S, Sabattini E, Stein H. Hodgkin's disease with monoclonal and polyclonal populations of Reed-Sternberg cells. N Engl J Med 1995;333(14):901-6.
78. Kanzler H, Kuppers R, Hansmann ML, Rajewsky K. Hodgkin and Reed-Sternberg cells in Hodgkin's disease represent the outgrowth of a dominant tumor clone derived from (crippled) germinal center B cells. J Exp Med 1996;184(4):1495-505.
79. Kuppers R, Rajewsky K, Zhao M, Simons G, Laumann R, Fischer R, et al. Hodgkin disease: Hodgkin and Reed-Sternberg cells picked from histological sections show clonal immunoglobulin gene rearrangements and appear to be derived from B cells at various stages of development. Proc Natl Acad Sci U S A 1994;91(23):10962-6.
80. Roth J, Daus H, Trumper L, Gause A, Salamon-Looijen M, Pfreundschuh M. Detection of immunoglobulin heavy-chain gene rearrangement at the single-cell level in malignant lymphomas: no rearrangement is found in Hodgkin and Reed-Sternberg cells. Int J Cancer 1994;57(6):799-804.
81. Kuppers R. Molecular biology of Hodgkin's lymphoma. Adv Cancer Res 2002;84:277-312.
82. Drexler HG. Recent results on the biology of Hodgkin and Reed-Sternberg cells. II. Continuous cell lines. Leuk Lymphoma 1993;9(1-2):1-25.

83. Muschen M, Rajewsky K, Brauninger A, Baur AS, Oudejans JJ, Roers A, et al. Rare occurrence of classical Hodgkin's disease as a T cell lymphoma. J Exp Med 2000;191(2):387-94.

84. Seitz V, Hummel M, Marafioti T, Anagnostopoulos I, Assaf C, Stein H. Detection of clonal T-cell receptor gamma-chain gene rearrangements in Reed-Sternberg cells of classic Hodgkin disease. Blood 2000;95(10):3020-4.

85. Rajewsky K. Clonal selection and learning in the antibody system. Nature 1996;381(6585):751-8.

86. Kuppers R, Zhao M, Hansmann ML, Rajewsky K. Tracing B cell development in human germinal centres by molecular analysis of single cells picked from histological sections. Embo J 1993;12(13):4955-67.

87. Kuppers R, Rajewsky K. The origin of Hodgkin and Reed/Sternberg cells in Hodgkin's disease. Annu Rev Immunol 1998;16:471-93.

88. Marafioti T, Hummel M, Anagnostopoulos I, Foss HD, Huhn D, Stein H. Classical Hodgkin's disease and follicular lymphoma originating from the same germinal center B cell. J Clin Oncol 1999;17(12):3804-9.

89. Stein H, Hummel M. Cellular origin and clonality of classic Hodgkin's lymphoma: immunophenotypic and molecular studies. Semin Hematol 1999;36(3):233-41.

90. Re D, Muschen M, Ahmadi T, Wickenhauser C, Staratschek-Jox A, Holtick U, et al. Oct-2 and Bob-1 deficiency in Hodgkin and Reed Sternberg cells. Cancer Res 2001;61(5):2080-4.

91. Saez AI, Artiga MJ, Sanchez-Beato M, Sanchez-Verde L, Garcia JF, Camacho FI, et al. Analysis of octamer-binding transcription factors Oct2 and Oct1 and their coactivator BOB.1/OBF.1 in lymphomas. Mod Pathol 2002;15(3):211-20.

92. Jundt F, Kley K, Anagnostopoulos I, Schulze Probsting K, Greiner A, Mathas S, et al. Loss of PU.1 expression is associated with defective immunoglobulin transcription in Hodgkin and Reed-Sternberg cells of classical Hodgkin disease. Blood 2002;99(8):3060-2.

93. Henderson A, Calame K. Transcriptional regulation during B cell development. Annu Rev Immunol 1998;16:163-200.

94. Wirth T, Pfisterer P, Annweiler A, Zwilling S, Konig H. Molecular principles of Oct2-mediated gene activation in B cells. Immunobiology 1995;193(2-4):161-70.

95. Cepek KL, Chasman DI, Sharp PA. Sequence-specific DNA binding of the B-cell-specific coactivator OCA-B. Genes Dev 1996;10(16):2079-88.

96. McKercher SR, Torbett BE, Anderson KL, Henkel GW, Vestal DJ, Baribault H, et al. Targeted disruption of the PU.1 gene results in multiple hematopoietic abnormalities. Embo J 1996;15(20):5647-58.

97. Oikawa T, Yamada T, Kihara-Negishi F, Yamamoto H, Kondoh N, Hitomi Y, et al. The role of Ets family transcription factor PU.1 in hematopoietic cell differentiation, proliferation and apoptosis. Cell Death Differ 1999;6(7):599-608.

98. Pongubala JM, Atchison ML. PU.1 can participate in an active enhancer complex without its transcriptional activation domain. Proc Natl Acad Sci U S A 1997;94(1):127-32.

99. Bargou RC, Leng C, Krappmann D, Emmerich F, Mapara MY, Bommert K, et al. High-level nuclear NF-kappa B and Oct-2 is a common feature of cultured Hodgkin/Reed-Sternberg cells. Blood 1996;87(10):4340-7.

100. Bargou RC, Emmerich F, Krappmann D, Bommert K, Mapara MY, Arnold W, et al. Constitutive nuclear factor-kappaB-RelA activation is required for proliferation and survival of Hodgkin's disease tumor cells. J Clin Invest 1997;100(12):2961-9.

101. Krappmann D, Emmerich F, Kordes U, Scharschmidt E, Dorken B, Scheidereit C. Molecular mechanisms of constitutive NF-kappaB/Rel activation in Hodgkin/Reed-Sternberg cells. Oncogene 1999;18(4):943-53.

102. Bours V, Bentires-Alj M, Hellin AC, Viatour P, Robe P, Delhalle S, et al. Nuclear factor-kappa B, cancer, and apoptosis. Biochem Pharmacol 2000;60(8):1085-9.

103. Izban KF, Ergin M, Huang Q, Qin JZ, Martinez RL, Schnitzer B, et al. Characterization of NF-kappaB expression in Hodgkin's disease: inhibition of constitutively expressed NF-kappaB results in spontaneous caspase-independent apoptosis in Hodgkin and Reed-Sternberg cells. Mod Pathol 2001;14(4):297-310.

104. Cabannes E, Khan G, Aillet F, Jarrett RF, Hay RT. Mutations in the IkBa gene in Hodgkin's disease suggest a tumour suppressor role for IkappaBalpha. Oncogene 1999;18(20):3063-70.

105. Emmerich F, Meiser M, Hummel M, Demel G, Foss HD, Jundt F, et al. Overexpression of I kappa B alpha without inhibition of NF-kappaB activity and mutations in the I kappa B alpha gene in Reed-Sternberg cells. Blood 1999;94(9):3129-34.

106. Jungnickel B, Staratschek-Jox A, Brauninger A, Spieker T, Wolf J, Diehl V, et al. Clonal deleterious mutations in the IkappaBalpha gene in the malignant cells in Hodgkin's lymphoma. J Exp Med 2000;191(2):395-402.

107. Schwering I, Brauninger A, Klein U, Jungnickel B, Tinguely M, Diehl V, et al. Loss of the B-lineage-specific gene expression program in Hodgkin and Reed-Sternberg cells of Hodgkin lymphoma. Blood 2003;101(4):1505-12.

108. Hertel CB, Zhou XG, Hamilton-Dutoit SJ, Junker S. Loss of B cell identity correlates with loss of B cell-specific transcription factors in Hodgkin/Reed-Sternberg cells of classical Hodgkin lymphoma. Oncogene 2002;21(32):4908-20.

109. Braeuninger A, Kuppers R, Strickler JG, Wacker HH, Rajewsky K, Hansmann ML. Hodgkin and Reed-Sternberg cells in lymphocyte predominant Hodgkin disease represent clonal populations of germinal center-derived tumor B cells. Proc Natl Acad Sci U S A 1997;94(17):9337-42.

110. Marafioti T, Hummel M, Anagnostopoulos I, Foss HD, Falini B, Delsol G, et al. Origin of nodular lymphocyte-predominant Hodgkin's disease from a clonal expansion of highly mutated germinal-center B cells. N Engl J Med 1997;337(7):453-8.

111. Ohno T, Stribley JA, Wu G, Hinrichs SH, Weisenburger DD, Chan WC. Clonality in nodular lymphocyte-predominant Hodgkin's disease. N Engl J Med 1997;337(7):459-65.

112. Chan WC. Cellular origin of nodular lymphocyte-predominant Hodgkin's lymphoma: immunophenotypic and molecular studies. Semin Hematol 1999;36(3):242-52.

Index